Recent Clinical Techniques, Results, and Research in Wounds

Series Editors

Melvin A. Shiffman
Mervin Low

More information about this series at http://www.springer.com/series/15695

Melvin A. Shiffman • Mervin Low
Editors

Burns, Infections and Wound Management

Springer

Editors
Melvin A. Shiffman
Tustin, CA
USA

Mervin Low
Newport Beach, CA
USA

ISSN 2524-4590 ISSN 2524-4604 (electronic)
Recent Clinical Techniques, Results, and Research in Wounds
ISBN 978-3-030-10685-0 ISBN 978-3-030-10686-7 (eBook)
https://doi.org/10.1007/978-3-030-10686-7

This Springer imprint is published by the registered company Springer Nature Switzerland AG
The registered company address is: Gewerbestrasse 11, 6330 Cham, Switzerland

Foreword[1]

It is a great honour for me to be invited to provide a foreword for the series of six books edited by Dr. Shiffman and Dr. Low, which cover a broad expanse of subjects relevant to and important in the care of patients with wounds.

Wounds have existed since the beginning of time and, until recent years, have received scant attention unless major conflicts developed which necessitated innovation in the treatment of patients with wounds. However, in recent years there has been an increasing interest in this subject as evidenced by the explosion of journals, meetings, societies and associations and initiatives that have been developed in this field.

The need for an academic underpinning of the subject of wound healing is without question. Research papers published in recent years have undoubtedly enhanced the scientific basis for wound healing. This, coupled with demographic changes in many countries around the world, has led to increasing numbers of patients developing wounds or wound healing problems. It is recognised that in the vast majority of geographies globally the number of patients with wounds is increasing in everything other than major burns where better health and safety initiatives have been an effective preventive strategy.

This series of books not only attempts to deal with subjects that are normally seen in wound healing text but also provides a huge amount of space to the management of wounds seen in surgical practice, both general and specialist surgery. The sections on infection are an attempt to deal with a very common but poorly managed clinical problem and one that requires urgent attention in view of the global challenge of antimicrobial stewardship. The tradition chronic wounds are also included and provide a medical as well as a nursing and paramedical focus on these subjects.

It is particularly pleasing to see books and chapters focused on specialised surgical practice as these are areas that are rarely covered in other educational products in this area. The opportunity for new therapies, measuring the range of effective and appropriate outcomes and the use of new technologies are all included.

For those of us who work in the area of wound healing, these books will unquestionably be an important reference source. For those readers who want to get an insight into this common, expensive and complex problem they will without doubt find the content of these books an important source of informed opinion and refer to the rapidly expanding evidence base that is developing in this subject area.

I would urge you to immerse yourself in these books. Read, reflect and consider how information that you have had access to can and will change your clinical practice.

Keith Harding
Clinical Innovation Cardiff (CIIC),
College of Biomedical and Life Sciences,
Cardiff University School of Medicine,
Heath Park, Cardiff,
UK

[1]P. S.

We, Melvin A. Shiffman and Mervin Low, are greatly enthralled by Keith Harding's willingness to write the Foreword for the books on wounds. Keith Harding is the Director of TIME Institute (Translation, Innovation, Methodology and Engagement) and Head of the Wound Healing Research Unit in the School of Medicine at Cardiff University. He is Clinical Lead for Wound Healing in the Cardiff and Vale NHS Trust. In September 2013 Harding was appointed Dean of Clinical Innovation at Cardiff University. From 2002 to 2005 he was Head of the Department of Surgery at Cardiff University. He is Editor-in-Chief of the *International Wound Journal*. Harding is a Past President of the European Tissue Repair Society. He was the first President of the European Pressure Ulcer Advisory Panel and first Recorder of the European Wound Management Association. He was Chair of the International Working Group on Wound Healing in Diabetic Foot Disease in 2003. He was Chair of the Expert Working Group that produced a range of International Consensus Documents from 2004 to 2011. Professor Harding was appointed a Commander of the Order of the British Empire in the 2013 New Year Honours for services to medicine and healthcare.

Preface

We are delighted to have the book on wounds extended into six volumes. There is so very much medical literature in journals and books that to cover the whole gamut of wounds would be virtually impossible. We tried to include as many of the experienced practitioners in wound care as possible, but many of them are too busy to spend the time committing to submitting a chapter.

The selection of topics in each of the volumes was decided by the number of authors responded to each of the subjects. As usual in editing a book, many authors who agreed to submit manuscripts finally were not available to complete the chapters. We contacted or tried to contact over 1500 authors and most of them did not respond or the responses were not as good as expected.

The volumes include:

1. Biofilm, Pilonidal Cysts and Sinuses
2. Burns, Infections and Wound Management
3. Pressure Injury, Diabetes and Negative Pressure Wound Therapy
4. Plastic and Thoracic Surgery, Orthopedics and Ophthalmology
5. Vascular Surgery, Neurosurgery, Lower Extremity Ulcers, Antimicrobials, Wound Assessment, Care, Measurement and Repair
6. Chronic Wounds, Wound Dressings and Wound Healing

There are many expert international contributors who have worked in various aspects of wound research as well as clinical practice. We have tried to have chapters that involved humans and in vivo results and avoided as much as possible animals and in vitro results. Chapter conclusions are those of the authors and may not be the same as those of the editors. At times the chapter may appear cumbersome, but the authors try to show some proof of their results. Language difficulties are common when translated into English so that grammar, spelling and sometimes words have to be corrected.

Hopefully, the reader will get information that adds to their care and treatment of patients. Researchers may gain knowledge of other researchers' progress and improve on the results or can continue their work in other directions. Controversy is many times a good thing since looking in other directions to prove or disprove a result can improve knowledge. We have a long way to go to be able to treat all wounds properly and successfully in as short a time as possible.

Tustin, CA, USA — Melvin A. Shiffman
Newport Beach, CA, USA — Mervin Low

Contents

Part I

Burns

Overview of Burns

Melvin A. Shiffman

1 Introduction

Burns can be one of the most devastating injuries, although ranging from first-degree burn that can be treated at home to third- and fourth-degree burns that can require extreme care both medically and surgically that can, hopefully, keep the patient alive but with major scars that may remain to be treated.

2 History

Cave paintings from more than 3500 years ago showed burns and their management [1]. The earliest Egyptian records on treating burns describe dressings prepared with milk from mothers of baby boys [2]. The 1500 BCE *Edwin Smith Papyrus* describes treatments using honey and the salve of resin [1]. Tea leaves were used by the Chinese as early as 600 BCE. Hippocrates described the use of pig fat and vinegar in 400 BCE, while Celsus used wine and myrrh in 100 CE [1]. Ambroise Paré was the first to describe different degrees of burns in the 1500s [3], and Guillaume Dupuytren developed the 6° classification of burns 1832 [4, 5].

M.A. Shiffman, M.D., J.D.
Private Practice, Tustin, CA, USA
e-mail: shiffmanmdjd@gmail.com

James Syme established the first burn unit in Edinburgh in 1843 [6]. He argued that mixing burn patients with postoperative patients would make him "chargeable with the highest degree of culpable recklessness." This logic motivated the Edinburgh Royal Infirmary leadership to set aside the former high school janitor's house for burn patients. This experiment was relatively short-lived, however, since burn patients were transferred to one of the "sheds" in 1848 to make way for an increased number of mechanical trauma casualties from railway accidents. Glasgow Royal Infirmary had from 1833 to 1933 accumulated 100 years of experience with over 10,000 burn patients and in 1883 established a separate burn ward. In Dunbar's report on these patients, he commented that in the pre-antiseptic era, only the worst burns would come to the hospital; there were a biphasic mortality pattern (with the highest number of deaths between postburn hours 12–24), a high incidence of streptococcal wound infection, the infrequency of skin grafting, and a frustratingly high mortality rate of 20–30% despite the introduction of antisepsis.

During World War I, Henry D. Dakin and Alexis Carrel developed standards for the cleaning and disinfecting of burns and wounds using sodium hypochlorite solutions, which significantly reduced mortality [1]. In the 1940s, the importance of early excision and skin grafting was acknowledged, and around

Recent Clinical Techniques, Results, and Research in Wounds (2017)
DOI 10.1007/15695_2017_20, © Springer International Publishing AG
Published Online: 24 October 2017

the same time, fluid resuscitation and formulas to guide it were developed. In the 1970s, researchers demonstrated the significance of the hypermetabolic state that follows large burns.

3 Types of Burns

1. Heat burns (thermal burns):
   Caused by fire, steam, hot objects, or hot liquids.
2. Cold temperature burns:
   Caused by skin exposure to wet, windy, or cold conditions.
3. Radiation burns:
   Caused by the sun, tanning booths, sunlamps, X-rays, or radiation therapy for cancer treatment.
4. Chemical burns:
   Caused by contact with household or industrial chemicals in a liquid, solid, or gas form.
5. Electrical burns:
   Caused by contact with electrical sources or by lightning.
6. Friction burns (abrasion and heat burns):
   Caused by contact with any hard surface such as roads ("road rash"), carpets, or gym floor surfaces.
7. Inhalation injuries:

Breathing in hot air or gases can injure the lungs.

4 Burn Degree [7, 8]

1. First-degree burns:
   Burns of the epidermis. Painful but no blisters and get better over 3–7 days
2. Second-degree burns:
   Superficial partial-thickness burns to the papillary layer. Pink, moist, and painful and forms blisters. Heal within 2–3 weeks without scarring
   Deep partial-thickness burns to the reticular layer. White, pink, or red but less painful and fairly dry. Slow capillary refill. Heal within 3–8 weeks with scarring
3. Third-degree burns (full-thickness burns):
   Injury to all the skin layers and subcutaneous layer. Leathery, no pain, and no capillary refill. Heal by epithelial migration from the periphery
4. Fourth-degree burns:
   Extend through the skin and subcutaneous tissues to injured muscle, ligaments, tendons, nerves, blood vessels, and bones. Black and necrotic

5 In this Article

5.1 Symptoms of Burns

The symptoms of burns depend on the cause and type of burn. They can include:

1. Red skin or pale and clammy skin.
2. Blisters with peeling.
3. Swelling.
4. Pain: The degree of pain is not related to the severity of the burn. The most serious burns can be painless.
5. Faintness.
6. Weakness.
7. Decreased alertness.
8. Dizziness.
9. Bluish lips and fingernails.
10. Muscle twitching.
11. Seizures.
12. White or charred skin.
13. Irregular heartbeat.
14. Shock.
15. Cardiac arrest.

6 Surface Area Assessment of Burns

Smart (1876) [9] noted that burn severity was determined by their size and depth as well as other bodily systems that were affected including airway.

6.1 Rule of Nines

The rule of nines was devised by Pulaski and Tennison in 1947 [10] and published by Wallace in 1951 [11].

The extent of burn injury to the skin can be estimated using the "rule of nines" (Fig. 1). This allocates approximate percentages to the major anatomical areas relative to the total body surface area (TBSA). The adult head and neck are allotted 9% of TBSA, each upper limb 9%, each lower limb 18%, each anterior and posterior surfaces of the trunk 18%, and perineum and urogenital structures 1%. The area of an adult palm and fingers is approximately 1% of TBSA, and

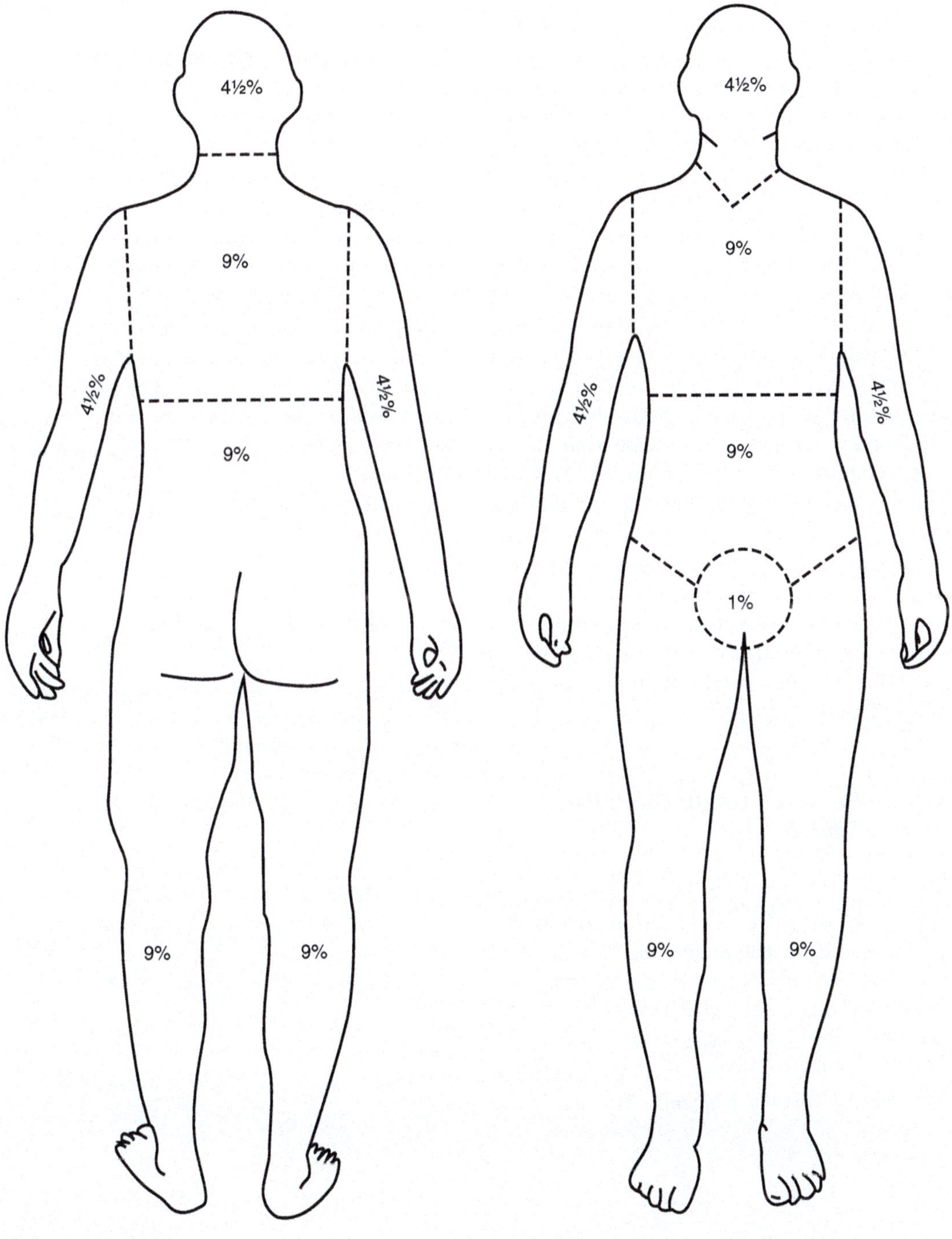

Fig. 1 Rule of nines

the total of multiple scattered areas of burn injury can be estimated using the open hand size as a guide.

6.2 Serial Halving

Serial halving is a prehospital assessment tool for burns. Using this method, the assessor decides if the area burned is greater than half of total body surface area (TBSA), between a quarter and half, between an eighth and a quarter, or less than an eighth. This can be useful in decisions about initial management and does not depend on knowledge of the proportion of the major anatomical areas relative to the TBSA.

Smith et al. (2005) [12] found no statistical difference between serial halving and the rule of nines as an initial assessment tool when determining dispositional. Serial halving has an inherent weakness when assessing certain sizes of burn. The rule of nines requires that the assessor knows and understands the proportionate areas of the body. The mathematics of percentages and fractions appeared to confuse some assessors. Simply stated, a burn from the wrist to the elbow is 50% of the arm, while a burn from the wrist to the mid-forearm is 25% of the arm. A burn from the feet to the nipple line is 75%.

6.3 Berkow Formula (Berkow's Table)

Berkow (1924) [13] described a method of estimating the extensiveness of lesions (burns and scalds) based on determining the percentage of total body surface affected by a burn. A method for the formula is derived from the rule of nines where certain body areas account for 9% each and the total body area is given a value of 99. The remaining 1% is the perineum. The age of the patient is taken into consideration when applying the Berkow formula. For example, the head of a 1-year-old child is proportionately larger than that of an adult; therefore, the 1-year-old's head would account for 19% of total body surface, while the head of an adult would account for 7%.

6.4 Lund and Browder Chart

A series of charts was produced by Lund and Browder in 1944 [14]. They are useful in the management of burns of children for estimating the total body surface area affected. It takes into consideration the age of the person, with decreasing percentage of body surface area (BSA) for the head and increasing percentage of BSA for the legs as the child ages. Children have smaller extremities but larger heads than adults.

More accurate assessment can be made using a Lund and Browder chart that maps the percentage total body surface area (TBSA) in a little more detail and includes some of the variations that occur with age, from birth to adulthood (Table 1).

The degree of burn can be drawn on Fig. 2.

7 Resuscitation Fluid

For calculation of resuscitation fluid, Jain (2014) [15] used the Berkow formula to determine the percent surface area burned.

A simplified version of the Parkland burn therapy fluid formula is described by

Table 1 Lund and Browder chart

Area	Age 0	Age 1	Age 5	Age 1	Age 15	Adult
1/2 of the head	9 1/2	8 1/2	6 1/2	5 1/2	4 1/2	3 1/2
1/2 of the thigh	2 3/4	3 1/4	4	4 1/2	4 1/2	4 3/4
1/2 of the lower leg	2 1/2	2 1/2	2 3/4	3	4 1/4	3 1/2

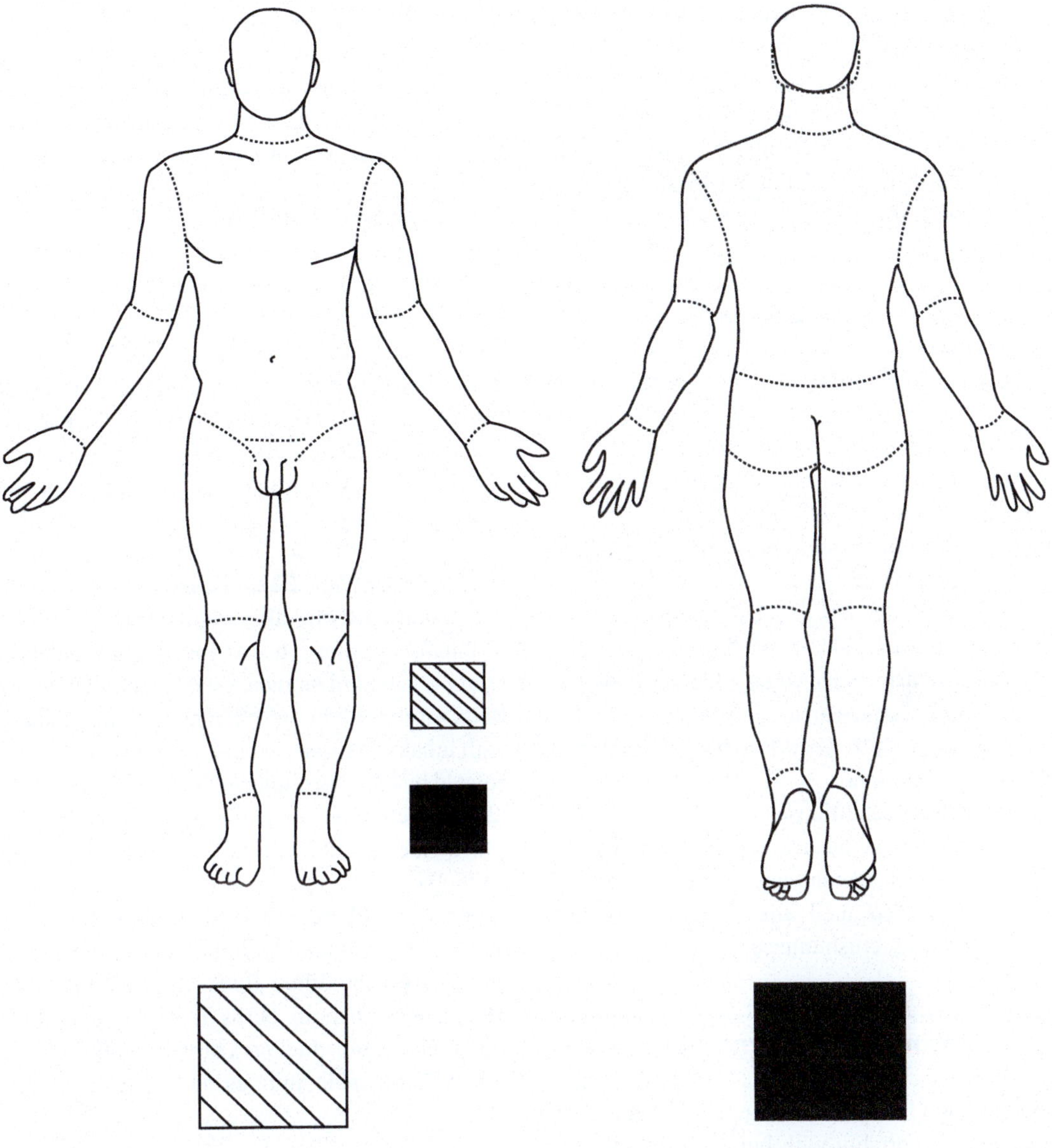

Fig. 2 Lund and Browder

Freshwater and Su (1979) [16]. The rule states that for the first 8 h after burn, the hourly rate of Ringer's lactate solution (in milliliters per hour) equals the patient's weight in pounds multiplied by the percent burn and divided by 9.

8 Indications for Referral to a Burns Unit [17]

1. All complex injuries should be referred.
2. A burn injury is more likely to be complex if associated with:

   (a) Extremes of age—under 5 or over 60 years
3. Site of injury:
   (a) Face, hands, or perineum
   (b) Feet (dermal or full-thickness loss)
   (c) Any flexure, particularly the neck or axilla
   (d) Circumferential dermal or full-thickness burn of limb, torso, or neck
4. Inhalational injury:
   (a) Any substantial injury, excluding pure carbon monoxide poisoning
5. Mechanism of injury:
   (a) Chemical injury >5% of total body surface area
   (b) Exposure to ionizing radiation
   (c) High-pressure steam injury
   (d) High-tension electrical injury
   (e) Hydrofluoric acid burn >1% of total body surface area
   (f) Suspicion of non-accidental injury
6. Large size (dermal or full-thickness loss):
   (a) Pediatric (<16 years old) >5% of total body surface area
   (b) Adult (≥16 years) >10% of total body surface area
7. Coexisting conditions:
   (a) Any serious medical conditions (cardiac dysfunction, immunosuppression, pregnancy)
   (b) Any associated injuries (fractures, head injuries, crush injuries)

9 Mortality in Burns

Schjerning (1884) [18] advanced the idea of the relation of mortality with burn size in 1884. He found that death always followed if two thirds of the body was burned, was to be expected if 50% of the body was burned, and generally occurred if a third of the body was burned.

9.1 Baux Score

The Baux score is a system used to predict the chance of mortality due to severe burns. The score is an index which takes into account the correlative and causal relationship between mortality and factors including advancing age, burn size and the presence of inhalational injury. Studies have shown that the Baux score is highly correlative with length of stay in hospital due to burns and final outcome.

9.1.1 Original Method

The original Baux score was proposed by Baux in 1961 [19]. Two factors were used. The first was the total body surface area affected by burning (usually estimated using the Wallace rule of nines or calculated using a Lund and Browder chart) and the second being the age of the patient. According to Roberts et al. (2012) [20], the Baux score continues to provide an indication of the risk of mortality.

9.1.2 Modified Baux Score

The modified score takes into account the effect of inhalation injury. It was found that inhalation injury resulted in an increase of around 17 on the Baux score, and this addition means that a patient with inhalation injury would have their score calculated by *body area affected* + *age of patient* + 17 [21]. Recent analysis of mortality in burn units worldwide has shown that for well-performing units the LD50 (the point at which 50% of patients would be expected to die) for major burns has significantly improved and the best units have a modified Baux score of 130–140. This means that all burns in children (except 100% TBSA full-thickness burns) should be considered survivable injuries and actively treated [22].

9.2 The Belgian Outcome in Burn Injury (BOBI)

The Belgian Outcome in Burn Injury (BOBI) prediction model consists of a 0–10 point score based on three major predictors for mortality: increasing age, total burned surface area, and the presence of inhalation injury [23]. This is an easy-to-use prediction model, which proved to be accurate in distinct populations with severe burn injury.

9.3 Charlson Comorbidity Index (CCI)

Heng et al. [24] reviewed the revised Baux score, Belgian Outcome in Burn Injury (BOBI) score, Abbreviated Burn Severity Index (ABSI), APACHE II score, Sequential Organ Failure Assessment (SOFA) score, and updated Charlson Comorbidity Index (CCI). Only the revised Baux score and the updated CCI were independently associated with shorter time to death. The data suggested that the revised Baux score and the updated Charlson Comorbidity Index (CCI) are independently associated with inpatient mortality in patients admitted to intensive care with burn injuries affecting ≥15% total burn surface area (TBSA). This emphasizes the importance of comorbidities in the prognosis of patients with severe burn injuries.

The Charlson Comorbidity Index (CCI) assesses the comorbidity risk associated to a series of conditions in order to offer medical specialists an informed decision-making process in terms of specific screenings or medical procedures [25]. The index accounts for the patient age and 16 conditions. This instrument is used to categorize comorbidities of patients and uses the International Classification of Diseases (ICD) diagnosis codes [26].

9.3.1 Charlson Comorbidity Index Scoring System

The CCI index predicts the 10-year mortality for patients presenting one or more of the conditions in the model. This is an index used in decision-making when a medical professional is presented with a treatment solution but needs to take into account the short- and long-term benefits of the treatment in a patient with other comorbidity conditions and should assess their long-term risk. Comorbidity is the term given to the presence of one or more additional conditions existing simultaneously, independently or not (with or without a causal effect), with a disease considered primary. It also suggests the effect of one or more additional conditions on the primary disease.

The age groups and each condition are awarded a specific number of points, some conditions weighing more than others, based on the adjusted risk of mortality (Table 2). The more points given, the more likely the predicted adverse outcome. The index then sums the points and offers a 10-year survival/mortality prognosis.

Table 2 Charlson Comorbidity Index scoring system

Score	Condition
1	Over 40 years of age: Divided into four age groups of different risk—under 50, between 50 and 59, between 60 and 69, and 70 or over Myocardial infarction: Patient or family Congestive heart failure Peripheral vascular disease peripheral artery occlusive disease and peripheral obliterative arteriopathy, including aortic aneurysm Cerebrovascular disease Dementia Chronic pulmonary disease Connective tissue disease Peptic ulcer disease Mild liver disease Diabetes without end organ damage (excludes diet controlled alone)
2	Hemiplegia Moderate or severe renal disease Diabetes with end organ damage or brittle diabetes Tumor without metastasis except over 5 years Leukemia Lymphoma
3	Moderate or severe liver disease
6	AIDS (not just HIV positive)

9.3.2 Calculating the Charlson Probability

This is the method through which the CCI score is transformed into a survival/mortality percentage: taking into account that C is the score result obtained by adding the points. For example, at a score of 6, the 10-year survival is 2.25%.

The list of comorbidities has been modified to 17 categories by Deyo et al. (1992) [27]. The list of specific ICD diagnosis codes that are used to identify different categories of comorbidity has been modified by Romano et al. (1993) [28] and updated from ICD-9-CM to work with ICD-10 coding by Quan et al. (2005) [29]. The original weights developed for use with the index have also been modified by Schneeweiss et al. (2003) [30].

There have been several variations to the index such as the Charlson-Deyo, Charlson-Romano, Charlson-Manitoba, and Charlson-D'Hoores comorbidity indices.

10 Treatment of Burns

The treatment of burns is dependent on the type and extent of the burns. A first-degree burn can be treated at home. The only symptom may be pain, and acetaminophen or ibuprofen may be used. The wounds are best treated with cool water for 5 min or longer to decrease the discomfort. If the patient still complains, lidocaine with aloe vera gel or cream may be used. At times, an antibiotic ointment with loose gauze can be applied especially on the knees, ankles, feet, spine, shoulders, elbows, and forearms. These will heal in 7–10 days.

With second-degree burns, there will be blisters and soreness. Pain medication such as acetaminophen or ibuprofen may be used. Running cool water on the region for about 15 min may help. Some blisters may burst and a wet or weeping appears. This can be treated with an antibiotic cream. Over time, thick, soft, scab-like fibrinous exudate may develop over the wound keeping the area clean, and bandaging it properly is required to prevent infection. Colloid (dextran or plasma) may be necessary. The wound heals in 3 weeks or longer. Rarely is a skin graft necessary.

Third-degree burns require hospitalization, and treatment is dependent on the extent of the area burned. There may not be significant pain except with dressing changes. If there is less than 15% of the body involved, fluid requirements are minimal and can be met with oral salt-soda solution containing 3 Gm of sodium chloride and 1.5 Gm of sodium bicarbonate [31].

In more extensive burns, the first 24 h should have colloid (whole blood), 0.5 mL per Kg body weight for each percentage of body surface burned, and electrolytes 1.5 mL per Kg body weight for each percentage of body surface burned. About 2000 mL of glucose should be administered. More than 50% burn is calculated as a 50% burn.

Extensively burned patients should have one half of the fluids in the first 8 h, and more colloids may be necessary. In the second 24 h, one half of the first 24 h of electrolytes and colloids should be infused with 2000 mL of glucose in water [31]. The rate of fluid administration depends on the blood pressure (if falling) and the urine output under 30 mL/h. If the urine output is more than 50 mL/h, the rate of administered should be slowed. The rate of infusion is slowed if the patient has respiratory involvement. The serum sodium level should not exceed 140 meq/L. From the 3rd to the 12th day, electrolyte imbalances occur and should be followed at least daily. When diuresis occurs, electrolyte-free water should be given in order to maintain the serum sodium at about 135 meq/L. Maintain the hematocrit at about 45%.

In extensively burned patients, the wounds should be cleaned thoroughly and debris and dead tissue removed. An occlusive dressing may be applied, but this may be conducive to infection because of the warmth and moisture. Changing dressings daily is painful, and morphine is usually required. The risks of general anesthesia may be necessary if the patient still cannot tolerate the dressing changes. Exposure of the area, if possible, allows the wound to be examined frequently for early detection of infection.

11 Complications

11.1 Metabolic Disturbances with Hypermetabolism

A burn of over 20% of the body is conducive to metabolic disturbances with hypermetabolism, increased gluconeogenesis, insulin resistance, increase in endogenous lipolysis, and loss of lean body mass [32, 33].

The nutritional requirements are particularly increased for glucose and proteins.

There is a maximal oxidation rate for glucose of 5 mg/kg/min for adults and children that should not be exceeded to avoid the development of fatty liver [34]. Protein requirements are increased to 1.5–2 g/kg/day.

Table 3 Calculation of caloric requirements in the patient with burn wounds can be assessed utilizing either the Curreri or Toronto formulas [35]

Curreri formula = 25 × body weight (kg) + 40 × % TBSA burned
Toronto formula = −4343 + 10.5 × % TBSA + 0.23 × previous 24 h caloric intake +0.84 × Harris-Benedict equation +114 × previous 24 h maximal temperature—4.5 × days postburn injury

Table 4 Derivation of IBW using the Devine formula and adjusted body weight (ABW)

Devine formula: Men—ideal body weight (in kilograms) = 50 + 2.3 kg per inch over 5 ft Women—ideal body weight (in kilograms) = 45.5 + 2.3 kg per inch over 5 ft
IBW (male) = 50 + (2.3 × (height [in inches]—60))
IBW (female) = 45.5 + (2.3 × (height [in inches]—60))
ABW = 0.25 × (actual body weight—IBW) + IBW

Enteral nutrition calculator may be used to calculate the appropriate tube feeding rate and supplemental protein required to meet a burn patient's nutritional needs. It provides the results of calculations using both the Curreri and Toronto formulas (Table 3). Protein requirements in the burn patient are estimated at 2 g/kg/day.

11.1.1 Determination of Ideal and Adjusted Body Weight

If the patient is greater than 20% above ideal body weight (IBW), the adjusted body weight should be used in the calculation of enteral nutrition rates for surgical and trauma patients. Derivation of IBW using the Devine formula and adjusted body weight (ABW) are shown in Table 4.

11.1.2 Trace Elements

Trace elements are lost in large amounts with the exudative losses in adults and children [36, 37]. The losses cause trace element deficiencies in patients with major burns, if not compensated (particularly selenium, zinc, and copper). Early substitution, with doses that represent six to ten times the recommended parenteral doses, is associated with improved wound healing and reduction of infective complications.

11.1.3 Further Treatment

Wolf et al. (2006) [38] found that propranolol, by attenuating the sympathetic response and its non-selective metabolic beta-2 blocking actions, strongly reduces catabolism and reduces cardiac workload in children and adults. Anabolic agents, such as insulin and oxandrolone, accelerate wound healing and shorten hospital stay. Oxandrolone started within 7 days of injury has been shown to improve long-term outcome in both adults and children in prospective randomized trials. Recombinant growth hormone (GH) probably has its place in the treatment of children (but not in adult burns patients) as children with burn injuries have a proven GH deficit.

The hypermetabolic state that may persist for years after a major burn can result in a decrease in bone density and a loss of muscle mass [39].

11.2 Multiple Organ Failure

Infective complications lead to multiorgan failure (MOF), poor outcome, and even death. Sheridan et al. (1998) [40] reported that burn patients dying in MOF did not have a high rate of positive blood cultures in the later phase of their care but succumbed during so-called "sterile" conditions. This finding was important as it underlined that infection is not always the immediate cause of death for this patient group. Some patients also develop sepsis, having had MOF of a different etiology. This led to the idea that burn injury and the inflammatory reaction secondary to it were important and significant contributors to the development of MOF in burn injury. Organ failure occurs in the lung (ARDS) and kidneys [41–43]. Mortality rates of patients with increasing number of organs failing are less than previously documented because of aggressive surgical approaches used in larger burn injuries and to a reduction in do not resuscitate (DNR) orders in some TBSA% ranges.

11.3 Delirium

Antipsychotic drugs are most effective in all types of delirium such as haloperidol

(0.5–10 mg), the dose to be reduced when symptoms improve, and alternatively or additionally olanzapine (5–10 mg) [44–46]. However, in delirium caused by alcohol or sedative hypnotic withdrawal, benzodiazepines are the treatment of choice, complemented in time by clonidine (600–1200 μg/day). Levomepromazine is not advocated to treat delirium in ICU patients.

11.4 Other Complications

A number of complications may occur, with infections being the most common [47]. In order of frequency, potential complications include pneumonia, cellulitis, urinary tract infections, and respiratory failure. Risk factors for infection include burns of more than 30% TBSA, full-thickness burns, extremes of age (young or old) or burns involving the legs, or perineum [48]. Anemia secondary to full-thickness burns of greater than 10% TBSA is common. Electrical burns may lead to compartment syndrome or rhabdomyolysis due to muscle breakdown. Pneumonia occurs commonly in those with inhalation injuries [49]. Blood clotting in the veins of the legs is estimated to occur in 6–25% of people. Keloids may form subsequent to a burn, particularly in those who are Hispanic, Asian, or African-American. Following a burn, children may have significant psychological trauma and experience post-traumatic stress disorder [50]. Scarring may also result in a disturbance in body image. In the developing parts of the world, significant burns may result in social isolation, extreme poverty, and child abandonment [51].

11.5 Prognosis

Deaths from burn injury increased with advancing age and burn size and the presence of inhalation injury. For patients under age 60 and with a TBSA between 0.1 and 19.9, the presence of inhalation injury increased the likelihood of death by nearly 24 times [52].

Table 5 Mortality rate by burn group size (TBSA) [52]

% TBSA	Mortality rate (%)
0.1–9.9	0.6
10–19.9	2.7
10–29.9	8.4
30–39.9	16.8
40–49.9	26.8
50–59.9	36.7
60–69.9	44.7
70–70.9	55.0
80–89.9	71.4

Table 5 shows the proportion of patients in each category of total burn size who died and the case fatality rate. This clearly increased with burn size. The burn size associated with a 50% case fatality (LD50) appears to be approximately 65–70% TBSA [52].

Conclusions

Care of the patient with burns is determined by the total body surface area that is burned and the degree of the burn as well as the age of the patient and whether there is concomitant lung injury from the burn. Secondary problems such as medical disorders can add to the patient's risks of mortality.

Proper and knowledgeable care of the burn and the patient will make all the difference in the world.

References

1. Herndon D (2012) A brief history of acute burn care management. In: Herndon D (ed) Total burn care, 4th edn. Saunders Elsevier, Edinburgh, p 24
2. Pećanac M, Janjić Z, Komarcević A, Pajić M, Dobanovacki D, Misković SS (2013) Burns treatment in ancient times. Med Pregl 66(5–6):263–267
3. Song D, Neligan PC (2012) Plastic surgery, 3rd edn. Saunders, Edinburgh, p 393
4. Dupuytren G (1833) Clinical Lectures in Surgery, Delivered at Hotel-Dieu in 1832. In: Doane AS, transl. Boston, Carter, Hendee, p 234–236
5. Wylock P (2010) The life and times of Guillaume Dupuytren, 1777–1835. Brussels University Press, Brussels, p 60

6. Cancio LC, Wolf SC (2012) A history of burn care. In: Jeschke MG, Kamolz LP, Sjöberg F, Wolf SE (eds) Handbook of burns. Springer-Verlag, Wien, pp 1–17
7. Khan A, Solan M. Burns: types, treatments, and more. www.healthline.com/health/burns. Accessed 24 Sep 2016
8. Blahd WH Jr, O'Connor M. Burns and electric shock—topic overview. http://www.webmed.com/first-aid/tc/burns-topic-overview. Accessed 24 Sep 2016
9. Smart C (1876) On burns by gunpowder and scalds by steam. Lancet 2(2769):421–422
10. Wallace rule of nines. Wikipedia, the free encyclopedia. https://en.wikipedia.org/wiki/Wallace_rule_of_nines. Accessed 8 Oct 2016
11. Wallace AB (1951) The exposure treatment of burns. Lancet 1(6653):501–504
12. Smith JJ, Malyon AD, Scerri GV, Burge TS (2005) A comparison of serial halving and the rule of nines as a pre-hospital assessment tool in burns. Br J Plast Surg 58(7):957–967
13. Berkow SG (1924) A method of estimating the extensiveness of lesions (burns and scalds) based on surface area proportions. Arch Surg 8:138–148
14. Lund CC, Browder NC (1944) The estimation of areas of burns. Surg Gynecol Obstet 79:352–358
15. Jain V (2014) Review of preventive & social medicine (including biostatistics). Jaypee Brothers Medical Publishers, New Delhi
16. Freshwater MF, Su CT (1979) The second rule of nines: a guide for resuscitation of burn patients. Ann Plast Surg 2(4):298
17. Hettiaratchy S, Papini R (2004) ABC of burns: Initial management of a major burn: II—assessment and resuscitation. BMJ 329(7457):101–103
18. Schjerning (1884) About the death as a result of burning and scalding from the court physician standpoint. 42:24–66, 273–300
19. Baux S (1961) Contribution a l'etude du traitement local des brulures thermique etendues. Paris, France, Thesis
20. Roberts G, Lloyd M, Parker M, Martin R, Philp B, Shelley O, Dziewulski P (2012) The Baux score is dead. Long live the Baux score: a 27-year retrospective cohort study of mortality at a regional burns service. J Trauma Acute Care Surg 72(1):251–256
21. Granger J, Estrada C, Abramo T (2009) An evidence-based approach to pediatric burns. Pediatr Emergency Med Pract 6(1):1–18
22. Osler T, Glance LG, Hosmer DW (2010) Simplified estimates of the probability of death after burn injuries: extending and updating the Baux score. J Trauma 68(3):690–697
23. Brusselaers N, Monstrey S, Blot S (2010) Predictive value of the Belgian outcome in burn injury (BOBI) prediction model. Burns 36(8):1318–1320
24. Heng JS, Clancy O, Atkins J, Leon-Villapalos J, Williams AJ, Keays R, Hayes M, Takata M, Jones I, Vizcaychipi MP (2015) Revised Baux score and updated Charlson comorbidity index are independently associated with mortality in burns intensive care patients. Burns 41(7):1420–1427
25. Charlson ME, Pompei P, Ales KL, MacKenzie CR (1987) A new method of classifying prognostic comorbidity in longitudinal studies: development and validation. J Chronic Dis 40(5):373–383
26. Frenkel WJ, Jongerius EJ, Mandjes-van Uitert MJ, van Munster BC, de Rooij SE (2014) Validation of the Charlson comorbidity index in acutely hospitalized elderly adults: a prospective cohort study. J Am Geriatr Soc 62(2):342–346
27. Deyo RA, Cherkin DC, Ciol MA (1992) Adapting a clinical comorbidity index for use with ICD-9-CM administrative databases. J Clin Epidemiol 45(6):613–619
28. Romano PS, Roos LL, Jollis JG (1993) Adapting a clinical comorbidity index for use with ICD-9-CM administrative data: differing perspectives. J Clin Epidemiol 46(10):1075–1079
29. Quan H, Sundararajan V, Halfon P, Fong A, Burnand B, Luthi JC, Saunders LD, Beck CA, Feasby TE, Ghali WA (2005) Coding algorithms for defining comorbidities in ICD-9-CM and ICD-10 administrative data. Med Care 43(11):1130–1139
30. Schneeweiss S, Wang PS, Avorn J, Glynn RJ (2003) Improved comorbidity adjustment for predicting mortality in Medicare populations. Health Serv Res 38(4):1103–1120
31. Artz CP, Soroff HS (1955) Modern concepts in the treatment of burns. J Am Med Assoc 159(5):411–417
32. Cunningham JJ (1990) Factors contributing to increased energy expenditure in thermal injury: a review of studies employing indirect calorimetry. JPEN J Parenter Enteral Nutr 14(6):649–656
33. Jeschke M, Norbury WB, Finnerty CC, Mlcak RP, Kulp GA, Branski LK, Gauglitz GG, Herndon B, Swick A, Herndon DN (2008) Age differences in inflammatory and hypermetabolic postburn responses. Pediatrics 121(3):497–507
34. Masters B, Aarabi S, Sidhwa F, Wood F (2012) High-carbohydrate, high-protein, low-fat versus low-carbohydrate, high-protein, high-fat enteral feeds for burns. Cochrane Database Syst Rev 1:CD006122
35. Burn Nutrition Calculator. http://www.surgicalcriticalcare.net/Resouces/burn_nutrition.php. Accessed 4 Oct 2016
36. Berger MM, Shenkin A (2007) Trace element requirements in critically ill burned patients. J Trace Elem Med Biol 21(Suppl 1):44–48
37. Berger MM, Baines M, Raffoul W, Benathan M, Chiolero RL, Reeves C, Revelly JP, Cayeux MC, Sénéchaud I, Shenkin A (2007) Trace element supplementation after major burns modulates antioxidant status and clinical course by way of increased tissue trace element concentrations. Am J Clin Nutr 85(5):1293–1300

38. Wolf SE, Edelman LS, Kemalyan N, Donison L, Cross J, Underwood M, Spence RJ, Noppenberger D, Palmieri TL, Greenhalgh DG, Lawless M et al (2006) Effects of oxandrolone on outcome measures in the severely burned: a multicenter prospective randomized double-blind trial. J Burn Care Res 27(2):131–139
39. Rojas Y, Finnerty CC, Radhakrishnan RS, Herndon DN (2012) Burns: an update on current pharmacotherapy. Expert Opin Pharmacother 13(17):2485–2494
40. Sheridan RL, Ryan CM, Yin LM, Hurley J, Tompkins RG (1998) Death in the burn unit: sterile multiple organ failure. Burns 24(4):307–311
41. Cumming J, Purdue GF, Hunt JL, O'Keefe GE (2001) Objective estimates of the incidence and consequences of multiple organ dysfunction and sepsis after burn trauma. J Trauma 50(3):510–515
42. Fitzwater J, Purdue GF, Hunt JL, O'Keefe GE (2003) The risk factors and time course of sepsis and organ dysfunction after burn trauma. J Trauma 54(5):959–966
43. Steinvall I, Bak Z, Sjoberg F (2008) Acute respiratory distress syndrome is as important as inhalation injury for the development of respiratory dysfunction in major burns. Burns 34(4):441–451
44. Lonergan E, Britton AM, Luxenberg J, Wyller T (2007) Antipsychotics for delirium. Cochrane Database Syst Rev 2:CD005594
45. Devlin JW, Skrobik Y (2011) Antipsychotics for the prevention and treatment of delirium in the intensive care unit: what is their role? Harv Rev Psychiatry 19(2):59–67
46. Burns A, Gallagley A, Byrne J (2004) Delirium. J Neurol Neurosurg Psychiatry 75(3):362–367
47. Herndon D (2012) Epidemiological, demographic, and outcome characteristics of burn injury. In: Herndon D (ed) Total burn care, 4th edn. Saunders, Edinburgh, p 23
48. King C, Henretig FM, King BR, Loiselle J, Ruddy RM (2008) In: Wiley JF II (ed) Textbook of pediatric emergency procedures, 2nd edn. Lippincott Williams & Wilkins, Philadelphia, p 1077
49. Brunicardi FC (2010) Burns. In: Brunicardi FC, Andersen D, Billiar T, Dunn D, Hunter J, Matthews J, Raphael E, Pollock RE (eds) Schwartz's principles of surgery, 9th edn. McGraw-Hill, New York
50. Roberts MC (2009) Handbook of pediatric psychology, 4th edn. Guilford, New York, p 421
51. Peck MD (2011) Epidemiology of burns throughout the world. Part I: distribution and risk factors. Burns 37(7):1087–1100
52. American Burn Association. 2015 National Burn Repository: Report of Data from 2005–2014. p. 10

Care and (First) Aid of Children with Burns

Martin G.A. Baartmans, Helene G. Stas, and Cornelis H. van der Vlies

1 Introduction

Nearly half of all burns are caused by accidents. Risk factors include psychiatric problems, addiction, and low socioeconomic status. Neglect and child abuse must always be considered for children with burns. Globally, burns are a serious public health problem. An estimated 265,000 deaths occur each year from fires alone. Almost half occur in the WHO Southeast Asia Region [1]. Approximately 1.25 million people are burned in the United States every year. Of these burn patients, 60,000–80,000 require hospitalization. Of those, 40% (30,000) are children younger than 15 years. About 4000 burn patients die each year and approximately 1000 of them are children [2]. In the Netherlands, 35,000 patients with burns are treated by GPs annually. 1700 patients are admitted to the hospital, of which 600 patients are treated in one of the burn centers. One third (200) of these patients are children. Hot liquids are the main cause of burns in young children up to the age of 4 (two thirds of all admitted children). In children of school-going ages, we encounter more burns caused by flames, particularly in boys. Additionally, there are seasonal burns during summer caused by barbecues and fireworks/flame burns at New Year's [3].

Care of children with burns is performed in a structural way (as it is done for every patient with a trauma). After the first care and stabilization, it is important to make an estimation of the degree of the burn, the total burned surface area (TBSA), and, if necessary, start rehydration [3].

It is crucial that all (para)medics of a referring hospital and/or ambulance are able to adequately provide first care for a child and refer it to a burn center. The guidelines of the Dutch Burns Foundation (2014) "First care of burn patients in the acute phase (1st 24 h) of a burn and referral to a burn center" or the European guideline may be used as reference [4, 5].

2 Degree of the Burn

In case of a burn, the skin is partly or fully damaged, caused by the effect of heat (hot liquids, fire/flame, or contact burn), a chemical substance, or electricity, during a certain time, above a certain critical temperature [6, 7].

2.1 First-Degree Burn

Skin is only red and painful, without disruption of the tissue or continuity, and therefore there is no wound. When determining the surface area of

M.G.A. Baartmans, M.D., Ph.D. (✉) • H.G. Stas
Department of Pediatrics, Maasstad Hospital, Rotterdam, The Netherlands
e-mail: BaartmansM@maasstadziekenhuis.nl

C.H. van der Vlies, M.D., Ph.D.
Department of Trauma and Burn Surgery, Maasstad Hospital, Rotterdam, The Netherlands

Recent Clinical Techniques, Results, and Research in Wounds (2017)
DOI 10.1007/15695_2017_21, © Springer International Publishing AG
Published Online: 24 October 2017

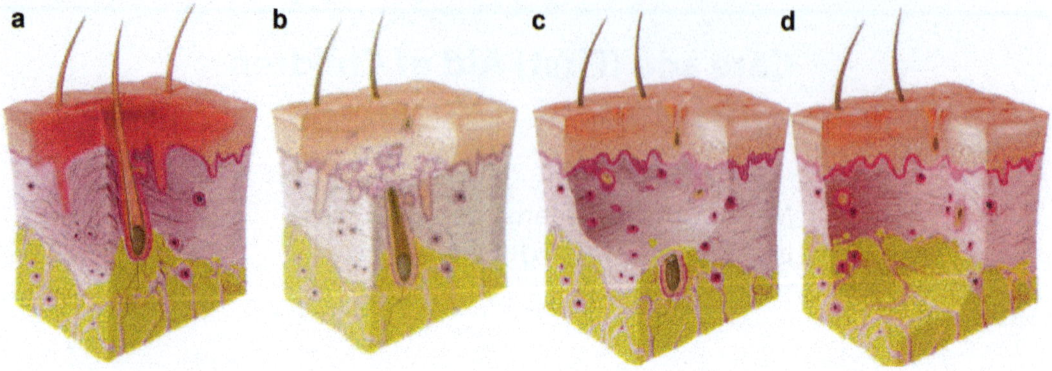

Fig. 1 Burn depths. (**a**) First-degree burns. (**b**) Superficial second-degree burns. (**c**) Deep, second-degree burns. (**d**) Third-degree burns (Used with permission from Dutch Burn Foundation)

a burn, this area is not included. A well-known example of a first-degree burn is a sun burn, where no blistering or fluid loss occurs. After a few days, the skin will start to peel and spontaneous healing occurs (Fig. 1).

2.2 Second-Degree Burns

In case of a second-degree burn or partial thickness burn, the epidermis and dermis are damaged. This dermal burn can be subdivided into superficial and deep dermal. This distinction is important for the expected healing time and scarring. In case of a superficial dermal burn, necrosis reaches to the superficial dermis.

The skin is painful, red, shiny, and moist and displays blisters. There are still lots of vital epithelial cells present in the bed of the burn, from which healing occurs within 14 days. Usually, there is no thickened scarring. However, discoloration of the skin may be permanent (Fig. 1).

2.3 Deep Dermal Burns

In case of deep dermal burns, necrosis reaches deep into the dermis. Here, the skin is pale. Vital epithelial cells can only be found in the remnants of the skin adnexa (hair follicles, sweat, and sebaceous glands). Reepithelialization may occur from this, but this will take longer than 2 weeks. Surgical treatment may be necessary. Both in conservative and surgical treatment of deep dermal burns, scarring may occur (Fig. 1).

2.4 Third-Degree Burns

In case of a full-thickness burn, also referred to as subdermal burn, necrosis reaches into the subcutis, and this always leads to scarring (Fig. 1). The skin has a waxlike feel or is tough like leather (eschar). There is no circulation and no capillary refill. The patient feels no pain from these burns due to destruction of the nerve fiber ends. These burns are often caused by fire (skin is black or brown) but may also be caused by hot liquid (skin is white or a redness that cannot be pushed down ("lobster redness").

3 Pathophysiology

In 1953, Jackson [8] described a burn model where the burn is subdivided into three zones: zone of coagulation (necrosis), stasis, and hyperemia. The zone of coagulation consists of dead necrotic tissue, from which no healing can occur. The zones of stasis and hyperemia still contain vital tissue. In case of poor circulation (local and/or systematic) or wound care (for instance due to dehydration or infections), these zones can deepen and transfer to the zone of coagulation. As a result, the burn cannot only deepen further, but the total body surface area burn may also expand. Healing of a burn is a dynamic process and is influenced by the care that is being provided.

In case of large burns with a TBSA >20% to 25%, the whole body consists of a zone of hyperemia due to which generalized edema may occur. In case of a burns with a TBSA >15%, a generalized response occurs due to the release of inflammatory mediators and neural stimulation. Consequently, changes may occur on various levels.

Due to increased capillary permeability, fluid loss and loss of protein in tissues and (generalized) edema occur with a chance of hypovolemia and circulatory shock. On a pulmonary level, respiratory distress syndrome may occur. Due to the release of stress hormones such as cortisol, catecholamines, and glucagon, a hypermetabolic state arises that may continue for a long time. There is an immune suppression, both on a cellular and humoral level. Due to increased permeability of the intestines, there is a risk of bacterial translocation, certainly a reason to start with enteral nutrition as soon as possible [9].

4 TBSA Calculation

Severity of burn is determined by extensiveness and location of the burn, the age and general condition, etiology, and additional injuries. Extensiveness is expressed in percentage of TBSA. Here, only second- and third-degree burns are included. Redness of first-degree burns is not included. TBSA can be calculated in multiple ways. The best known method is the rule of nine [10]. This assumes adult proportions, where the body is subdivided into zones of 9% or a multitude of this. For instance, the head and neck are 9%, an arm is 9%, front and back of the torso each 18%, and a leg is 18% as well. For the genitalia, 1% is calculated separately. For a child younger than 10 years old, other proportions apply with a relatively large head and smaller legs.

Surface of the head and neck is 18% and each leg 14% of the total surface area for a child up to the age of 1 year old. After the first year, the surface area of the head and neck reduces with 1% per year and that of each leg increased with 0.5%. Around the age of 10, the child has reached adult proportions.

A second method is the hand method [11]. Here, the palmar side of the hand with closed fingers of the patient is used as a measurement for 1% of the total body surface area. In the burn centers, modified methods are used, such as the Lund and Browder chart [12].

TBSA is often overestimated. This may be due to a number of factors, such as redness (first-degree burn) or the incorrect application of the surface corrections for children [13].

5 Cooling Burns

After stopping the burning process, the residual heat in the skin must be discharged to prevent deepening of the burn. Cool acute burns between 10 and 20 min if this does not hinder other interventions. Preferably cool with water underneath a running faucet (at approx. 15–30 °C) and adjust the temperature to what the patient experiences as comfortable. Cooling should ideally be started immediately, but also after a delay of up to 3 h, cooling can be considered to alleviate pain [4, 14–16]. In case of chemical burns, rinsing occurs during 45 min in order to dilute the concentration of the substance. Hypothermia due to cooling too long or too cold may increase mortality [17]. After cooling, cover the wound and provide pain medication [7, 18]. After adequate cooling with running water, cooling blankets have no added value and are not recommended. Due to their powerful heat-extracting capacity, the danger of hypothermia in children is significant, and the chance of secondary deepening of the burn due to vasoconstriction is also present. Only use cooling blankets as an alternative when no water is available. After cooling, the patient must be covered dry and sterile (warm). Burn wound covering, may be done by clean/sterile cloths; at home, one may also use plastic cling film immediately on the wound and then cover it with cloths [4].

6 First Care of Children with Burns (Primary Survey)

Care of burn patients does not initially differ with that of trauma patients, and also in burn patients, attention is first paid to vital functions according to the ABCD principle (Fig. 2) [19, 20].

EMERGENCY MANAGEMENT OF BURNS

GUIDELINE EMERGENCY MANAGEMENT OF BURNS*

A. Airway maintenance with cervical spine control
B. Breathing and ventilation
C. Circulation with haemorrhage control
D. Disability - neurological status - **Alert / Voice / Pain / Unresponsive**
E. Exposure and environmental control
Calculate percentage **T**otal **B**urn **S**urface **A**rea (TBSA)
F. Fluid resuscitation proportional to burn size
Adults: ≥ 15% TBSA - Children: ≥ 10% TBSA
Ringer's lactate solution or NaCl 0.9%: 4 ml/kg / % TBSA / 24 hr
(Give 1/2 this amount in the first 8 hours post burn)
In children extra fluids: glucose / NACL (24 hr)
100 ml/kg < 10 kg + 50 ml/kg 10-20 kg + 20 ml/kg > 20 kg
Urine output:
Adults 0.5 ml/kg/hr
Children (< 30 kg) range 1-2 ml/kg/hr
G. Get lab - Vital functions, catheters and radiology
Give medication (pain control)
H. History
A - **Allergies**
M - **Medications**
P - **Past illnesses**
L - **Last meal**
E - **Events/Environment related to injury**

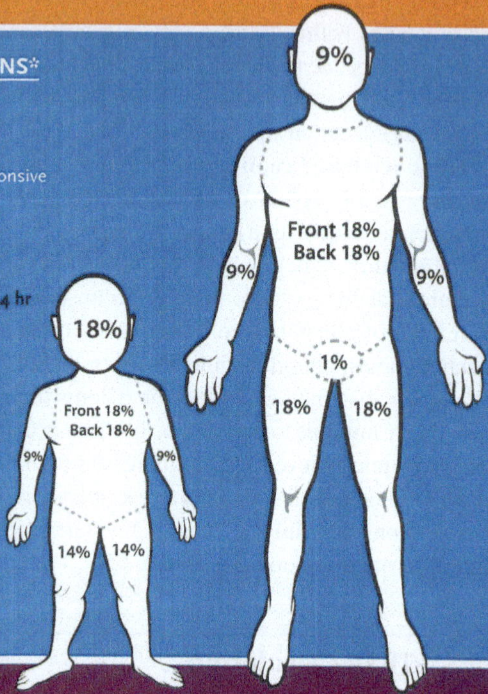

CALCULATE % TBSA

Wallace rule of nines

Child 1 year old: head 18% - leg 14%

For children over the age of one year, for each year above one, add 0.5% to each leg and subtract 1% for the head. This formula should be used until the adult rule of nines values are reached.

TBSA - Hand rule:
Patients palm with fingers and thumb = 1% body surface area

TBSA - Lund & Browder chart

SURFACE AREA	1 year	1 - 4 years	5 - 9 years	10 - 14 years	15 years
Head	19	17	13	11	9
Neck	2	2	2	2	2
Trunk front	13	13	13	13	13
Trunk back	13	13	13	13	13
Right Buttock	2.5	2.5	2.5	2.5	2.5
Left Buttock	2.5	2.5	2.5	2.5	2.5
Genitalia	1	1	1	1	1
Right upper arm	4	4	4	4	4
Left upper arm	4	4	4	4	4
Right lower arm	3	3	3	3	3
Left lower arm	3	3	3	3	3
Right hand	2.5	2.5	2.5	2.5	2.5
Left hand	2.5	2.5	2.5	2.5	2.5
Right tigh	5.5	6.5	8	8.5	9
Left tigh	5.5	6.5	8	8.5	9
Right leg	5	5	5.5	6	6.5
Left leg	5	5	5.5	6	6.5
Right foot	3.5	3.5	3.5	3.5	3.5
Left foot	3.5	3.5	3.5	3.5	3.5

Referral criteria to burn centre

- TBSA ≥ 10% in Adults
- TBSA ≥ 5% in children and the elderly
- Deep Burns ≥ 5% TBSA
- Burns with inhalation injury, associated Injury or pre-existing diseases
- Electric or Chemical burns
- Burns in functional areas (face, hands, feet, large joints, genitals and perineum)

Before transfer to burn centre/hospital

- Do not apply creams or ointments to the burns
- Cover the burn (tulle, metalline or sterile drapes)
- Elevate extremities with burns
- Transport the patient with facial burns in (half-)sitting position
- Consider escharotomy at deep circular burns

* Emergency Management of Severe Burns (EMSB) dutch publication 2017, The Education Committee of the Australian and New Zealand Burn Association Limited – ACN 054089520

BURN CENTRES

BWC Beverwijk: +31 (0)251 26 55 55
BWC Groningen: +31 (0)50 524 52 45
BWC Rotterdam: +31 (0)10 291 19 11

DUTCH BURNS FOUNDATION

www.brandwondenzorg.nl
+31 (0)251 27 55 55
dutch burns foundation

Fig. 2 Emergency management of burns (Used with permission from Dutch Burn Foundation)

6.1 Airway and Inspection of the Cervical Spinal Column

Exposure to hot gases, steam, or smoke may damage the airways. Hot air causes edema, particularly above the vocal chords. In case of fire in enclosed spaces, smoke may have particularly been inhaled by unconscious patients. This may also be the case due to the chimney effect (the smoke and heat rise and stream past the airways) when clothing catches fire. Facial burns may cause serious edema with obstruction of the airways. Scorched nasal hair, soot in the throat or sputum and nose, hoarse voice, and stridor could point to inhalation injuries. Even though there are no clear signs of respiratory distress under such conditions, administering 10–15 L of oxygen via a non-rebreathing mask is always necessary. Children have narrow airways due to which a small amount of edema may already cause a significant increase of the resistance. Therefore, it is important to intubate on time, possibly preventive in case of doubt about proper accessibility of the airways.

In case of suspected carbon monoxide intoxication, 100% oxygen is administered.

Additional injury in children with hot liquid burns is rare, but depending on the trauma mechanism, the cervical spinal column must, in case of suspicion, be protected until certainty can be given regarding stability of the neck.

6.2 Breathing

After the airways have been secured, the breathing must be assessed with regard to labored breathing, effectiveness, and systematic effects of respiratory failure. In order to assess breathing, thorax excursions are first inspected and thorax auscultated and tapped. Circular burns may inhibit thorax expansion. Relieving incisions (escharotomy) may be necessary. Additionally, respiratory failure may be caused by smoke inhalation and carbon monoxide intoxication (Table 1). One must be mindful of the fact that the saturation measured with the pulse oximeter displays normal values in case of carbon monoxide intoxication and is therefore not reliable.

Table 1 Symptoms in case of carbon monoxide intoxication

COHb levels (%)	Symptoms
0–10	Minimal (normal levels of heavy smokers)
10–20	Vomiting and headache
20–30	Drowsiness and lethargy
30–40	Confusion and agitation
40–50	Coma and respiratory depression
>50	Death

Source [3]

6.3 Circulation and Bleeding Control

Circulation is assessed by means of heart frequency, capillary refill, and blood pressure (non-burned parts). In case of severe burns, hypovolemia occurs within several hours due to systematic capillary leak. In case of hypovolemia in acute phase, attention must also be paid to other causes, such as internal or external blood loss.

Intravenous access must be acquired as soon as possible with two properly functioning intravenous drips. Additionally, blood must be taken (cross matching, Hb Ht glucose). Because in this stage a calculation of the TBSA has not yet been made, a fluid bolus (10 mL/kg) with Ringer's lactate is administered. Colloids are now contraindicated.

6.4 Disability/Neurological Condition

All patients will receive a brief neurological assessment via AVPU scale or Glasgow coma scale (GSC). Pupillary response is also assessed. Keep in mind that patients may be confused due to hypoxia or hypovolemia.

6.5 Exposure/Undressing the Patient and Controlling (Environmental) Temperature

The patient's body must be fully investigated, including the back in order to assess the depth of burns, extensiveness (TBSA), and presence of circularly burns, for which escharotomy is necessary.

Burn patients and particularly children are prone to hypothermia, which may be hastened by cooling with (too) cold water or inexpert use of cooling blankets. Hypothermia may cause secondary deepening of the burns due to occurring hypoperfusion. Therefore, adequate fluid resuscitation, wound covering, and keeping the patient warm are very important.

6.6 Fluids/Administration of Fluids

When the TBSA is calculated, the fluid need is determined with the Parkland formula.

Total fluid = 4 mL × %TBSA × kg body weight (Fig. 2)

This formula calculates the fluid requirement from the moment the burn has occurred. In children, intravenous resuscitation takes place in case of TBSA >10%. Adults are intravenously resuscitated if their burned body surface area exceeds 15%. Compared to adults, children have a relatively large body surface, and therefore they will also receive maintenance fluids in addition to supplementation for the burns. For resuscitation, a crystalloid solution (Ringer's lactate) is used, and for maintenance infusion, glucose saline solutions are used. Colloids are not used for initial fluid resuscitation. Albumin supplementation starts 12–16 h post-burn. This is dosed according to the formula albumin 20%: 0.5 × TBSA % × weight (KG)/24 = mL/h. In order to control adequate resuscitation, the most important measurement for the diuresis is target diuresis for children 1–2 mL/kg/h. Additionally, it is important to monitor vital parameters such as pulse and blood pressure. For a correct monitoring of diuresis, a urinary catheter is used for children with a TBSA >10%. In order to prevent overfilling, the amount of rehydration fluid must be reduced during the rehydration phase when the diuresis is excessive.

6.7 Gets and Gifts

After initial stabilization, the necessary diagnostic must be performed, such as blood pressure and indicatory radiological examination such as X-ray photos or ultrasound. In case of severe burns, a feeding tube and urinary catheter are indicated.

Burns can be extremely painful, which means that adequate pain alleviation must always be provided. This could be done with nasal opiates, such as fentanyl. In case of less severe burns, proper bandaging already alleviates the pain, and paracetamol and NSAIDs may be administered rectally. Patients with severe burns can best be treated intravenously with opiates. Pain medication must be administered on the basis of patient's pain. During the care, it must be regularly assessed whether the pain medication is still sufficient. Subsequently, maintenance medication starts. Administering pain medication via intramuscular or subcutaneous route is not recommended, due to poor absorption with regard to peripheral vasoconstriction.

Additionally, in a later phase, when vasodilation and edema forming may occur, increased absorption from these areas may cause intoxication. In case of restlessness and pain, hypoxia must also be considered. When hypoxia has been excluded, a sedative such as benzodiazepines may be given. During the rehydration phase, caution is required with NSAIDs due to the possible negative effect on diuresis and renal function.

A burn is a wound where tetanus prophylaxis is indicated. Children vaccinated according to the RVP (Dutch vaccination program) are protected up to the age of 20.

7 Secondary Survey

After life-threatening conditions have been treated, a complete examination follows, and more information is acquired with regard to the accident via the child, the parents, the ambulance paramedics, family, or witnesses of the accident. Allergies, medications, past medical history, last meal, events

Table 2 Wound treatment of smaller burns

Depth wound	Aspect wound/moistness	Wound covering material
First-degree burn	No wound, redness, possible swelling	Moisturizing lotion
Second-degree burn	Intact blister	Vaseline gauze, silicone tule
	Non-intact blister, pink, shiny wound bed	Hydrofiber, hydrocolloids, silicone tule, alginate or foam bandages
Third-degree burn	Smaller wounds, white/brown/black (charred) and demarcation wall	Silver-containing burns (hydrofiber AG/ hydrocolloid AG/foam bandages AG)

Source [21]

(AMPLE) leading to (including trauma mechanism, temperature agents, contact duration).

Additional injuries are less common in children but cannot be excluded. Therefore, thorough physical examination must be conducted including acting on the basis of the findings.

In addition to medical care for the child with burns, the psychosocial aspect must also be considered, with attention for the guilt that parents or a responsible caregiver may be experiencing.

Finally, it must not be forgotten that every child has its own social and emotional developmental stage. The fear and stress caused by the burn may result in nutrition and behavioral problems, among others. It is therefore necessary that both the child and the parents/caregivers are properly guided in this process.

8 Burn Treatment

8.1 First-Degree Burns

These can be treated with moisturizing lotion or cream and analgesics.

8.2 Second-Degree Burns

Small intact blisters that are not in the way can be kept intact. The fastest reepithelialization takes place in this gel-like environment [21, 22]. Blisters in functional areas and tense blisters can be aspirated, where the roof of the blister may be used as organic wound cover. These (closed) blisters only need to be protected. If the blisters are not intact, the blister roofs must be removed. In case of second-degree burns with open blisters, gel-forming wound covers (for instance, Aquacel®) are recommended) [23].

8.3 Small Third-Degree Burns

These can be treated with a wound cover or silver-containing bandages. In case of nonprogressive healing, refer the patient to a burn center for further treatment and skin transplant. Silver sulfadiazine is an antibacterial means, primarily indicated for infected wounds or in case of a large wound surface. Silver sulfadiazine can halt epithelial outgrowth and is preferably not used for superficial burns (Table 2).

In case of referral to a hospital or burn center, the wound must be covered warmly and cleanly with film, metaline sheets, clean cloths, or tule. The use of topical salves such as silver sulfadiazine does not apply, because this hinders a proper assessment of the burn in the second- or third-line treatment.

9 Preparing for Transport

When in doubt whether a patient meets the criteria for transport, consultation may occur with one of the three burn centers. In case of transport, the referral form may be used, available on the website of the Dutch Burn Foundation (www.brandwonden.nl) or local burn center.

When suspicion of inhalation injury or facial burns exists, intubation occurs upon indication or after consultation. Non-intubated patients with burns in the neck and facial area are transported sitting upright. Affected extremities are placed as high as possible, in order to prevent worsening of edema by means of gravity.

Burn wounds must be, covered sterilely and cooling down must be prevented. Cooling blankets are not suitable as wound cover and must be replaced by sterile bandages before transport. Burns covered with salves may be difficult to assess without removing the salve. Therefore, it is not recommended to cover wounds with salves when the patient is referred to a burn center for assessment. It is recommended to document all objective information, the team members involved in the care, and the applied treatment.

10 Child Abuse and Burns

Recent retrospective Dutch research has shown that for approximately 10% of children who have been admitted in a burn center, guidance and/or supervision at home was implemented after discharge due to neglect or child abuse [24].

In addition to intentionally inflicted injury, burns can also arise due to unsafe home situations, such as carelessness or neglect. Just as children with accidental burns, victims of child abuse are nearly always younger than 10 years old and usually younger than 2 years old [25].

Hot liquid burns are, just as in accidental burns, the most frequently occurring type of burn. Uniform wound depth, clear demarcation line on the skin, the absence of splash marks, and burns in unusual locations, such as the buttocks, are suspicious signs of non-accidental burn injuries. Submersion is sometimes used as punishment, for instance, during toilet training. Sometimes, central parts of the buttocks have been spared, the so-called donut configuration, because of contact with the cooler surface of the bathtub. If an extremity is held in a hot liquid, this could give the appearance of a sock or glove with a clear water or demarcation line. Sometimes, typical patterns are recognizable of spared skin areas such as caused by a clenched fist or toes.

Contact burn is the second most occurring cause of non-accidental burns and can be caused by many different kinds of objects. These burns are usually isolated and have a recognizable pattern of the surface of the hot object. Most often occurring location of accidental burns are palms of the hands and the inside of the fingers. Burns on the dorsal side of hands and burns with a clear demarcation are more suspicious for non-accidental burns. Intentionally inflicted burns from cigarettes are often circular, 7–8 mm in diameter, deeply burned, and with a clear demarcation. Sometimes, multiple impressions are visible [3].

Although awareness regarding child abuse appears to be increasing, the relationship between the burns and child abuse is often not recognized. In case of burns where child abuse or neglect plays a role, there is generally a high risk of repetition, high morbidity, and relatively high mortality [26]. Each first responder should consider child abuse or neglect as a cause for a child with burns.

References

1. World Health Organization. Facts about injuries. http://www.who.int/mediacentre/factsheets/fs365/en/. Accessed 20 Mar 2017
2. Herndon DN (2012) Special considerations of age the pediatric burned patient. In: Herndon DN (ed) Total burn care, 4rd edn. Saunders Elsevier, London, p 405
3. Baartmans MGA, Stas HG, Dokter J, Boxma H (2008) De opvang van kinderen met brandwonden. Tijdschr Kindergeneeskd 76(6):282–290
4. Directive initial burn patients. http://brandwondenstichting.nl/professionals/richtlijn. Accessed 20 Mar 2017
5. European Burns Association (2015) European Practice Guidelines for Burn Care. http://euroburn.org/wp-content/uploads/2016/04/EBA-Guidelines-Version-3-2015.pdf. Accessed 20 Mar 2017
6. Lewis GM (2012) Evaluation of the burn wound management decisions. In: Herndon DN (ed) Total burn care, 4th edn. Saunders Elsevier, London, pp 125–127
7. Hettiaratchy S, Dziewulski P (2004) ABC of burns: pathophysiology and types of burns. BMJ 328:1427–1429
8. Jackson DM (1953) The diagnosis of the depth of burning. Br J Surg 40:588–596
9. Kramer GC (2012) Pathophysiology of burn shock and burn edema. In: Herndon DN (ed) Total burn care, 4th edn. Saunders Elsevier, London, pp 103–112
10. Knaysi GA, Crikelair GF, Cosman B (1968) The role of nines: its history and accuracy. Plast Reconstr Surg 41(6):560–563
11. Amirsheybani HR, Crecelius GM, Timothy NH, Pfeiffer M, Saggers GC, Manders EK (2001) The

natural history of the growth of the hand: I. Hand area as a percentage of body surface area. Plast Reconstr Surg 107:726–733
12. Lund CC, Browder NC (1944) The estimation of areas of burns. Surg Gynaecol Obstet 79:352–358
13. Baartmans MG, van Baar ME, Boxma H, Dokter J, Tibboel D, Nieuwenhuis MK (2012) Accuracy of burn size assessment prior to arrival in Dutch burn centres and its consequences in children: a nationwide evaluation. Injury 43(9):1451–1456
14. Davies JW (1982) Prompt cooling of burned area: a review of benefits and the effector mechanisms. Burns Incl Therm Inj 9:1–6
15. Jandera V, Hudson DA, deWet PM, Innes PM, Rode H (2000) Cooling the burn wound: evaluation of different modalities. Burns 26:256–270
16. Osgood PF, Szyfelbein SK (1989) Management of burn pain in children. Pediatr Clin North Am 36:1001–1013
17. Latenser BA (2009) Critical care of the burn patient: the first 48 hours. Crit Care Med 37(10):2819–2826
18. Muehlberger T, Ottomann C, Toman N, Daigeler A, Lehnhrdt M (2010) Emergency pre-hospital care of burn patients. Surgeon 8(2):101–104
19. Turner N (ed) (2017) Advanced paediatric life support, 5th Dutch edn. Bohn Stafleu van Loghum, Houten, Netherlands
20. Emergency Management of Severe Burns (EMSB) (2015) Meeting of the Education Committee of the Australian and New Zealand Burn Association Limited, 17 and 18 March, Bangladesh
21. Oen-Coral I, Dokter J, van der Vlies C, Boxma H (2010) Katern dermatologie. Modern Med 11:375–379
22. Jonkman MF (1989) Epidermal wound healing between moist and dry, Thesis, Rijks Universiteit, Groningen, Netherlands
23. Dokter J, Boxma H, Oen IM, van Baar ME, van der Vlies CH (2013) Reduction in skin grafting after the introduction of hydrofiber dressings in partial thickness burns: a comparison between a hydrofiber and silver sulphadiazine. Burns 39(1):130–135
24. Bousema S, Stas HG, van de Merwe MH, Oen IM, Baartmans MG, van Baar ME, Dutch Burn Repository group, Maasstad Hospital Rotterdam (2016) Epidemiology and screening of intentional burns in children in a Dutch burn centre. Burns 42(6):1287–1294
25. Burn injuries in child abuse (2001) Portable guidelines to investigate child abuse. US Department of Justice. https://www.ncjrs.gov/pdffiles/91190-6.pdf. Accessed 20 Mar 2017
26. Chester DL, Jose RM, Aldlyami E, King H, Moiemen NS (2006) Non-accidental burns in children—are we neglecting neglect? Burns 32:222–228

Learning from the Management of Carbapenemase-Producing Organisms at a Regional Burns Centre

Louise Teare and Katheryn Hobbs

1 What Are Carbapenemase-Producing Organisms (CPOs) and Why Are They Important?

CPOs are bacteria which have acquired genes that produce resistance to carbapenem antibiotics. Resistance is mediated by plasmids, a small DNA molecule within a cell that is physically separated from chromosomal DNA and can replicate and exist independently in the environment. In this form, plasmids may be transmitted from person to person by direct contact on unwashed hands or indirectly on inadequately decontaminated equipment going from one patient to another.

Klebsiella Producing Carbapenemase (KPC) is one example of a CPO. The gene encoding the KPC enzyme resides on transmissible plasmids which can be transferred to other *Enterobacteriaceae* bacteria, e.g. from *Klebsiella pneumoniae* to *Escherichia coli.* KPC enzymes are a particular concern because of limited therapeutic options and associated high mortality rate. In recent times, KPC nosocomial-associated outbreaks have been reported [1], and this organism has become a priority for infection prevention and control.

L. Teare, MBBS, FRCPath, MBA (✉)
K. Hobbs, RN (Paeds), MSc
Department of Infection Prevention and Control, Mid Essex Hospitals NHS Trust, Chelmsford, UK
e-mail: Louise.teare@meht.nhs.uk

Many carbapenemase-producing *Enterobacteriaceae* are resistant to multiple antibiotic classes, with only colistin remaining active against >90% of all producers. However, colistin resistance may occur and is frequent in some isolates of the internationally disseminated *K. pneumoniae* clone sequence type (ST) 258 [2]. This was first detected in New York hospitals in the 2000s and disseminated rapidly to other neighbouring states. Later on, KPC *K. pneumoniae* occurred in Israel, Latin America, Greece and China.

In 2009, the New Delhi metallo-beta-lactamase (NDM) was described. Many of the early cases in the UK were linked to having health care in India or Pakistan where resistant bacteria had been detected in seepage or communal tap waters [3, 4]. A point prevalence survey analysed data from a carbapenemase-producing *Enterobacteriaceae* outbreak in Israel to determine asymptomatic carriage [5]. Samples were collected from 298 patients. Sixteen patients (5.4%) had a CPO identified. Eighteen percent of those colonised had received carbapenem antibiotics previously. The rectum was found to be the most sensitive screening site detecting 15/16 carriers. Multivariate analysis showed that length of stay, diaper use and vancomycin administration were significantly related to carriage.

In Ireland, CPO was first reported in 2009 [6]. Between January and May 2011, ten cases were reported in three hospitals. Reported cases were predominantly linked to critical care units. In June

Recent Clinical Techniques, Results, and Research in Wounds (2017)
DOI 10.1007/15695_2017_22, © Springer International Publishing AG
Published Online: 24 October 2017

2011 a 4-week national pilot survey [7] took place in 40 Irish critical care units (37 adult and three paediatric) to examine the prevalence of rectal carriage of CPO and inform national CPO screening guidelines. A total of 760 screening swabs were taken over the study period. CPO was not detected in any of the participating critical care units.

The UK's first known carbapenemase-positive enterobacterial isolate was detected in 2003, and until 2007, data from the Public Health England Antibiotic Resistance Monitoring and Reference Laboratory[2] confirmed fewer than five cases per year. In stark contrast, there have been marked year-on-year increases since 2008 with more than 1000 cases in 2013 and more than 1600 in 2014 (Table 1).

While early UK KPC isolates were often linked with overseas travel, there has now been spread within some UK hospitals. This has involved not only the transmission of plasmids encoding KPC enzymes between different bacterial strains, principally *K. pneumoniae*, but also spread to *E. coli* and *Enterobacter* spp. Many of these isolates have been identified from faecal screens rather than infections. Areas in the UK where CPO is considered endemic and where outbreaks have been experienced include London, Leeds, Manchester, Merseyside, Cheshire and Sheffield.

In 2013 the Department of Health introduced the CPO 'toolkit' [8]. This recommended ongoing laboratory surveillance and infection prevention measures to screen at-risk groups. KPC media was developed for CPO screening samples, and advice was given to test all significant Gram-negative organisms against carbapenems. It is against this background that this chapter describes how a UK regional burns unit dealt with its first cases of CPO.

2 Clinical Cases

Our regional burns centre treats 1500 patients per annum with over 700 in-patient admissions. It exists within a large district general hospital, but is self-contained with four intensive care beds, four high-dependency beds, a dedicated theatre, eight adult beds and a children's burns ward with eight beds. There are dedicated burns outpatient area and rehabilitation facilities. Until the summer of 2015, the

Table 1 Increase in isolates of CPO in the UK

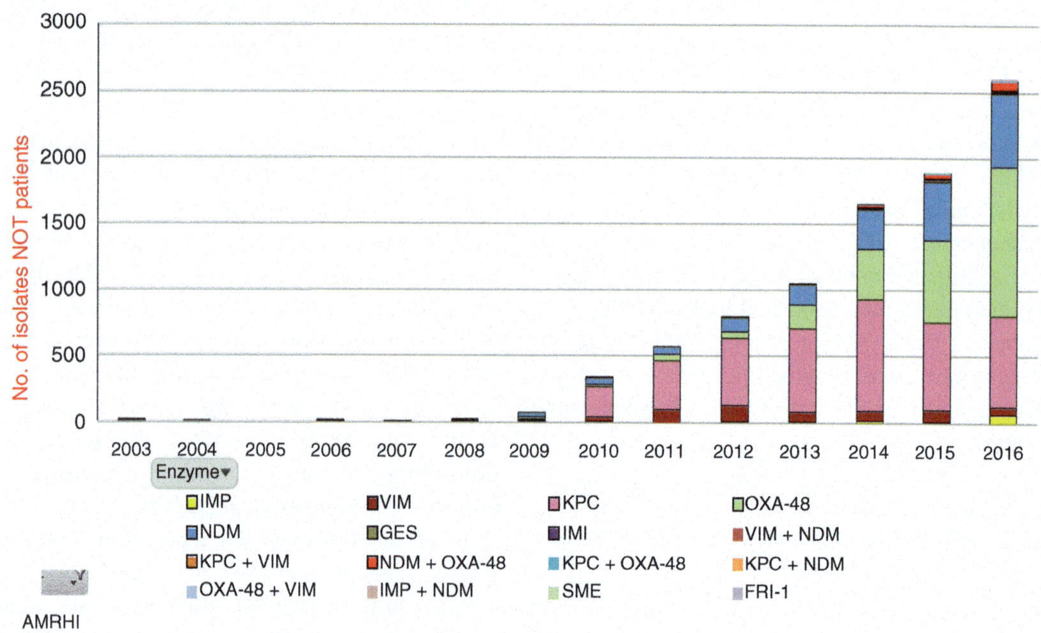

Source: Public Health England Antibiotic Resistance Monitoring and Reference Laboratory

unit had not knowingly looked after a patient colonised or infected with a CPO.

Case 1 sustained a 25% total body surface area burn in the Indian subcontinent where she had been hospitalised for several weeks prior to repatriation to the UK. On the same day, Case 2 was admitted to the room next door to patient A after sustaining a small burn. Case 2 was British, but born in India. Both patients had swabs taken on admission and coincidentally; both had carbapenemase-resistant *Klebsiella pneumoniae* isolated from burn wound swabs. Case 1 had a number of other organisms as well, and full results are summarised in Table 2. Typing results indicated that the strains of *Klebsiella pneumoniae* isolated from Cases 1 and 2 were different and did not represent cross infection.

Four months later, Cases 3 and 4 were admitted. Both had been involved in a fire in Eastern Europe and managed at different hospitals for 4 weeks. Case 3 had sustained 80% total body surface area burns, and Case 4 30%. Admission sampling results of Cases 3 and 4 are summarised in Table 3.

Table 2 Organisms colonising and infecting Cases 1 and 2 on admission swabs

	Resistance mechanism/type	Antibiotic sensitivity profile
Case 1		
Providencia stuartii	NDM	Sensitive to aztreonam, ciprofloxacin, tazocin
Pseudomonas aeruginosa	VIM	Only sensitive to colistin
Klebsiella oxytoca	NDM	Only sensitive to colistin
Klebsiella pneumoniae	Oxa-48 and NDM	Sensitive to colistin and tigecycline
Proteus mirabilis	ESBL	Only sensitive to aztreonam
Escherichia coli (2 types)	Oxa-48 and NDM	Sensitive to meropenem and amikacin
Enterobacter cloacae		Sensitive to meropenem, amikacin, ciprofloxacin
Gentamicin-resistant MRSA	Spa type t064	Sensitive to tigecycline and linezolid
Acinetobacter baumannii	Oxa-23, Oxa-51	No sensitive antibiotics identified
Enterococcus faecium	VRE	Sensitive to tigecycline and linezolid
Case 2		
Klebsiella pneumoniae	Oxa-48 and NDM	

Table 3 Organisms colonising and infecting Cases 3 and 4

	Resistance mechanism/type	Antibiotic sensitivity profile
Case 3		
Pseudomonas aeruginosa	Negative for carbapenemase-producing gene ESBL positive	
Klebsiella pneumoniae	NDM	Pan resistant
Proteus mirabilis	Negative for carbapenemase-producing gene	
Escherichia coli	Oxa-48	
Acinetobacter baumannii	Oxa-40, Oxa-51	*Only sensitive to tobramycin Identical to strain isolated from Case 4
Case 4		
Klebsiella pneumoniae		Sensitive to meropenem, ciprofloxacin
Enterobacter aerogenes	ESBL positive	Sensitive to meropenem, ciprofloxacin
Acinetobacter baumannii	Oxa-40, Oxa-51	*Only sensitive to tobramycin Identical to strain isolated from Case 3
Escherichia coli		Fully sensitive
Enterococcus faecium	VRE	Sensitive to tigecycline and linezolid

3 Discussion

It is widely recognised that healthcare-associated infection caused by multidrug-resistant bacteria is a worldwide problem of profound importance because of the limited treatment options. There has been experience in Brazil of CPOs causing outbreaks. Goncalves et al. described two outbreaks of KPC-producing *Klebsiella pneumoniae* in a Brazilian adult ICU [10]. Their paper indicates that traditional control measures on their own were inadequate to halt the outbreaks and that an organisational approach is essential.

Following the identification of CPOs from Cases 1 and 2, a CPO management team was formed. The focus was to put systems in place to avoid spread to other parts of the hospital and prevent CPOs becoming endemic in our organisation.

Case 1 was in our hospital for 11 weeks. She required three trips to theatre for debridement and allografting of her chronically infected granulating wounds.

This was followed by further wound excision and autografting. At no time did Case 1 become clinically infected and only required antibiotics for surgical prophylaxis. On three occasions she was given colistin, tigecycline and aztreonam on induction to cover all her resistant organisms.

Case 2 was only in hospital for 24 h and was then managed as an outpatient.

Case 3 died of a pan-resistant *Klebsiella pneumoniae* septicaemia within 48 h of admission.

Case 4 did well. She was with us for 3 weeks. Her burns healed, although she remained colonised with carbapenemase-producing *Acinetobacter baumannii.*

3.1 The CPO Management Team Identified the Following Priority Areas

3.1.1 Management of Staff Looking After Patients with CPO

Nurses looking after patients positive for CPO were dedicated to their management for the duration of their shift as far as possible. Any other member of staff including doctors, nurses, therapists, dieticians, healthcare assistants, estates staff and cleaners were required to wear scrubs if entering a CPO positive patient room. They were required to shower and change on leaving if having physical contact with the patient. We decided that provided staff had showered (including hair wash) and changed after being on the unit, they were 'safe' to work elsewhere.

3.1.2 Theatre Visits

Patients colonised or infected with CPOs requiring theatre went last on the list. After each such case, the theatre was cleaned using 1000 ppm hypochlorite solution followed by 6% hydrogen peroxide vapour fogging.

3.1.3 Outpatients

Patients A and B both required ongoing management in the outpatients department. Patient were seen on their own at the end of the day using isolation precautions and the area cleaned and fogged as described above.

3.1.4 Environmental Contamination

Garvey et al. report their experience in dealing with a burns patient infected with CPOs and the decontamination methods employed to render a burns shock room safe for reuse [11]. The shock room was cleaned after being vacated, but environmental sampling cultured multiple CPOs. A second decontamination was undertaken comprising a detergent, steam and hypochlorite clean of 2000 ppm followed by hydrogen peroxide misting (12%). No CPOs were cultured after subsequent environmental sampling. Their take-home message is that a burns patient harbouring CPOs contaminates the surrounding environment heavily and standard cleaning is insufficient to clear the environmental bioburden.

3.1.5 Education

We were particularly concerned to ensure that all staff clearly understood the problem associated with CPOs and the risks in allowing spread. We ensured this topic was regularly included in safety huddles and educational programmes.

Staff were constantly reminded that genes encoding resistance reside on transmissible plasmids that can be transferred to other patients via inadequately cleaned hands and equipment.

All grades and types of healthcare workers were included in our educational programme. We particularly focused on those spending long periods with patients in isolation. All were given the opportunity of discussing the issues further and having CPO screening. Only one member of staff took this up. He was negative.

3.1.6 'It Doesn't Mean Me'

On occasions we became aware that staff didn't think the rules we set applied to them. Sustaining the educational message for all staff groups was found to be a challenge, but essential to persist with.

3.1.7 Do Not Relax Guard

Case 1 improved clinically and it was vital not to relax our guard. CPOs continued to be widely isolated from her and also environmental samples around her bed. She was discharged after an 11-week inpatient stay to be seen twice weekly in outpatients. As with Case 2, this patient was seen on her own at the end of the day with 1000 ppm hypochlorite cleaning and hydrogen peroxide vapour fogging after each visit. As on the ward, staff wore surgical scrubs and showered with hair washes after seeing her.

There were 4 months between our experience with patients A and B and the admission of patients C and D. No transfer information had been given to our service about previous microbiology results for patients C and D. In spite of this, the burns team went into immediate 'CPO mode' because of the geographical location and knowledge that CPOs are endemic in that area. Control measures initiated immediately included dedicated nursing in isolation facilities with all staff entering the room wearing scrubs, changing and showering immediately after leaving the room if having physical contact.

3.1.8 Terminal Cleaning Process

In association with the CPO management plan, a terminal cleaning process was developed as follows:

- Terminal cleaning using 1000 ppm hypochlorite
  - Routine nursing staff cleaning
  - Routine domestic staff cleaning
- Normal 6% hydrogen peroxide vapour fogging with cupboard doors open
- Repair and refurbishment of ward as necessary
- Change of shower heads
- Repeat routine ward cleaning by nurses and domestic staff as appropriate
- Repeat ward hydrogen peroxide vapour fogging
- Pillows and mattresses used by patients to be destroyed. Also mattress on shower trolley
- Sign off by domestic service manager, lead nurse, estates representative and a member of the Infection Prevention Team
- Staff involved to wear scrubs and shower after being on the ward
- Changing of air filters
- Inclusion of the mortuary in the CPO management process, to ensure no onward transmission in that facility

4 Effective Triggers of the CPO Management Plan

Astute and prompt triggering of a CPO management plan is essential if CPOs are not to become endemic in an organisation. Have a low threshold for assuming CPO positive until proven otherwise. It is likely that if we had not done this, spread would have occurred in our hospital. Surveillance can run alongside this approach, but should not replace it. Surveillance is often initiated in outbreak settings with the aim of detecting unknown reservoirs. This strategy is based on an assumption that colonised patients may perpetuate transmission and that early identification with isolation will control. The clinical relevance and subsequent impact of IPC measures based on active surveillance cultures remains to be determined. To date, screening of patients for multidrug-resistant Gram-negatives, including CPOs, has relied primarily on culture. The main drawback to culture is the prolonged turnaround time of at least 24–72 h. PCR-based assays with rapid turnaround time and high sensitivity are an attractive alternative [9], but a low positive predictive value of the test raises serious concerns regarding the meaning of a positive result if the sole purpose of the test is to screen for CPO.

5 Conclusion and Learning

Our experience with patients colonised and infected with CPO highlights the value of a multidisciplinary team working together, for example, ward staff working closely with the Infection Prevention and Control Team, estates, and microbiology and cleaning departments. The experience allowed us to develop a template for managing patients from CPO endemic areas. This covered both inpatient and outpatient areas.

As a result of measures put in place, we were able to avoid spread of CPO to any other patient, staff or visitor.

Our main learning is that we have *'Got to get the basics right'*. This includes:

- Effective cleaning of the environment
- Effective hand hygiene using the 'five moments' between and before each patient contact
- Effective decontamination of each item of equipment going from one patient to another
- Confidence that when admitting patients with both resistant and sensitive organisms we will not spread them around
- The importance of CPOs being considered in empirical antibiotics for any patient from an endemic area

Whilst high standards of cleaning were maintained at all times, in spite of this contact plates from environmental samples such as the bedside table, trunking behind the bed, bin lid and parent bed showed an excess of 100 cfu/mL of bacteria.

Managing CPOs is an ongoing issue for hospitals. This problem will increase over time and a robust strategy to deal with the issue is essential. CPOs may occur at any time. They may occur singly or in large numbers. We developed a well-documented terminal cleaning strategy on discharge of CPO patients to include changing of shower heads and air filters. We realised the profound importance of organisational education to increase the profile, awareness and understanding of CPO. Once in place a robust carbapenemase resistance strategy needs to be ready for testing at any time.

References

1. Morris D, Boyle F, Morris C, Condon I, Delannoy-Viellard A-S, Power L, Khan A, Morris-Downes M, Finnegan C, Powell J, Manahan R, Burns K, O'Connell N, Boyle L, O'Gorman A, Humphreys H, Brisse S, Turton J, Woodford N, Cormican M (2012) Inter-hospital outbreak of Klebsiella pneumoniae producing KPC-2 carbapenemase in Ireland. J Antimicrob Chemother 67:2367–2372
2. Carbonase-producing enterobacteriaceae in the UK 2003–2011 (2011) Health Protection Report. 5(24). http://webarchive.nationalarchives.gov.uk/20140714084352/http://www.hpa.org.uk/HPR/archives/2011/news2411.htm. Accessed 3 Mar 2017
3. Kumarasamy KK, Toleman MA, Walsh TR, Bagaria J, Butt F, Balakrishnan R, Chaudhary U, Doumith M, Giske CG, Irfan S, Krishnan P, Kumar A, Maharjan S, Mushtaq S, Norrie T, Paterson D, Pearson A, Perry C, Pike R, Rao B, Ray U, Sarma J, Sharma M, Sheridan E, Thirunarayan MA, Turton J, Upadhyay S, Warner M, Welfare W, Livermore DM, Woodford N (2010) Emergence of a new antibiotic resistance mechanism in India, Pakistan, and the UK: a molecular, biological, and epidemiological study. Lancet Infect Dis 10:597–602
4. Walsh TR, Weeks J, Livermore DM, Toleman M (2011) Dissemination of NDM-1 positive bacteria in the New Delhi environment and its implications for human health: an environmental point prevalence study. Lancet Infect Dis 11:355–362
5. Wiener-Well Y, Rudensky B, Yinnona AM, Kopuita P, Schlesingera Y, Broideb E, Lachisha T, Raveh D (2010) Carriage rate of carbapenem-resistant Klebsiella pneumoniae in hospitalised patients during a national outbreak. J Hosp Infect 74:344–349
6. Roche C, Cotter M, O'Connell N, Crowley B (2009) First identification of class A carbapenemase-producing Klebsiella pneumoniae in the Republic of Ireland. Euro Surveill 14:19163
7. Burns K, Morris D, Murchan S, Cunney R, Smyth E, Power M, Schaffer K, Collins C, Sheahan A, Cormican M, Fitzpatrick F (2013) Carbapenemase-producing Enterobacteriaceae in Irish critical care units: results of a pilot prevalence survey, June 2011. J Hosp Infect 83(1):71–73
8. Stokle L (2013) Acute trust toolkit for the early detection, management and control of carbapenemase-producing Enterobacteriaceae. Public Health England, London. https://www.gov.uk/government/uploads/system/uploads/attachment_data/file/329227/Acute_trust_toolkit_for_the_early_detection.pdf. Accessed 3 Mar 2017

9. Rossi GI, Ferreira ML, Araujo BF, Campos PA, Royer S, Batistão DW, Souza LP, Brito CS, Urzedo JE, Gontijo-Filho PP, Ribas RM (2016) Outbreaks of colistin-resistant and colistin-susceptible KPC-producing Klebsiella pneumoniae in a Brazilian intensive care unit. J Hosp Infect 94:322–329
10. Garvey MI, Bradley CW, Jumaa P (2016) Environmental decontamination following occupancy of a burns patient with multiple carbapenemase-producing organisms. J Hosp Infect 93:136–140
11. Kontopidou F, Giamarellou H, Katerelos P, Maragos A, Kioumis I, Trikka-Graphakos E, Valakis C, Maltezou HC, Group for the Study of KPC-producing Klebsiella pneumoniae infections in intensive care units (2014) Infections caused by carbapenem-resistant Klebsiella pneumoniae among patients in intensive care units in Greece: a multi-centre study on clinical outcome and therapeutic options. Clin Microbiol Infect 20:O117e23

A Hemostatic Technique Using Silicone Gel Dressing for Burn Surgery

Akinori Osuka and Masashi Ueyama

1 Introduction

Significant bleeding remains challenging in tangential excision of burn wounds [1, 2]. Although various techniques to reduce intraoperative blood loss have been described, there is an absence of uniformity and consistency in their application [3]. The blood loss in burn surgery is estimated to be more than 100 mL per percentage body surface area excised (Fig. 1) [4, 5]. However, tangential excision can be applied to partial-thickness burns; patients with extensive burns might require fascial excision to avoid massive blood loss because the bleeding from the perforator vessels can be easily stopped with electric cautery. On the other hand, the oozing from the dermal is difficult to control, especially in the large debridement area. We often face the dilemma of whether to perform tangential excision to preserve the dermis layer or fascial excision to minimize bleeding [6]. To minimize blood loss in tangential excision, we developed a hemostatic technique using silicone gel dressings [7, 8].

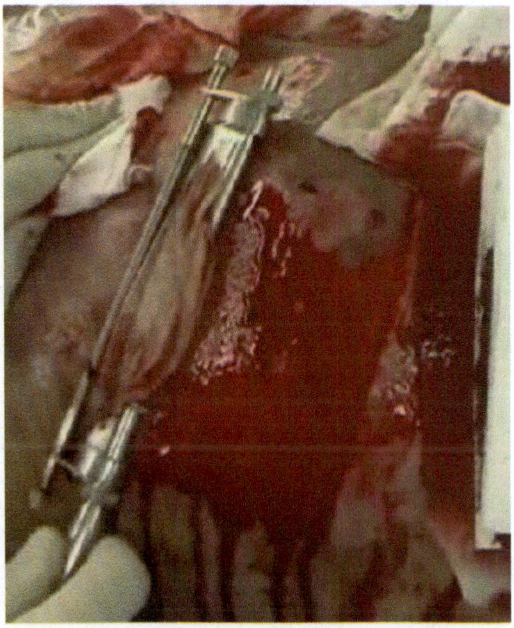

Fig. 1 Massive bleeding during tangential excitation

2 Technique

The method used to control intraoperative bleeding from tangential excision is shown in Fig. 2. Burn wounds on limbs are tangentially excised under tourniquet control. After tangential excision with knives, the wounds are rinsed with warm saline. Soon after that, the wounds are sprayed with thrombin and with 1:100,000 adrenalin solution and wrapped tightly with the silicone gel dressing and bandage for a full 5 min

A. Osuka, M.D., Ph.D. (✉) • M. Ueyama, M.D., Ph.D.
Department of Trauma, Critical Care Medicine and Burn Center, Nagoya, AICHI, Japan
e-mail: osuka-ngy@umin.ac.jp

Recent Clinical Techniques, Results, and Research in Wounds (2017)
DOI 10.1007/15695_2017_23, © Springer International Publishing AG
Published Online: 24 October 2017

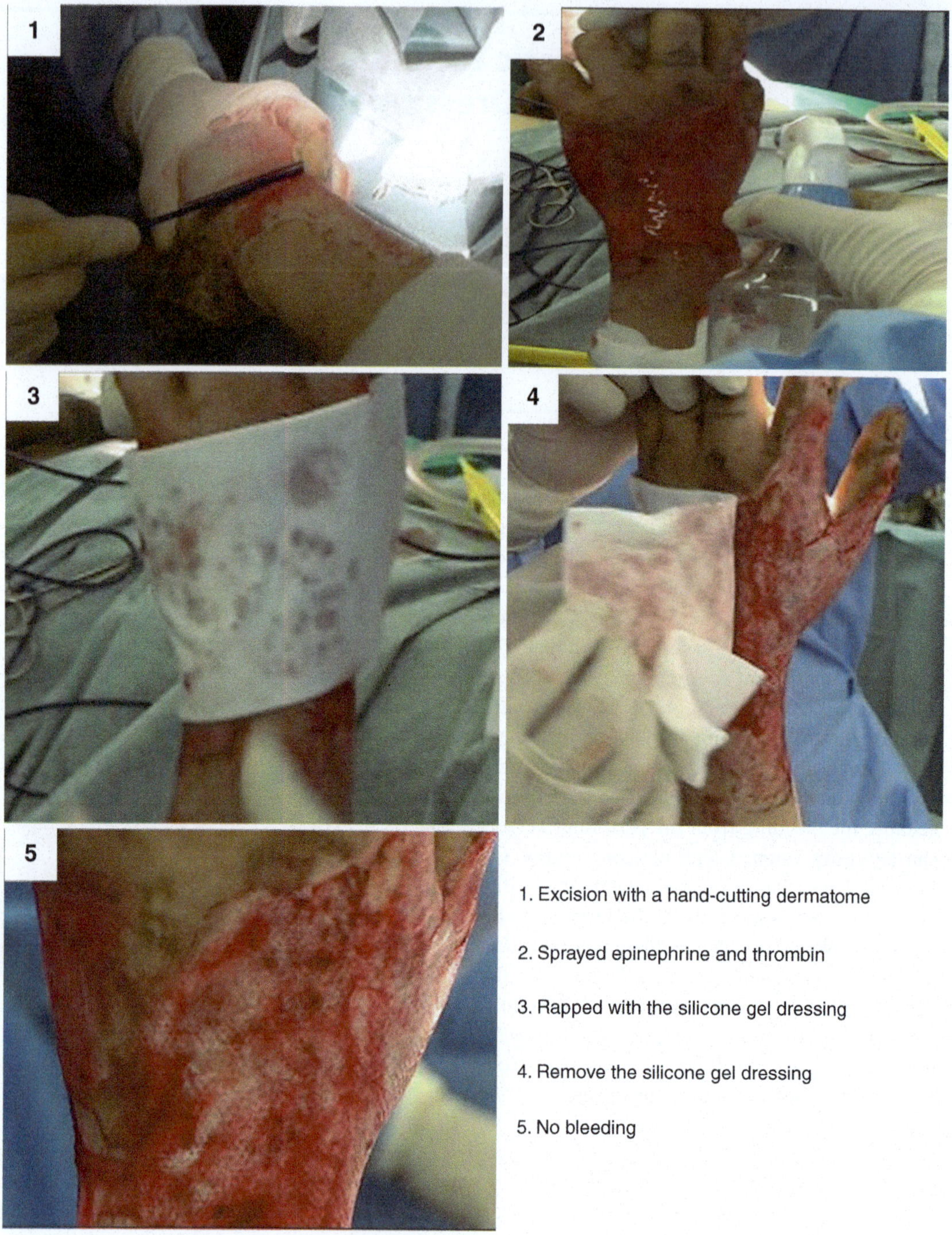

Fig. 2 Tangential excitation using silicone gel dressing

before deflation of the tourniquet (Fig. 3). When the silicone gel dressings are removed, the hemostasis is almost completed. Any major bleeders should be cauterized, and dermal oozing can be stopped for another 5 min compression with the silicone gel dressing following thrombin spray.

It is difficult to apply this silicone gel dressing technique to round-shaped areas such as the head

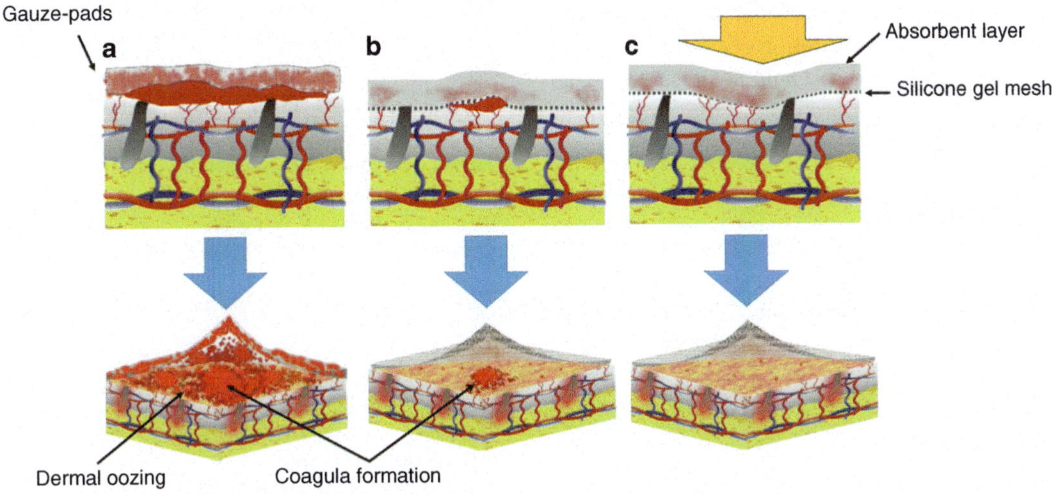

Fig. 3 The mechanism behind the procedure toe stop bleeding during tangential excision. (**a**) Conventional procedure includes thrombin- and epinephrine-soaked gauze pads. Dermal oozing usually occurs when the gauze pads are removed because removal of the pads with coagula can cause rebleeding from the excised wound bed. (**b**) Silicone gel dressing with inadequate compression. Some coagula formation can occur. When the coagulum is removed, additional dermal oozing can occur. (**c**) Our new procedure with silicone gel dressing and adequate compression (indicated by the *arrow*). The silicone gel dressing sticks to the wound and absorbs blood into the absorbent layer through the silicone gel mesh with no formation of coagula. No additional dermal oozing occurs because of the less irritation when the silicone gel dressing is removed [8]. Used with permission

or to concave–convex surfaces such as the area around the spine or collarbone.

We usually use viscoelastic foam mattress that can be compressed suitably over round and concave–convex surfaces. When we need the second round of compression, pushing with the fingers may be the best way, because the ooze point is already small and surgeon's fingers, of course, compress adequately.

3 Discussion

Tangential excision debrides the burned skin while preserving the underlying viable dermis, which makes skin grafting better than fascial excision. In large burn surgeries, it is a challenging problem to stop the oozing from the dermal surface. Tangential excision can cause more bleeding and prolong the duration of the operations. Hemostatic methods for major bleeders are astriction (binding) and cauterization of major bleeders, and cauterization creates more burn tissue. For oozing from dermal, hemostatic technique usually used is probably compression with epinephrine- and/or thrombin-soaked gauze pads. Removal of the gauze pads results in rebleeding because of the irritation caused by peeling away the gauze pads. Gauze pads rarely adhere to the excision site without creating space between the pads and the site, which allows the formation of coagula.

The silicone gel dressing itself does not have the capability to stop the bleeding. The merits of the silicone gel dressing are its adhesiveness, low irritation, and high absorbability. These help us compress the wounds adequately, which makes the thrombin work on hemostasis. The structure of the silicone gel dressing allows it to adhere gently to the skin around the wounds, and any exudates including blood are absorbed by means of its silicone adhesion technology. The point of this technique is to avoid creating any blood coagulum before attaching the silicone gel dressings.

By using the silicone gel dressing technique, we could achieve significant reduction of blood loss compared with conventional techniques or other reports [3, 5]. Because this technique is easy, the simple substitution of silicone gel dressings for gauze pads can help us preserve the dermis, shorten the duration of the surgery, and reduce transfusion requirement [8].

Conclusions

The application of the silicone gel dressing during tangential excision and grafting resulted in a remarkable reduction in blood loss and transfusion requirements.

References

1. Budny PG, Regan PJ, Roberts AH (1993) The estimation of blood loss during burns surgery. Burns 19(2):134–137
2. Steadman PB, Pegg SP (1992) A quantitative assessment of blood loss in burn wound excision and grafting. Burns 18(6):490–491
3. Sterling JP, Heimbach DM (2011) Hemostasis in burn surgery—a review. Burns 37(4):559–565
4. Gomez M, Logsetty S, Fish JS (2001) Reduced blood loss during burn surgery. J Burn Care Rehabil 22(2):111–117
5. Cartotto R, Musgrave MA, Beveridge M, Fish J, Gomez M (2000) Minimizing blood loss in burn surgery. J Trauma 49(6):1034–1039
6. Osuka A, Kuroki Y, Nakajima S, Sakai T, Kojima H, Yamada M, Okuma S, Onishi S, Ueyama M (2014) Damage control strategy for extensive burn injury -tangential excision or fascial excision. Japanese J Burn Inj 40(1):19–25
7. Osuka A, Kuroki Y, Nakajima S, Sakai T, Kojima H, Yamada M, Okuma S, Onishi S, Ueyama M (2014) Haemostatic technique using a novel silicone gel dressing for tangential excisions in burn surgery. Burns 40(1):165–166
8. Osuka A, Kuroki Y, Ueyama M (2016) A haemostatic technique using silicone gel dressing for burn surgery. Int Wound J 13(6):1354–1358

Skin Graft Fixation in Severe Burns: Use of Topical Negative Pressure

Christian Smolle, Petra Brinskelle, Andreas Steiner, Michael Schintler, and Lars-Peter Kamolz

1 Introduction

Burns are common and devastating injuries, often accompanied by severe physical and psychological impairment. Advances in burn care have effected a steady decline of burn mortality rates during the past decades [1]. While until the mid-twentieth century, the burn eschar was left to be digested by bodily and bacterial enzymes, the 1970s brought the early excision of the burns. This paradigm change in the approach to burn wounds resulted in a dramatic increase of survival rates after burn injuries [2].

Nowadays, extensive burns remain a challenge for burn surgeons for two main reasons: on the one hand, large areas of tissue loss require rapid coverage with autologous skin transplants, while on the other hand, there is a limited availability of donor sites [3]. The chance of complete graft take decreases with increasing percentage of burned total body surface area (TBSA). While in burns smaller than 35% TBSA take rates average 95%, the mean take rate in burns exceeding 35% TBSA is much lower [4].The chance of survival is closely related to the success of early skin grafting. Not only does a restored skin barrier prevent from further fluid and temperature loss and life-threatening hypothermia. Untreated burn wounds represent the ideal habitat for microorganisms and consequently act as origin for bloodstream infections. Today, septic complications are the most common cause of death after burns [2]. Prolonged and incomplete graft healing furthermore facilitates the development of hypertrophic scars and contractures which further impair the functional and aesthetic outcome of the injury [5].

High skin graft take rates are of utmost importance and determine the course of the recovery process to significant extent. Topical negative pressure (TNP) has found various applications in wound management since its introduction in the 1990s [6]. Due to its healing-promoting properties, it was soon proposed as method for skin graft fixation [7]. In acute burns, TNP dressings have been found superior to gauze bandages with regard to burn wound progression [8]. Skin graft fixation in burns using TNP helped to achieve good wound healing results [9].

2 General Effects of Topical Negative Pressure (TNP)

TNP wound therapy was first described by Morykwas and Argenta in 1997 [10, 11]. The TNP dressing consists of a reticulated open-cell polyurethane foam that is fit into the wound and sealed toward the surrounding with an adhesive occlusive drape. Negative pressure is then applied through a specialized tubing system and a suction

C. Smolle, M.D. (✉) • P. Brinskelle • A. Steiner
M. Schintler • L.-P. Kamolz
Division of Plastic, Aesthetic and Reconstructive Surgery, Department of Surgery, Medical University of Graz, Graz, Austria
e-mail: christian.smolle@klinikum-graz.at

Recent Clinical Techniques, Results, and Research in Wounds (2017)
DOI 10.1007/15695_2017_24, © Springer International Publishing AG
Published Online: 24 October 2017

Table 1 Effects of TNP on wounds

	Effects of TNP
Perfusion	• Increased perfusion • Perfusion decrease at the wound margins, increase approximately 2 cm to the periphery, normal levels 5 cm to the periphery • Increase of perfusion greater in muscle than in adipose tissue
Edema	• Reduced edema (observed clinically) • TNP-treated tissue shows increased fluid storage potential
Proliferation	• Enhanced granulation tissue formation • Reduced concentrations of antiproliferative enzymes • Increased concentrations of matrix metalloproteinase inhibitors
Wound microbiome	• Inhibits bacteria proliferation • Inhibits formation of biofilms • Antibacterial effects are enhanced when silver-impregnated foam is used

device. Subsequently wound exudate is removed, and the wound tissue is exposed to mechanical forces exerted by the subatmospheric pressure [6]. Since its upcoming the technique has been used for wounds of various etiologies, and different mechanisms and effects on wound healing have been discovered. Firmly established are the effects of TNP on local blood flow, formation of granulation tissue, and its regulatory influence on the microbiome of the wound [12]. Table 1 provides an overview over the known effects of TNP on wound healing.

3 Tissue Perfusion and Edema Reduction

The effects of TNP on microcirculation have been investigated in various models. Many of the wound-healing-promoting properties of TNP are being deduced on its perfusion-altering properties.

In an early animal trial with pigs, random-pattern flap survival was significantly increased (by 20% on average) when −125 mmHg TNP was applied. This effect was mainly interpreted as the result of improved microcirculation. The effect has been seen to be pressure dependent. At −125 mmHg TNP, blood flow increased, whereas it was decreased at −400 mmHg [10]. This increase in blood flow seems to be accompanied by morphologic changes in the tissue, including increased vascular diameter, increased angiogenesis, and enhanced endothelial proliferation [13]. The changes in blood flow are, however, unevenly distributed across the wound and also depend on the type of tissue. There is a zone of relative hypoperfusion close to the wound margins, while approximately two centimeters from the wound perfusion increases to its maximum before returning to baseline levels again in the periphery. In musculature the zone of relative hypoperfusion is comparably small, while there is a strong increase in perfusion. In subcutaneous tissue, the increase in blood flow is less pronounced, and the zone of relative hypoperfusion is larger. Blood flow at the wound edges increases multifold when TNP is discontinued—an effect that is most likely the result of reactive hyperemia [14, 15]. There is evidence that negative pressures between −80 mmHg and the clinical standard of −125 mmHg can be considered as equivalent regarding wound perfusion [16]. Recent research explored novel and potentially promising indications for TNP treatment with regard to tissue perfusion. TNP doubled microvascular blood flow in normal, ischemic, and reperfused myocardium in pigs [17].

Although it is not yet fully understood how TNP causes improved microcirculation, it seems feasible that the applied subatmospheric pressure creates an interstitial fluid gradient and reduces edema. Thus the extrinsic cause for impaired vascular perfusion is removed [10]. So far this hypothesis however lacks profound scientific foundation—also because tissue edema is notoriously difficult to quantify. Nonetheless, a reduction of edema can be observed clinically [6, 11, 18], and recent findings also suggest that TNP-treated tissue is “dryer” than untreated and has greater fluid storage potential [19].

4 Tissue Proliferation and Cellular Response

According to Wolff's law established in the late 1800s, all living tissues react to mechanical stresses in dynamic fashion. While pressure results in tissue atrophy with only few exceptions (e.g., epiphyseal cartilage), tensile forces promote tissue proliferation. Similarly also TNP exerts tractive effort on the wound surface. For example, full-thickness skin defects in pigs treated with −125 mmHg TNP were completely filled with granulation tissue after 8 days. During that time, wounds treated with −25 mmHg were filled up to 20% with granulation tissue, and wounds treated with −500 mmHg were filled up to just 6% with granulation tissue. At this pressure also a significant thickening of the wound walls occurred, resulting in artificial deepening of the defect [20]. On the other hand, also improper handling of TNP dressings can have deleterious consequences: when an air leak was simulated in −125 mmHg TNP dressings, experimental wounds in pigs increased almost twofold in size [20]. On the molecular level, TNP seemed to reduce concentrations of pro-matrix metalloproteinase-9 (pro-mmp-9) as well as the active enzyme mmp-9 in chronic and acute wounds. Mmp-9 is a type IV collagenase, and high levels are associated with prolonged wound healing. TNP also helped to maintain a low ratio of mmp-9 to the tissue inhibitor of metalloproteinases 1 (TIMP-1) in the wound. A low ratio of mmp-9/timp-1 is associated with improved wound healing [21].

5 Effects on Wound Microbiome

TNP is often referred to as a mean for maintaining a clean wound surface by removing exudates. However, also regulatory effects on the wound microbiome seem to exist. A significant reduction of bacteria counts in experimental wounds in pigs occurred after application of −125 mmHg TNP for 4 days [10]. It seemed as if the application of TNP had the ability to prevent systemic spread of local infections. In a murine burn wound sepsis model, full-thickness scalds contaminated with *Pseudomonas aeruginosa* inocula received either wet-to-dry dressings or TNP therapy. After 2 weeks of treatment, 33% of TNP-treated mice had survived compared to 10% in the wet-to-dry dressings group [22].

Observations from in vitro models support the aforementioned findings: reduced growth rates and loss of the ability to create biofilms were observed when *Staphylococcus aureus* was cultured under −125 mmHg negative pressure conditions [23]. TNP application to biofilm forming *P. aeruginosa* for 2 weeks resulted in a small but statistically significant reduction of bacterial counts compared to untreated controls. Silver-impregnated TNP foam speeded this process up, and the difference reached significance after only 24 h [24]. The synergistic effects of silver-impregnated foam and TNP application however depended on the bacterial strains used. Application of silver foam alone already led to a significant reduction of *S. aureus* and MRSA counts, whereas the effects on *P. aeruginosa* and *Staphylococcus epidermidis* were negligible until TNP is added [25].

6 Treatment of Acute Burns with TNP

According to Jackson's [26] original definition of tissue damage in burn wounds, a burn consists of three concentric zones: the innermost coagulation zone is characterized by irreversible tissue damage. Next to it there is the hypoperfused zone of stasis, where both viable and necrotic cells are present, which is followed by the zone of hyperemia that is characterized by active edema formation. The zone of stasis and the zone of hyperemia are at risk for necrosis but potentially salvageable if perfusion can be kept upright. When progressive edema and local inflammation further impair vascular flow in these two zones, thrombotic obliteration of the affected vessels results in necrosis of formerly viable tissue [27].

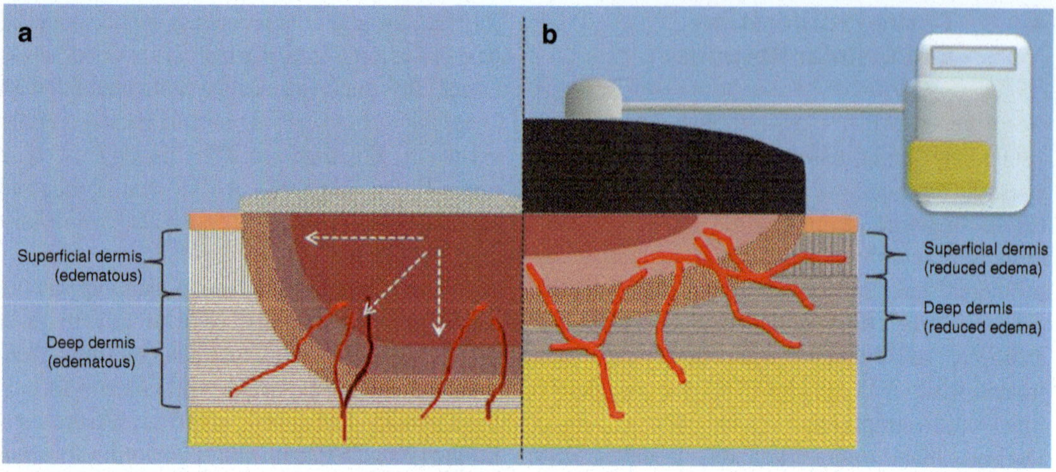

Fig. 1 Theory of TNP effects on burn wounds: (**a**) Edema forms in tissues around the burn wound and impairs perfusion through compression of vasculature which results in deepening of a burn. (**b**) TNP dressings reduce edema and alter perfusion which counteracts burn wound progression

The process of burn wound progression usually occurs during the first 3–5 days after trauma. During this time frame, a burn that has initially been diagnosed to be superficial may progress in size and depth to a deep dermal or full-thickness skin defect requiring surgery and skin grafting. Consequently burn wound progression significantly adds to the initial morbidity of the injury [28].

Due to its perfusion-altering effects, TNP has been ascribed the potential of counteracting burn wound progression [8, 29]. The effects of TNP on acute burns have been studied both in animals [30] and humans [8, 29, 31]. The main influence of TNP on burn wounds seems to lie in the reduction of burn wound edema which in turn increases blood flow (Fig. 1) [8, 29].

7 Observations from Animal Trials

Application of −125 mmHg TNP on burn wounds in pigs for 6 h resulted in a significantly decreased maximum depth of cellular death below the wound surface when compared to controls treated with sterile dressings. Thereby it seemed as if TNP had greatest efficacy when applied early after the injury [30]. The tissue-preserving effect of TNP is probably based in part on its ability to restore the integrity of damaged collagen fibers. Burns are accompanied by denaturation of collagen strands within the damaged tissue. It is likely that the surface tension exerted by unfolded collagen fibers causes a fluid gradient from the vasculature to the extracellular space [32, 33]. Explants of burned skin from pigs treated with −125 mmHg TNP in situ presented with a fluid storage capacity similar to that of unsevered tissue when put into a water bath. This finding was attributed to the mechanical compression of dermal structures that prevents fluid influx in situ. This in turn probably reduced swelling and further unfolding of damaged collagen [19].

8 Clinical Observations

Clinical studies investigated the use of TNP to prevent burn wound progression in hand burns [8, 29]. Burn wound perfusion was the primary endpoint and monitored using indocyanine green angiography (ICGA). The technique allowed for objective qualitative and quantitative measurement of vascular perfusion. Indocyanine green dye was injected intravenously, and vascular dye uptake in the region of interest was recorded with a specialized video camera using dynamic laser-fluorescence angiography. The maximum recorded pixel intensity was assessed to quantify wound perfusion. ICGA accurately predicts survival in the zone of ischemia [34] and can be used to identify areas requiring surgical intervention [35, 36].

In the studies published [8, 29], patients with bilateral second-degree hand burns were assigned to the study protocol within 6 h after trauma. The more severely injured hand received −125 mmHg TNP therapy, while the other was treated with sulfadiazine cream and conventional gauze dressings. For sufficient and easy coverage of the treated hand, a special TNP glove was used (Fig. 2). ICGA measurements were carried out upon admission and daily thereafter. If burn wound progression necessitated surgery, conservative treatment was discontinued. Surgical therapy consisted of a combination of tangential excision and split-thickness skin grafting or dermabrasion and autologous keratinocyte application.

In conventionally treated hands, vascular perfusion as assessed with ICGA was significantly decreased on days 1–3 after trauma relative to baseline levels. In TNP-treated hands, vascular perfusion could be maintained, i.e., did not decrease compared to baseline levels [8, 29]. Also dye uptake, meaning the time from intravenous injection of indocyanine green dye to maximum pixel intensity recorded, was significantly slower in controls than in treated hands [8, 29]. In addition, skin grafting was required less often in TNP-treated hands. Clinically an impressive reduction of edema was observed [8].

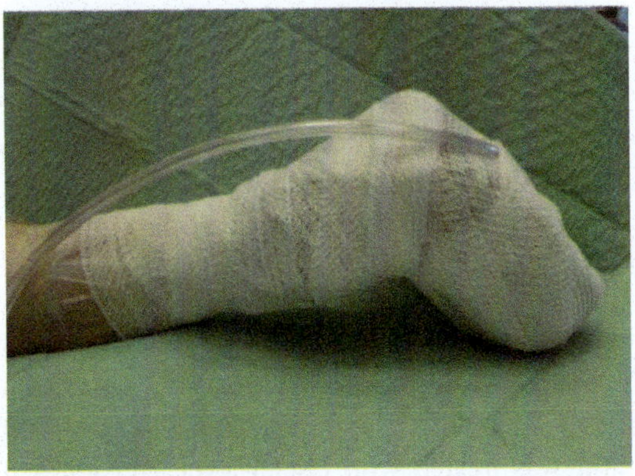

Fig. 2 TNP glove is used to immobilize the hand in intrinsic plus position

According to case studies, TNP may also have beneficial effects on frostbites. Poulakidas et al. [37] treated an adult male with frostbites to one foot. Although the wounds were in a detrimental state upon admission and TNP therapy was initiated 72 h after trauma, all wounds had healed after 4 weeks. In children with frostbites to the hands, TNP therapy helped to prevent the loss of digits. Follow-up X-rays revealed that full integrity of epiphyseal cartilages could be preserved. Therefore, TNP therapy may be a method to prevent long-term complications in pediatric frostbites [38].

9 Skin Engraftment and TNP to Enhance Skin Graft Take Rates

During the first days after grafting, the skin transplant is nourished by diffusion of nutrients from the wound bed. In this phase of treatment, the parts of the transplant that are not in contact with the wound bed will not take, i.e., die off. After 48–72 h, the vessels from the wound bed connect to existing graft vasculature, and reperfusion sets in [39, 40]. During the following days, the autochthonous graft vasculature is successively replaced by sprouting vessels from the wound bed, and the skin graft is incorporated [41, 42]. Seroma or hematoma formation underneath the graft may hinder successful engraftment, and shearing forces may disrupt the early vascular connections between transplant and wound bed. Local infection often has detrimental consequences and may result in complete graft loss. Desiccation must be avoided by all means [43].

TNP combines all features required for ideal skin graft treatment in one application: immobilization of the graft and ensuring close contact to the wound bed, maintenance of a moist wound milieu, and reduction of bacterial load [6]. Possibly TNP alters diffusion of nutrients from the wound bed to the skin graft [44]. First clinical experiences with TNP for skin graft fixation have been made by Schneider et al. [7]. The authors found that TNP was especially useful in difficult recipient areas and is applicable to a wide range of wounds. Results from later clinical studies support this rationale.

In an early case study, the use of TNP dressings for split-thickness skin graft fixation in chronic leg ulcers was described. After only 5 days of treatment, take rates ranged from 95 to 100% [45]. Because there was no representative control group, no conclusions could be drawn concerning the superiority of TNP over conventional dressings. A later report compared conventional dressings and TNP for skin graft fixation in wounds of different etiology in 61 consecutive patients. Although there were no differences concerning take rates, patients in the TNP arm of the study required re-grafting significantly less often [43]. A retrospective analysis compared the outcome of meshed split-thickness skin grafts in 74 leg ulcers before and after implementation of TNP dressings. The mean take rate in the TNP-treated group (93%) was significantly higher than that of the group managed with conventional dressings (67%). No severe side effects of TNP were reported; however, occasional discomfort occurred in TNP-treated areas when suction was applied, and some patients reported sleeping problems because of the noises of the electric pump [46].

Currently, few randomized controlled trials exist that compare TNP and conventional skin graft bolster dressings. Moisidis et al. [47] reported increased or equal take rates in 75% of TNP-treated grafts compared to conventional dressings. In a subjective evaluation, TNP-treated grafts were also considered qualitatively equal or better in 85% of the cases [47]. A randomized, double-masked, controlled trial reported significantly better take rates, significantly shorter hospitalization times, and significantly fewer reoperations in skin-grafted patients treated with TNP [48]. In a recent analysis of patients receiving skin grafts for burn wound coverage or secondary reconstruction, equally significant higher take rates were seen when TNP was used. TNP-treated grafts also healed faster, so they required dressings for a significantly shorter period of time [49].

TNP can also be used to prepare wound beds for skin grafting. While full-thickness skin grafts have advantages over split-thickness skin grafts—including better skin pliability, lower shrinking tendency, and better color match—high take rates cannot be achieved as reliably. Preconditioning of wound beds with TNP prior to full-thickness skin grafting resulted in average take rates of 95% even in large wounds [50].

10 Technique

Various methods to enhance graft take in burns have been proposed, including fibrin sealant [51], medical honey [52], or amniotic membrane [53]. Large burns requiring skin grafting represent a prime indication for TNP wound therapy in a way for two reasons: (1) especially second-degree burns go along with significant water evaporation, and (2) local and generalized edema compromise vascular perfusion of the wound bed [8, 54]. With the knowledge that TNP dressings allow for wound drainage, enhance perfusion of burn wounds through edema reduction, and improve skin graft take rates, TNP has been applied for skin graft fixation in burns on several occasions [3, 9, 55–59].

11 Experiences with TNP for Skin Graft Fixation in Burn Patients

Table 2 gives an overview over the results of clinical studies and case reports published on the topic. In general, good experiences have been made with the technique, and in all studies, the reported take rates were above 90% even in the severely burned [9, 55–59].

Schintler et al. [55] were the first to describe the use of TNP for skin graft fixation in extensive burns. A 6-year-old boy with 40% TBSA deep flame burns on the neck, the trunk, and the right arm was treated with fascial-level excision and

Table 2 Results of studies on application of TNP for skin graft fixation in burns

Study	Patients	Mean Baux score, age, and burned TBSA (BTBSA)	Grafted TBSA covered with TNP	Take rate (tr) survival rate (sr)	TNP-related complications	Additional benefits of TNP therapy
Roka et al. (2007) [56]	*n* = 29; 15 male, 14 female	Baux: 78.6 (sd ± 24.4) Age: 59.4 (sd ± 21.5) years BTBSA: n.a.	20.2% (sd ± 13.0)	tr: n.a. sr: 97%	None reported	Continuous wound drainage, splinting effect, yet early mobilization possible
Kamolz et al. (2014) [9]	*n* = 37; 18 male, 19 female	Baux: 88.6 (sd ± 24.4) Age: 59.4 (sd ± 21.5) years BTBSA: n.a.	>25%	tr: >95% sr: 97%	None reported	Wound drainage, local edema reduction
Hoeller et al. (2014) [57]	*n* = 60; 36 male, 24 female	Baux: n.a. Age: 8 (sd ± 6) years BTBSA: 4.5% (range 3.0–12.0%)	3.5% (range 2.0–6.0%)	tr: 95% sr: 100%	Extensive bleeding requiring revision (no influence on tr)	Fixation of grafts in physically very active non-compliant infants, early mobilization
Fischer et al. (2016) [58]	*n* = 12; gender n.a.	Baux: n.a. Age: 35.5 (range 18–63) years BTBSA: 29.6% (range 15–60%)	n.a. (total TNP-treated TBSA, donor sites, and skin grafts, 35.1%)	tr: 97% sr: 100%	Acute kidney injury after TNP installation, causal relation unlikely	Possibility of wound exudate collection to estimate fluid loss and requirements
Case studies						
Schintler, et al. (2005) [55]	1 male	Baux: n.a. Age: 6 years BTBSA: 40%	40%	tr: 100% survived	Leakages in the TNP system could be easily resealed	Early mobilization, good overall condition of treated patient, wound exudate collection
Psoinos et al. (2009) [59]	1 female	Baux: n.a. Age: 8 months BTBSA: 6%	4%	tr: 100% survived	None reported	TNP prevents wound contamination in perianal areas, can be used for donor site coverage

TNP topical negative pressure, *n.a.* not available, *sd* standard deviation

split-thickness skin grafts meshed 1:2. All grafted areas were treated with TNP for 5 days; 7 days after surgery take rate was 100% (Figs. 3 and 4). Throughout the whole course of the therapy, the patient was alert and in an unexpectedly good general condition [55].

Roka et al. [56] as well as Kamolz et al. [9] further explored the use of TNP for skin graft fixation in larger cohorts. Roka described a cohort of 29 patients with second- to third-degree burns and a mean Baux score of 78.6%, while Baux scores exceeded 100 in six patients. The mean grafted TNP-treated TBSA was 20.2%, and the median time of TNP treatment was 4 days. The survival rate was 97%—one male with a Baux score of 121 succumbed to his injuries, while one female with a Baux score of 127 however survived. There was no data available on take rates, but it was noted that all survivors could be discharged with completely healed wounds after a mean hospitalization time of 46.6 days [56]. The cohort of 37 patients described by Kamolz [9] received TNP dressings for at least 25% grafted TBSA. Although Baux scores in this cohort were higher (mean 88.6, above 100 in eight patients) and treatment modalities did not differ significantly from those of Roka et al., hospitalization time (46.6 days) and survival rate (97%) remained the same. Of 37 patients, 36 could be discharged, and the skin graft take rate was 95% and above in all cases (Fig. 5) [9]. Notably, in neither study any TNP-related complications such as severe wound site infections were described [9, 56].

Hoeller et al. [57] reviewed 60 pediatric burn patients who had received TNP for skin graft fixation. The mean burned TBSA was 4.5%, and children of all age groups—infants (<24 months), toddlers/preschoolers (2–6 years), school-age

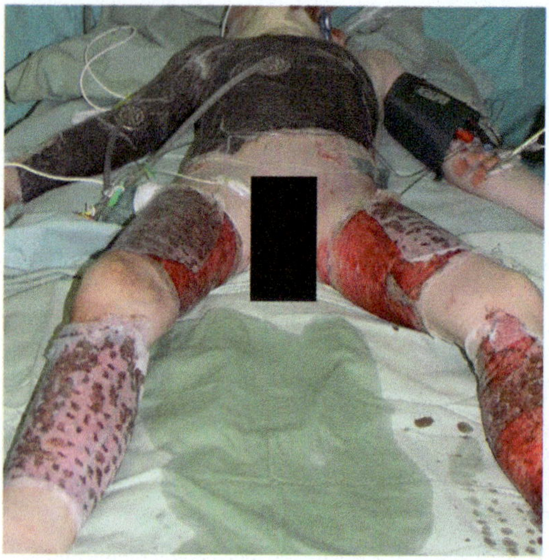

Fig. 3 Boy treated with TNP dressings after skin grafting. Donor sites were covered with biosynthetic dermal replacements

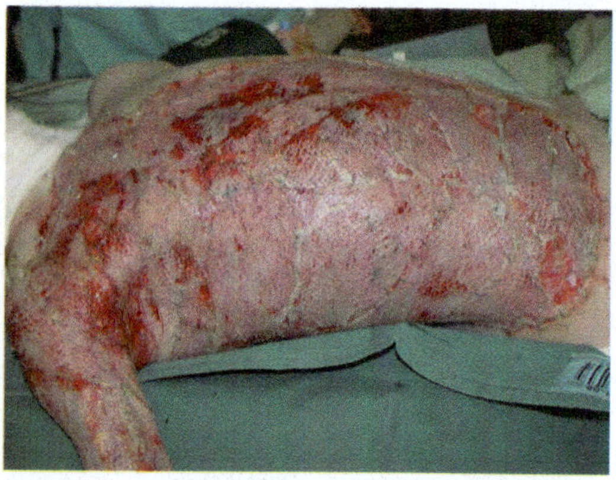

Fig. 4 Take rate is almost 100% in the same patient (Fig. 3) 5 days postsurgery

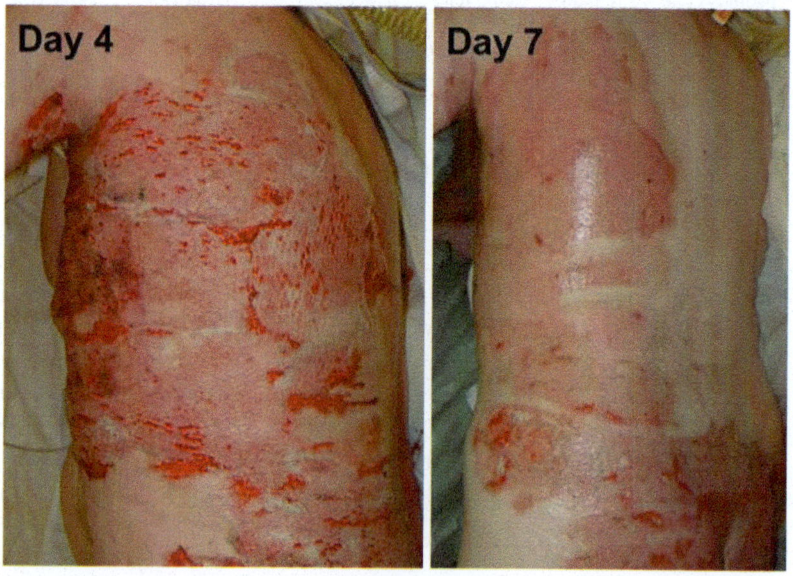

Fig. 5 Eighty-six-year-old female with a 20% second-degree to third-degree burn to her trunk (Baux score 106). Good initial graft take after 4 days of TNP treatment resulted in completely healed wounds on day 7 postsurgery

children (6–13 years), and adolescents (>13 years)—were analyzed. With 3.5% the mean TNP-treated TBSA was comparably small. After a median TNP application time of 5 days, the mean take rate was 96%. It was found that smaller grafted TBSA resulted in better take rates. In contrast the amount of TNP-treated TBSA had no influence on take rates. Three major complications were noted. In two cases major bleeding occurred hours after TNP installation which led to termination of therapy. Take rate was 95% in both cases though. In one case a bigger part of the skin graft became necrotic leading to the worst take rate in the cohort of 70%. Minor alterations were observed in 17 cases, of which one was contamination of a TNP system with stool after installation in the anogenital region. Nevertheless the mean take rate in this subgroup was 80%.

Psoinos et al. [59] reported a case of an 8-month-old female who sustained scalds averaging 6% TBSA to her lower back and the buttocks. Four percent of the wound area, mainly located in the gluteal region, required excision and skin grafting. After 5 days of TNP treatment, take rate was 100%. In this case TNP application was found especially useful to avoid fecal contamination of the grafted areas on the buttocks. Instead of the conventional foam dressing, gauze was used as wound filler material.

In another study with 12 patients, skin graft recipient sites as well as donor sites were covered with TNP dressings resulting in an average TNP-treated TBSA of 35.1%. Average graft take rate was 97%, and all patients survived. Although this data was available only for four patients, the reported median epithelialization time of donor sites after TNP treatment was 11 days. No major side effects were described. However, one patient developed acute kidney injury during the course of TNP treatment [58].

12 Method of Application

After depth-adapted burn wound debridement, split-thickness skin grafting is performed. Mesh grafts are fixed to the wound surface with staples. When Meek grafts are used, the silken carrier sheets are tacked down accordingly [3]. The grafts are then covered with sterile fatty gauze or other non-adherent dressings such as soft silicone wound contact layer [55]. This is done to prevent adherence of the TNP foam to the skin graft. The sterile polyurethane TNP foam dressing is clipped in shape to fit the wound dimensions and placed atop the non-adherent dressing. Most manufacturers provide foam dressings of various sizes [58], and for coverage of the entire hand, also special TNP gloves are available (Fig. 2) [8]. The entire area is covered with the occlusive transparent drape that is usually provided with the foam. Alternatively any available occlusive drape can be used, like Opsite [49]. An opening is cut into the film for the suction tubing, and a continuous pressure between −75 and −125 mmHg is applied (Fig. 6).

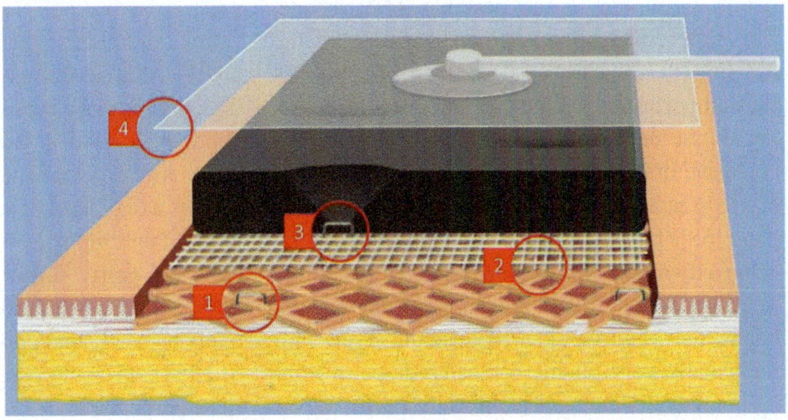

Fig. 6 Sequence of TNP application. (1) After stapling the skin grafts to the wound site. (2) They are covered with non-adherent dressings, i.e., fatty gauze. (3) The foam dressing is applied and tacked down if necessary. (4) The whole area is sealed with occlusive drape, and suction is applied

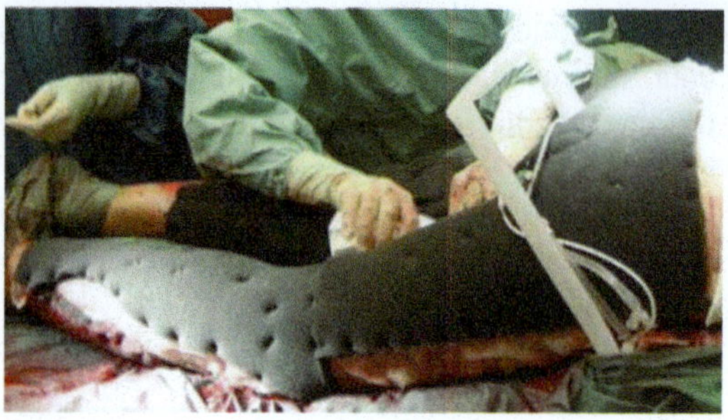

Fig. 7 Large TNP foam dressings are held in place with staples

When large areas have to be covered or when the wound lies in a region of complex contour that is subject to repeated motion—such as the axilla, the groins, or the circumference of the arm—the foam is stapled to the wound surface (Fig. 7). If more than one foam piece is required to cover the wound, the individual foam pieces are connected to one another with staples.

Large TNP dressings or multiple wound surfaces may necessitate the use of more than one negative pressure pump [9, 56]. In some cases it may be feasible though to connect TNP dressings on wound sites that are separated by viable skin to one another with thin polyurethane foam strips. To prevent direct contact with the skin and consequent maceration, the strips are wrapped up in occlusive drape. With this technique negative pressure can be distributed evenly to all wound sites, and resources can be saved [60].

When a tight seal cannot be achieved right away, it has proven useful to apply negative pressure temporarily with surgical suction units before switching to the portable TNP device. This proceeding allows for investigation of the dressing for leakages and also effectively removes the first portion of wound exudate from the dressing [9]. Some favor the technique of stapling the occlusive drape to the skin in the wound periphery to guarantee its adherence in mobile body parts [58]. In most cases a sufficient seal can be achieved without this approach though [9].

Application of TNP dressings to the fingers, hands, toes, and feet can be difficult. Even with the usually very pliable occlusive drape, a tight seal may be hard to achieve in web spaces. When special TNP gloves are not readily available, a good method to overcome those difficulties is the "sterile glove technique." Here a conventional sterile surgical glove is used instead of the occlusive drape. After the foam dressing has been applied, the hand or foot is dressed with a sterile glove. In small defects a single tight-fitting glove often suffices to seal the dressing. In larger defects, the glove dressing may require completion with a piece of occlusive drape proximally. An opening for the TNP suction tubing is created as usual. When using this technique, the proximal rubber band of the glove should always be removed because it has been seen to cause pressure marks. The fingertips of the glove can be cut off to monitor perfusion of the digits. When applied with care, this technique is very efficient, and strangulation of digits is unlikely. The method is, however, not recommended in patients with preexisting vascular diseases [61].

13 Additional Benefits of TNP for Skin Graft Fixation in Burns

The TNP foam becomes rigid when negative pressure is applied. In certain body parts, this makes an additional splint unnecessary because enough suspension is provided by the dressing. Burned hands can effectively be immobilized in the intrinsic plus position solely by using TNP gloves (Fig. 2) [8, 29].

Despite their splint-like effect, TNP dressings retain part of their flexibility also after negative pressure activation. This allows for active mobilization of joints also during the early stages of therapy [3]. Successful early mobilization with TNP dressings in place is possible in adults as well as in children [9, 55–57]. Especially in babies and toddlers, where compliance cannot be expected and there is a high level of activity, mobilization can be allowed unscrupulous with TNP dressings holding the skin grafts firmly in place. Portable TNP devices furthermore give children who would normally be bed bound opportunity to play outside the bed [57]. In some cases it may be necessary to spare particular body regions from TNP application to facilitate mobilization. In circular burns to the lower limbs, sparing the popliteal fossa may increase the range of motion. To further soften the dressings, negative pressure can be reduced to −50 mmHg or turned off temporarily [58].

Because the TNP system removes blood and exudates from the wound surface and stores it in a container, a relatively clean dressing can be guaranteed for a longer period of time. As a result dressing changes are required less often. The dressing can be left in place from 4 up to 7 days [50, 56]. The fluid captured in the container also allows for indirect evaluation of the wound. A significant amount of blood in the container may indicate hemorrhage, and purulent fluid could be an early sign for wound infection [56].

Additionally, the fluid output of the TNP system can be used as an orientation for fluid requirements. When wound healing progresses and the skin barrier is restored by reepithelialization emerging from the skin grafts, the amount of drainage fluid gradually decreases [55]. To estimate total evaporative fluid loss, skin grafts as well as donor sites may be covered with TNP dressings. In general, the fluid output of grafted areas is smaller than that of conservatively managed burn wounds or that of donor sites [8, 58].

TNP dressings are comparably expensive. In the long run, TNP may however have financial advantages over conventional wound dressings. Since TNP dressings have to be changed less often, less analgesics, sedatives, and also qualified health-care personnel are needed [56]. Higher initial take rates also decrease the risk for complications as well as the need for re-grafting. Complications and frequent reoperations go along with longer hospitalization times which in turn result in higher treatment costs [43, 47]. Consequently the higher costs of TNP therapy are likely to be compensated by better outcome [9, 56].

14 Discussion

With the use of TNP dressings as bolster, high skin graft take rates above 90% can be achieved in adults [9, 56, 58] as well as in children with severe burns [55, 57, 59]. Even in patients with Baux scores exceeding 100, high take rates can be achieved reliably [9, 56]. TNP dressings are especially useful for fixation of large skin grafts in body regions of inferior take rate, such as the gluteal region, the lower back, or the posterior aspect of the thorax [3]. There is no information available on the ideal duration of TNP application. However, most authors reported application times between 4 and 6 days until the first dressing change with satisfactory results [9, 55–57].

Despite the vast evidence that TNP interferes actively with wound healing processes, no significant side effects are known. In the treatment of burns, hardly any TNP-related complications have been described, and in all of them, a direct association to the wound dressings was questionable. By and large the reported events did not affect the final outcome, and all complications could be salvaged [57, 58].

The studies on TNP application for skin graft fixation in burns lack a representative control group in all cases. Still, randomized controlled trials on TNP for skin graft fixation in wounds of different etiology showed the beneficial effects of TNP on take rates, even when the dressing had to be improvised [49]. Concerning the quality of data, objective methods for wound assessment were not used in most of the cases.

Two studies [9, 56] used specialized burn size assessment software (BurnCase 3D, RISC Software GmbH, Linz, Hagenberg, Austria [62]) for estimation of grafted TBSA as well as take rates and thus provided objective data.

Not only the healing of skin grafts but also take rates of dermal substitutes can be improved by using TNP. The use of TNP has been seen to allow for earlier skin grafting in substitutes requiring a two-step procedure, such as Integra®. This in turn reduced the length of hospital stay and should on the long run decrease the risk for complications due to faster wound healing [63].

Currently TNP gauze dressings experience a revival with wound healing results similar to those of the usual foam dressings [59, 64]. Gauze dressings use smaller negative pressures of about −80 mmHg. In surgical wounds of different etiology, TNP gauze dressings produce an overall volume reduction of 15.1% per week—a value comparable to that of the foam alternative [64]. There is also evidence that gauze dressings produce less pain and discomfort around the wound site than foam dressings [65]. This makes TNP gauze a user-friendly alternative to foam dressings worthwhile considering. With regard to burns, TNP gauze dressings have been applied for skin graft fixation with good success in a pediatric burn patient [59]. It remains to be seen how TNP gauze will impact future burn wound management. First results are encouraging though.

Conclusions

TNP dressings can be used for skin graft fixation to reliably achieve take rates above 90% in severe burns. The application rarely leads to complications, and reported adverse events are manageable. Additional benefits of TNP comprise a splinting effect in extremity burns, a reduced need for dressing changes, the possibility of early mobilization without the risk of graft shear, and a good acceptance by patients.

References

1. Smolle C, Cambiaso-Daniel J, Forbes AA, Wurzer P, Hundeshagen G, Branski LK et al (2017) Recent trends in burn epidemiology worldwide: a systematic review. Burns 43:249–257
2. Kamolz LP (2010) Burns: learning from the past in order to be fit for the future. Crit Care 14:106
3. Lumenta DB, Kamolz LP, Frey M (2009) Adult burn patients with more than 60% TBSA involved-meek and other techniques to overcome restricted skin harvest availability—the Viennese concept. J Burn Care Res 30:231–242
4. Thourani VH, Ingram WL, Feliciano DV (2003) Factors affecting success of split-thickness skin grafts in the modern burn unit. J Trauma 54:562–568
5. Finnerty CC, Jeschke MG, Branski LK, Barret JP, Dziewulski P, Herndon DN (2016) Hypertrophic scarring: the greatest unmet challenge after burn injury. Lancet 388:1427–1436
6. Schintler MV (2012) Negative pressure therapy: theory and practice. Diabetes Metab Res Rev 28(Suppl 1):72–77
7. Schneider AM, Morykwas MJ, Argenta LC (1998) A new and reliable method of securing skin grafts to the difficult recipient bed. Plast Reconstr Surg 102:1195–1198
8. Kamolz LP, Andel H, Haslik W, Winter W, Meissl G, Frey M (2004) Use of subatmospheric pressure therapy to prevent burn wound progression in human: first experiences. Burns 30:253–258
9. Kamolz LP, Lumenta DB, Parvizi D, Wiedner M, Justich I, Keck M, Pfurtscheller K, Schintler M (2014) Skin graft fixation in severe burns: use of topical negative pressure. Ann Burns Fire Disasters 27:141–145
10. Morykwas MJ, Argenta LC, Shelton-Brown EI, McGuirt W (1997) Vacuum-assisted closure: a new method for wound control and treatment: animal studies and basic foundation. Ann Plast Surg 38:553–562
11. Argenta LC, Morykwas MJ (1997) Vacuum-assisted closure: a new method for wound control and treatment: clinical experience. Ann Plast Surg 38:563–576
12. Morykwas MJ, Simpson J, Punger K, Argenta A, Kremers L, Argenta J (2006) Vacuum-assisted closure: state of basic research and physiologic foundation. Plast Reconstr Surg 117:121s–126s
13. Chen SZ, Li J, Li XY, Xu LS (2005) effects of vacuum-assisted closure on wound microcirculation: an experimental study. Asian J Surg 28:211–217
14. Wackenfors A, Sjögren J, Gustafsson R, Algotsson L, Ingemansson R, Malmsjö M (2004) Effects of vacuum-assisted closure therapy on inguinal wound edge microvascular blood flow. Wound Repair Regen 12(6):600
15. Wackenfors A, Gustafsson R, Sjögren J, Algotsson L, Ingemansson R, Malmsjö M (2005) Blood flow responses in the peristernal thoracic wall during vacuum-assisted closure therapy. Ann Thorac Surg 79:1724–1730
16. Borgquist O, Ingemansson R, Malmsjö M (2010) Wound edge microvascular blood flow during negative-pressure wound therapy: examining the effects of pressures from -10 to -175 mmHg. Plast Reconstr Surg 125:502–509
17. Lindstedt S, Malmsjö M, Ingemansson R (2007) Blood flow changes in normal and ischemic myocardium during topically applied negative pressure. Ann Thorac Surg 84:568–573
18. Banwell PE, Musgrave M (2004) Topical negative pressure therapy: mechanisms and indications. Int Wound J 1:95–106
19. McGee MP, Morykwas M, Campbell D, Hoge K, Argenta L (2014) Interstitial-matrix edema in burns: mechanistic insights from subatmospheric pressure treatment in vivo. Wound Repair Regen 22:96–102
20. Morykwas MJ, Faler BJ, Pearce DJ, Argenta LC (2001) Effects of varying levels of subatmospheric pressure on the rate of granulation tissue formation in experimental wounds in swine. Ann Plast Surg 47:547–551
21. Mouës CM, van Toorenenbergen AW, Heule F, Hop WC, Hovius SER (2008) The role of topical negative pressure in wound repair: expression of biochemical markers in wound fluid during wound healing. Wound Repair Regen 16:488–494
22. Liu Y, Zhou Q, Wang Y, Liu Z, Dong M, Wang Y, Li X, Hu D (2014) Negative pressure wound therapy decreases mortality in a murine model of burn-wound sepsis involving Pseudomonas aeruginosa infection. PLos One 9:e90494

23. Li T, Wang G, Yin P, Li Z, Zhang L, Liu J, Li M, Zhang L, Han L, Tang P (2015) Effect of negative pressure on growth, secretion and biofilm formation of Staphylococcus aureus. Antonie Van Leeuwenhoek 108:907–917
24. Ngo QD, Vickery K, Deva AK (2012) The effect of topical negative pressure on wound biofilms using an in vitro wound model. Wound Repair Regen 20:83–90
25. Valente PMD, Deva A, Ngo Q, Vickery K (2016) The increased killing of biofilms in vitro by combining topical silver dressings with topical negative pressure in chronic wounds. Int Wound J 13:130–136
26. Jackson DM (1953) The diagnosis of the depth of burning. Br J Surg 40:588–596
27. Singh V, Devgan L, Bhat S, Milner SM (2007) The pathogenesis of burn wound conversion. Ann Plast Surg 59:109–115
28. Johnson RM, Richard R (2003) Partial-thickness burns: identification and management. Adv Skin Wound Care 16:178–187
29. Haslik W, Kamolz LP, Andel H, Meissl G, Frey M (2004) The use of subatmospheric pressure to prevent burn wound progression: first experiences in burn wound treatment. Zentralbl Chir 129(Suppl 1):s62–s63
30. Morykwas MJ, David LR, Schneider AM, Whang C, Jennings DA, Canty C, Parker D, White WL, Argenta LC (1999) Use of subatmospheric pressure to prevent progression of partial-thickness burns in a swine model. J Burn Care Rehabil 20:15–21
31. Molnar JA, Simpson JL, Voignier DM, Morykwas MJ, Argenta LC (2005) Management of an acute thermal injury with subatmospheric pressure. J Burns Wounds 4:e5
32. McGee MP, Morykwas M, Shelton J, Argenta L (2012) Collagen unfolding accelerates water influx, determining hydration in the interstitial matrix. Biophys J 103:2157–2166
33. McGee MP, Morykwas MJ, Argenta LC (2011) The local pathology of interstitial edema: surface tension increases hydration potential in heat-damaged skin. Wound Repair Regen 19:358–367
34. Fourman MS, Phillips BT, Crawford L, McClain SA, Lin F, Thode HC, Dagum AB, Singer AJ, Clark RA (2014) Indocyanine green dye angiography accurately predicts survival in the zone of ischemia in a burn comb model. Burns 40:940–946
35. Kamolz LP, Andel H, Auer T, Meissl G, Frey M (2006) Evaluation of skin perfusion by use of indocyanine green video angiography: rational design and planning of trauma surgery. J Trauma 61:635–641
36. Kamolz LP, Andel H, Haslik W, Donner A, Winter W, Meissl G, Frey M (2003) Indocyanine green video angiographies help to identify burns requiring operation. Burns 29:785–791
37. Poulakidas S, Cologne K, Kowal-Vern A (2008) Treatment of frostbite with subatmospheric pressure therapy. J Burn Care Res 29:1012–1014
38. Poulakidas SJ, Kowal-Vern A, Atty C (2016) Pediatric frostbite treated by negative pressure wound therapy. J Burn Care Res 37(5):e489–e492
39. Lindenblatt N, Calcagni M, Contaldo C, Menger MD, Giovanoli P, Vollmar B (2008) A new model for studying the revascularization of skin grafts in vivo: the role of angiogenesis. Plast Reconstr Surg 122:1669–1680
40. Lindenblatt N, Platz U, Althaus M, Hegland N, Schmidt CA, Contaldo C, Vollmar B, Giovanoli P, Calcagni M (2010) Temporary angiogenic transformation of the skin graft vasculature after reperfusion. Plast Reconstr Surg 126:61–70
41. Calcagni M, Althaus MK, Knapik AD, Hegland N, Contaldo C, Giovanoli P, Lindenblatt N (2011) In vivo visualization of the origination of skin graft vasculature in a wild-type/gfp crossover model. Microvasc Res 82:237–245
42. O'Ceallaigh S, Herrick SE, Bennett WR, Bluff JE, Ferguson MWJ, McGrouther DA (2007) Perivascular cells in a skin graft are rapidly repopulated by host cells. J Plast Reconstr Aesthet Surg 60:864–875
43. Scherer LA, Shiver S, Chang M, Meredith JW, Owings JT (2002) The vacuum assisted closure device: a method of securing skin grafts and improving graft survival. Arch Surg 137:930–933
44. Wang X, Zhang Y, Han C (2014) Topical negative pressure improves autograft take by altering nutrient diffusion: a hypothesis. Med Sci Monit 20:61–63
45. Sposato G, Molea G, Di Caprio G, Scioli M, La Rusca I, Ziccardi P (2001) Ambulant vacuum-assisted closure of skin-graft dressing in the lower limbs using a portable mini-VAC device. Br J Plast Surg 54:235–237
46. Körber A, Franckson T, Grabbe S, Dissemond J (2008) Vacuum assisted closure device improves the take of mesh grafts in chronic leg ulcer patients. Dermatology 216:250–256
47. Moisidis E, Heath T, Boorer C, Ho K, Deva AK (2004) A prospective, blinded, randomized, controlled clinical trial of topical negative pressure use in skin grafting. Plast Reconstr Surg 114:917–922
48. Llanos S, Danilla S, Barraza C, Armijo E, Piñeros JL, Quintas M, Searle S, Calderon W (2006) Effectiveness of negative pressure closure in the integration of split thickness skin grafts: a randomized, double-masked, controlled trial. Ann Surg 244(5):700
49. Petkar KS, Dhanraj P, Kingsly PM, Sreekar H, Lakshmanarao A, Lamba S, Shetty R, Zachariah JR (2011) A prospective randomized controlled trial comparing negative pressure dressing and conventional dressing methods on split-thickness skin grafts in burned patients. Burns 37:925–929
50. Landau AG, Hudson DA, Adams K, Geldenhuys S, Pienaar C (2008) Full-thickness skin grafts: maximizing graft take using negative pressure dressings to prepare the graft bed. Ann Plast Surg 60(6):661
51. Branski LK, Mittermayr R, Herndon DN, Jeschke MG, Hofmann M, Masters OE, Norbury WB, Traber DL, Tangl S, Redl H (2011) fibrin sealant improves graft adherence in a porcine full-thickness burn wound model. Burns 37:1360–1366
52. Emsen IM (2007) A different and safe method of split thickness skin graft fixation: medical honey application. Burns 33:782–787

53. Mohammadi AA, Johari HG, Eskandari S (2013) Effect of amniotic membrane on graft take in extremity burns. Burns 39:1137–1141
54. Lamke LO, Liljedahl SO (1971) Evaporative water loss from burns, grafts and donor sites. Scand J Plast Reconstr Surg 5:17–22
55. Schintler M, Marschitz I, Trop M (2005) The use of topical negative pressure in a paediatric patient with extensive burns. Burns 31:1050–1053
56. Roka J, Karle B, Andel H, Kamolz L, Frey M (2007) Use of V.A.C. therapy in the surgical treatment of severe burns: the Viennese concept. Handchir Mikrochir Plast Chir 39:322–327
57. Hoeller M, Schintler MV, Pfurtscheller K, Kamolz LP, Tripolt N, Trop M (2014) A retrospective analysis of securing autologous split-thickness skin grafts with negative pressure wound therapy in paediatric burn patients. Burns 40:1116–1120
58. Fischer S, Wall J, Pomahac B, Riviello R, Halvorson EG (2016) Extra-large negative pressure wound therapy dressings for burns - initial experience with technique, fluid management, and outcomes. Burns 42:457–465
59. Psoinos CM, Ignotz RA, Lalikos JF, Fudem G, Savoie P, Dunn RM (2009) Use of gauze-based negative pressure wound therapy in a pediatric burn patient. J Pediatr Surg 44:e23–e26
60. Low OW, Chong SJ, Tan BK (2013) The enhanced total body wrap—the new frontier in dressing care for burns. Burns 39:1420–1422
61. Kamolz L-P, Lumenta DB (2013) Topical negative pressure therapy for skin graft fixation in hand and feet defects: a method for quick and easy dressing application—the 'sterile glove technique'. Burns 39:814–815
62. Parvizi D, Giretzlehner M, Wurzer P, Klein LD, Shoham Y, Bohanon FJ, Haller HL, Tuca A, Branski LK, Lumenta DB, Herndon DN, Kamolz LP (2016) BurnCase 3D software validation study: burn size measurement accuracy and inter-rater reliability. Burns 42:329–335
63. Jeschke MG, Rose C, Angele P, Füchtmeier B, Nerlich MN, Bolder U (2004) Development of new reconstructive techniques: use of Integra in combination with fibrin glue and negative-pressure therapy for reconstruction of acute and chronic wounds. Plast Reconstr Surg 113:525–530
64. Campbell PE, Smith GS, Smith JM (2008) Retrospective clinical evaluation of gauze-based negative pressure wound therapy. Int Wound J 5:280–286
65. Fraccalvieri M, Ruka E, Bocchiotti MA, Zingarelli E, Bruschi S (2011) Patient's pain feedback using negative pressure wound therapy with foam and gauze. Int Wound J 8:492–499

Tissue Expanders in Post-Burn Alopecia: With or Without Galeotomies

Dalia Mohamed Mofreh El Sakka

1 Introduction

When a constant mechanical stress is applied to the skin over time, two phenomena occur:

1. Mechanical creep: The cell is stretched in response to the applied stress.
2. Biological creep: In the form of cell proliferation due to disruption of gap junctions and increased tissue surface area. Growth of the tissue by cell proliferation restores resting tension of the stretched tissue to baseline [1].

The use of silastic tissue expanders extends this natural principle with actual increase in the amount of skin available, along with increased vascularity in the expanded skin [2].

2 Types of Tissue Expanders (Fig. 1)

Tissue expanders are balloons made of silicone and filler ingredients, molded into a pre-shaped prosthesis, which can be filled with saline through a valve system. The standard tissue expanders available from the manufacturing companies are usually circular, rectangular, or crescentic in shape and are usually made in commonly required volumes/capacities from 50 to 1000 mL. Rectangular expanders generate the most usable tissue, although the shape of the expander should be tailored to the reconstructive needs [3].

Many advances have been made in tissue expansion since first used by Neumann [4]. It requires the placement of a silicone balloon filled with serial injections of sterilized solution over a period of weeks to months. It is widely used in reconstructive surgery for the reconstruction of various defects and deformities [5]. Tissue expansion has been used in hair restoration surgery and especially in post-burn alopecia [6]. Similarly, pre-expanded scalp flaps (scalp reduction) have also been mentioned in the literature [7]. Tissue expansion provides hair-bearing skin following the excision of non-hair-bearing/scarred/burned skin. Although follicular unit grafting can be performed, the graft does not usually provide adequate hair density, with results depending on the condition of the recipient skin. In most cases, there is a loss of fatty layers of the scalp, or the skin-grafted areas are generally not very good recipient areas [8]. The placement, volume, and shape of tissue expanders depend on the geometry of the defect and the available hair-bearing areas. Precise preoperative planning, therefore, is of utmost importance. There is generally less tissue laxity on the scalp than on the face and neck. Furthermore, the scalp exhibits regional differences in tissue laxity,

D.M.M. El Sakka, M.D.
Department of Plastic and Reconstructive Surgery, Faculty of Medicine, Menofia University, Menouf, Menofia, Egypt
e-mail: delsakka@yahoo.com

Recent Clinical Techniques, Results, and Research in Wounds (2017)
DOI 10.1007/15695_2017_25, © Springer International Publishing AG
Published Online: 24 October 2017

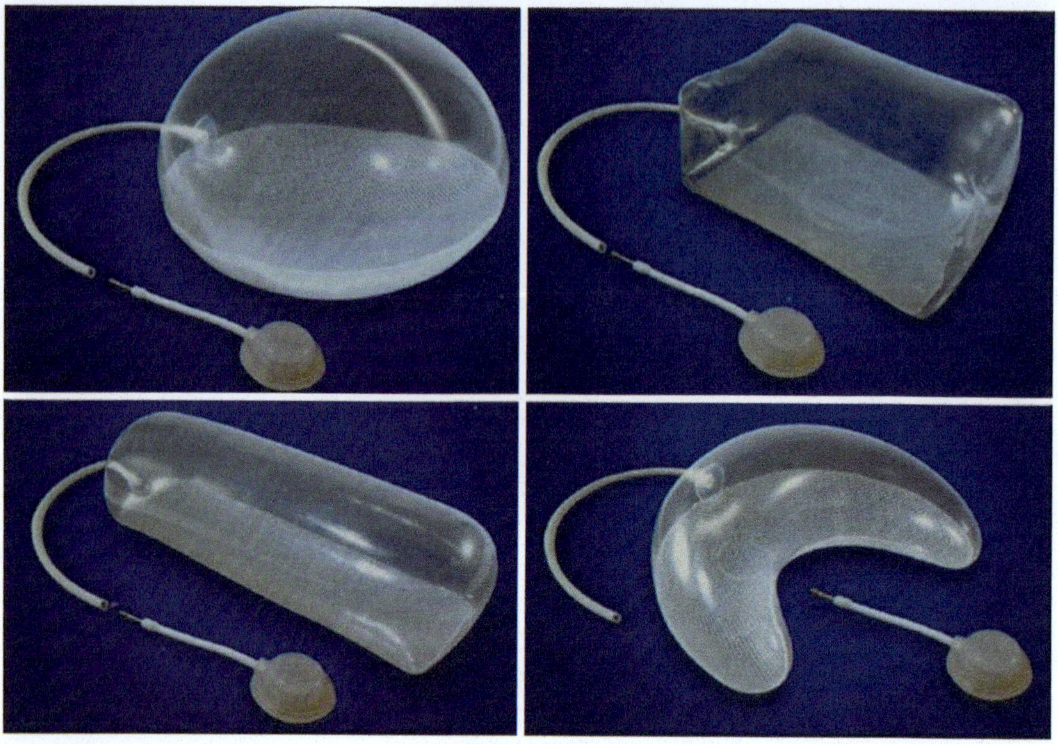

Fig. 1 Different types of tissue expanders

the tissue of the frontotemporal and occipital regions being looser or more distensible than that of the vertex [9].

3 Anatomy of the Galea

The galea aponeurotica is the strong membranous tendon of the occipitofrontalis muscle. It is attached to the tissue layer and is separated from the periosteum by the subgaleal space. Anteriorly, it is attached to the skin just above the supraorbital ridges and posteriorly to the superior nuchal ridge. Movement of the overlying skin is restricted by its attachment to this inelastic tendon sheath. This lack of local tissue distensibility may restrict reconstructive options [10].

Although scalp expansion by tissue expander without galeotomies may be achievable, this often results in significant wound margin tension and consequently, a high incidence of expander extrusion [11, 12]. Several parallel, relaxing linear incisions made in the galea via the subgaleal space enable this inelastic tendon sheath to stretch and constitute one method of increasing local tissue distensibility.

4 Patients

This study included 30 patients with post-burn alopecia, admitted to the Plastic and Reconstructive Surgery Department of the Menofia University Hospital, in the period from September 2010 to November 2014. The Ethics Committee approval was obtained prior to initiating the study, and all subjects signed an informed consent form. In all cases, the tissue expander was placed in the subgaleal plane: galeotomies were performed in 10 of these patients (Group A), and their results were compared with the other 20 patients in whom expanders were placed without galeotomies (Group B). Most of the alopecia patients were children, aged from 2 to 16 years.

5 Technique

5.1 Choice of Expander

1. Size: Base diameter of expander should be 2–2.5 times the diameter of the defect to be covered.
2. Shape: Mostly depends on location.

5.2 Anesthetic

A dilute epinephrine-containing anesthetic solution was infiltrated into the area to be expanded to promote hemostasis and facilitates surgical dissection.

5.3 Incision

Under general anesthesia, an incision was made at the junction of the hair-bearing and non-hair-bearing scalp.

5.4 Pocket

Dissection was done in the subgaleal plane in the normal, hair-bearing scalp that was to be expanded. Pocket was large enough for expander to lie flat without creases, but not so large to prevent migration or excessive movement of the expander. After creating an adequate pocket, the expander was inserted directly in 20 cases (Group B).

5.5 Galeotomies in Group A (Ten Cases)

Exclusively parallel linear incisions spaced 2 mm apart were made through the full depth of the galea, first using a #15 scalpel blade and then well-honed Metzenbaum (blunt tip) scissors with one blade above and one blade below the galea, pushing the scissors against the galea to separate and cut it without causing too much damage to vessels. Clear visualization of the under surface of the galea is essential (Fig. 2). As this was a relaxing incision, it was perpendicular to the desired direction of flap expansion. Since incision into the overlying subcutaneous tissue risks significant hemorrhage due to transection of blood vessels, this was avoided. The aim of these parallel incisions was to increase tissue distensibility.

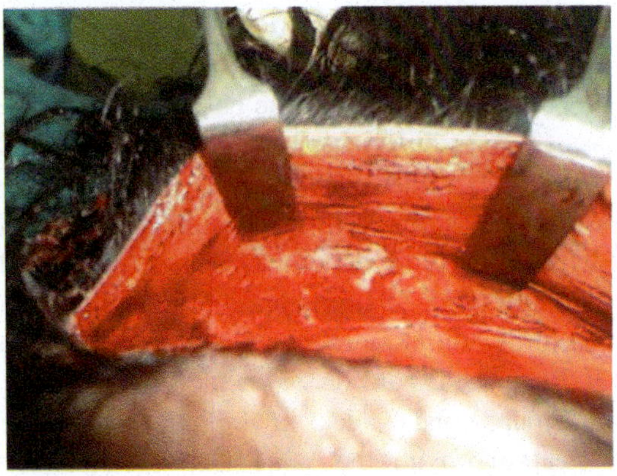

Fig. 2 Galeotomies in Group A. Under direct visualization, linear incisions were made in through the full depth of the galea using a #15 scalpel blade

Complete hemostasis using bipolar diathermy was achieved. Then the expander was placed in the pocket, and the ports were left outside to facilitate inflation. Suction drain was inserted for at least 24 h to ensure that there was no blood collection.

Incision was closed in two layers after injecting 5–10 mL of saline into the expander through the port to fill dead space and properly position expander without surface folds. First-layer closure was achieved by suturing the galea and the second layer by suturing skin to skin. A light dressing was applied to the wound for 2 days.

5.6 Follow-Up

Wound assessment and removal of the suction drain was carried out 1–2 days after surgery, and antibiotic spray and ointment were applied until suture removal. In all cases, expansion was started 14 days after surgery to allow the postoperative edema to subside and, secondly, to allow any problems with the flap to become evident. Most complications regarding wound healing would have manifested by this time.

6 Expansion Process

In both groups, on the same burned area, for the same size of defect and using the same size and shape of expander, such as a 250 mL rectangular expander, saline was injected weekly in Group A and every 10–14 days in Group B. We could inject up to 45–50 mL in one sitting with ease in Group A but no more than 20–25 mL in Group B. Required expansion was achieved in 4 weeks in Group A and 6 weeks in Group B on the same defect and with the same size of expander. Complete expansion was complete when enough soft tissue was available to cover the defect. The expander was left in situ for a further 2 weeks after the last injection to allow the expanded skin to stay stretched to that level (stress relaxation).

7 Reconstruction

Reconstruction was undertaken when expander was inflated to the desired volume; the alopecia scalp skin was then excised. The expander was removed, and the expanded skin of the scalp was advanced and rotated to resurface the defect.

8 Results

A total of 30 patients with post-burn alopecia underwent scalp expansion by subgaleal expander insertion; galeotomies were performed in 10 of these patients (Group A) but not in the other 20 patients (Group B). There were 19 females (63.33%) and 11 males (36.66%). The most common age group was 2–8 years and included 21 patients (70%). The most common site for alopecia was the parietal-temporal region with 17 cases (56.66%) followed by the frontal area in 10 patients (33.33%) and lastly the occipital area in 3 patients (10%). The rectangular expander was most frequently used in scalp reconstruction in 18 cases (60%) followed by the crescent-shaped one in 10 patients (33.3%) and lastly the round one in 2 patients (6.66%). In this preliminary study, required expansion was achieved in 4 weeks in Group A and 6 weeks in those patients in whom the expander was placed in the subgaleal plane without galeotomies (Group B), for the same burned area, same size of defect, and using the same size of expander. At each expansion session, up to 45–50 mL of saline was injected in Group A without inducing pain, compared to no more than 20–25 mL of saline in Group B, injected with difficulty and pain. Achieving desired expansion was a slow and painful process in Group B. We observed that in Group B the incidence of expander exposure, either early (from incision line) or late (from thinning and skin breakdown) (Figs. 3, 4, and 5), was very high (10 out of 20, i.e., 50% of Group B) and 33.3% of all patients. However, we did not have dehiscence or expander exposure in Group A (Figs. 6, 7, and 8). We did not observe thinning or hair loss except for the expected redistribution

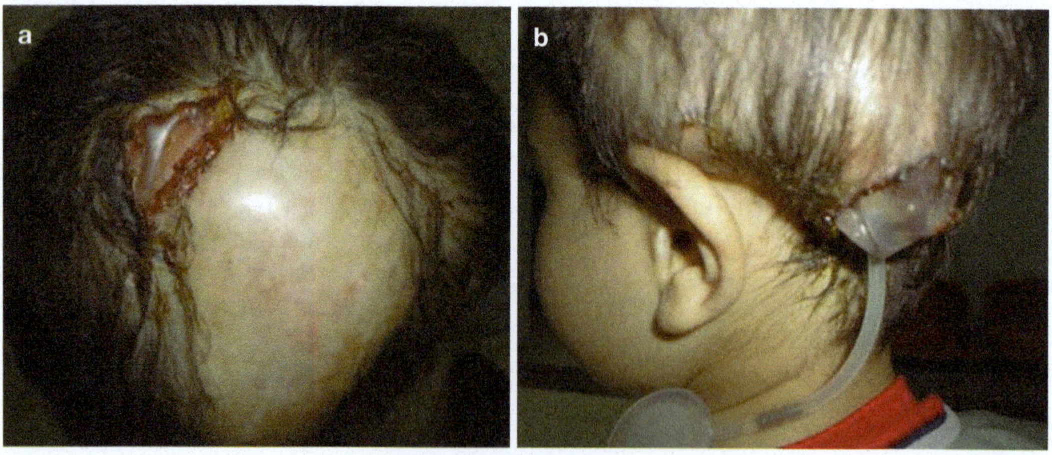

Fig. 3 (**a**, **b**) Male child aged 3 years in Group B with expander extrusion

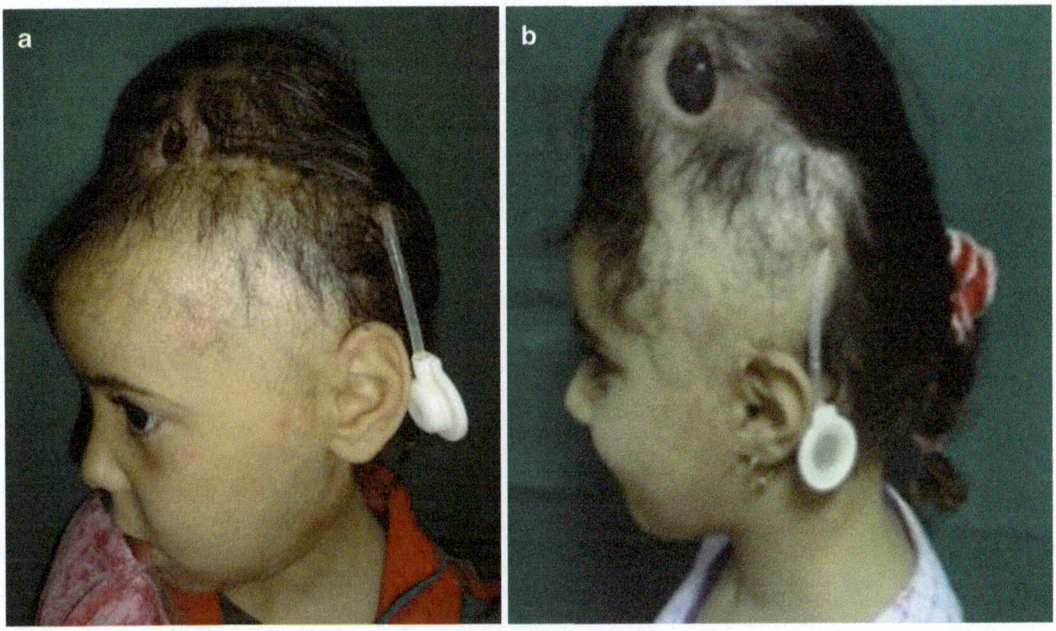

Fig. 4 (**a**, **b**) Female child aged 4 years in Group B with expander extrusion

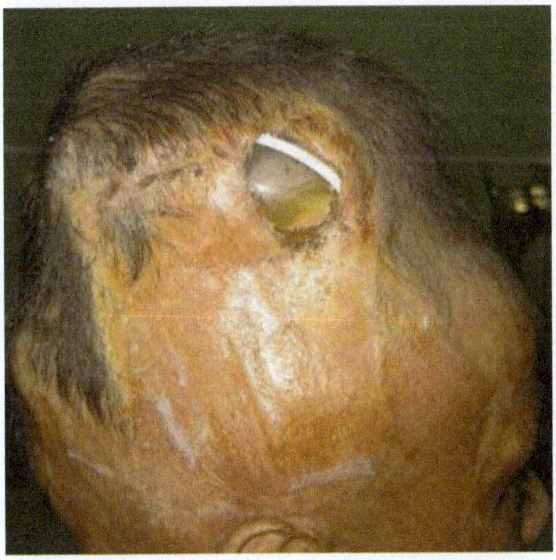

Fig. 5 Male child aged 5 years in Group B with expander extrusion

and thinning during the expansion process, which was observed in both groups (with and without galeotomies). No case of infection was noted in either group.

9 Discussion

The scalp is the second most visible part of the human anatomy after the face. Tissue expansion is widely used in plastic and reconstructive surgery. It is a valuable addition to the armamentarium of the hair restoration surgeon [13]. Tissue expansion produces a mechanical stretching resulting in localized ischemia of the expanded skin and, hence, promotes angiogenesis [14]. Expanding normal skin using tissue expanders has become the method of choice for post-burn alopecia in children, with excellent results [15].

A few case reports outline the results of follicular unit transplantation in burn scars. However, the results depend on the density of the grafted area. The density in turn depends on various factors such as scar tissue vascularity, amount of underlying fatty tissue, and smoking. Even after multiple sessions, it might not be possible to obtain reasonable hair density [16]. In these cases, tissue expansion could provide an excellent alternative. Similarly, in cases of skin grafts to the cranium, there would be virtually no underlying soft tissue so follicular unit transplantation

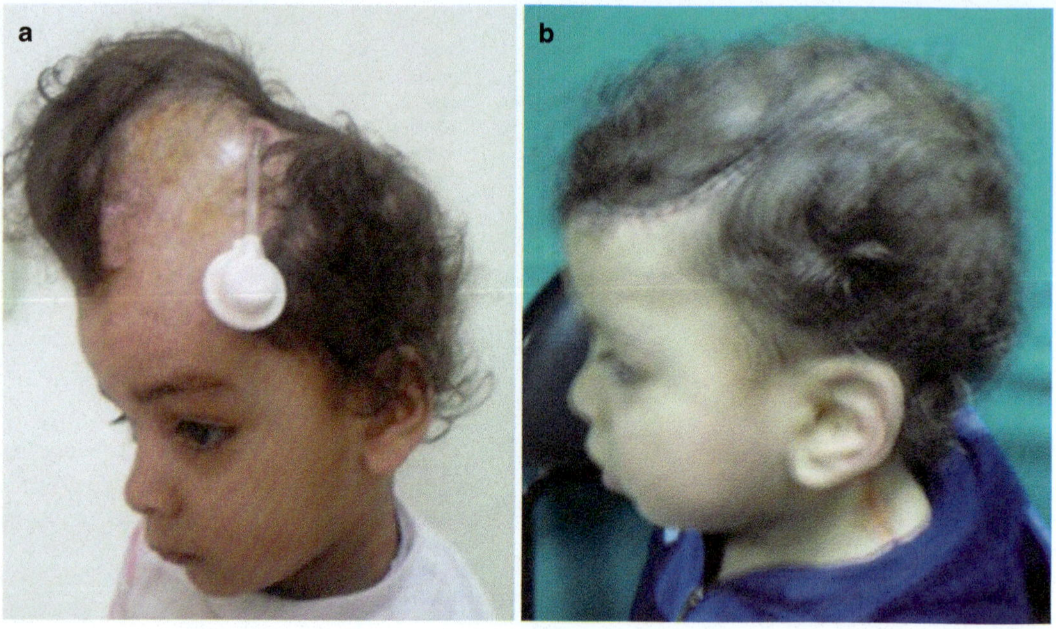

Fig. 6 Male child aged 3 years in Group A. (**a**) Complete expansion in 4 weeks without expander extrusion. (**b**) Postoperative

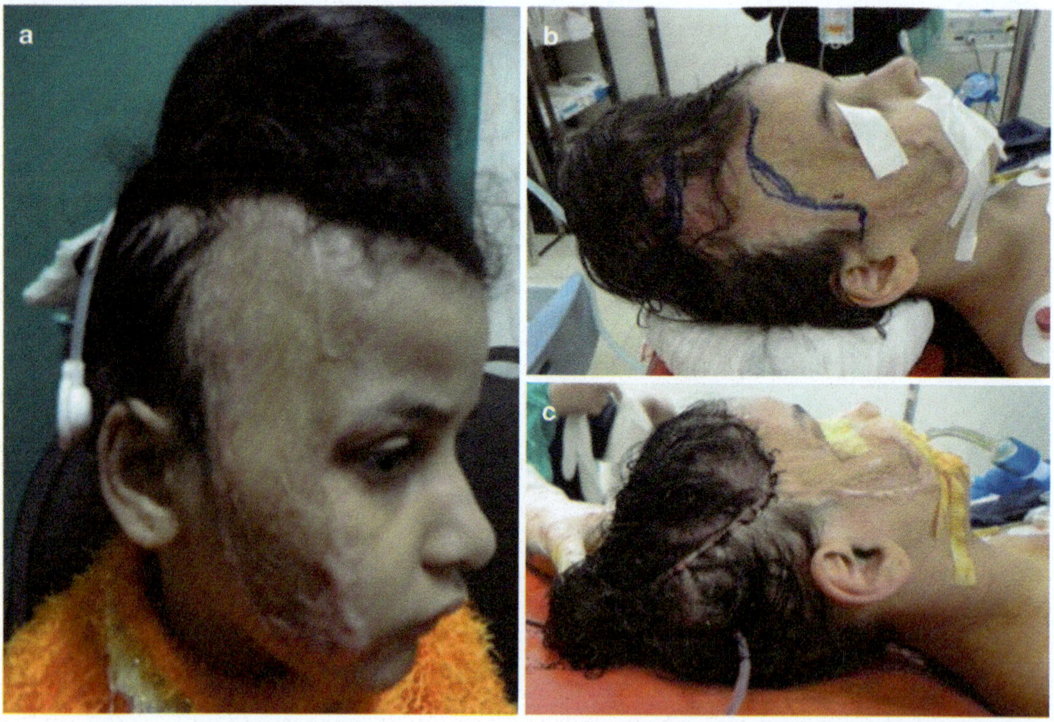

Fig. 7 Female child aged 8 years in Group A. (**a**) Complete expansion in 4 weeks without expander extrusion. (**b**) Intraoperative. (**c**) Postoperative

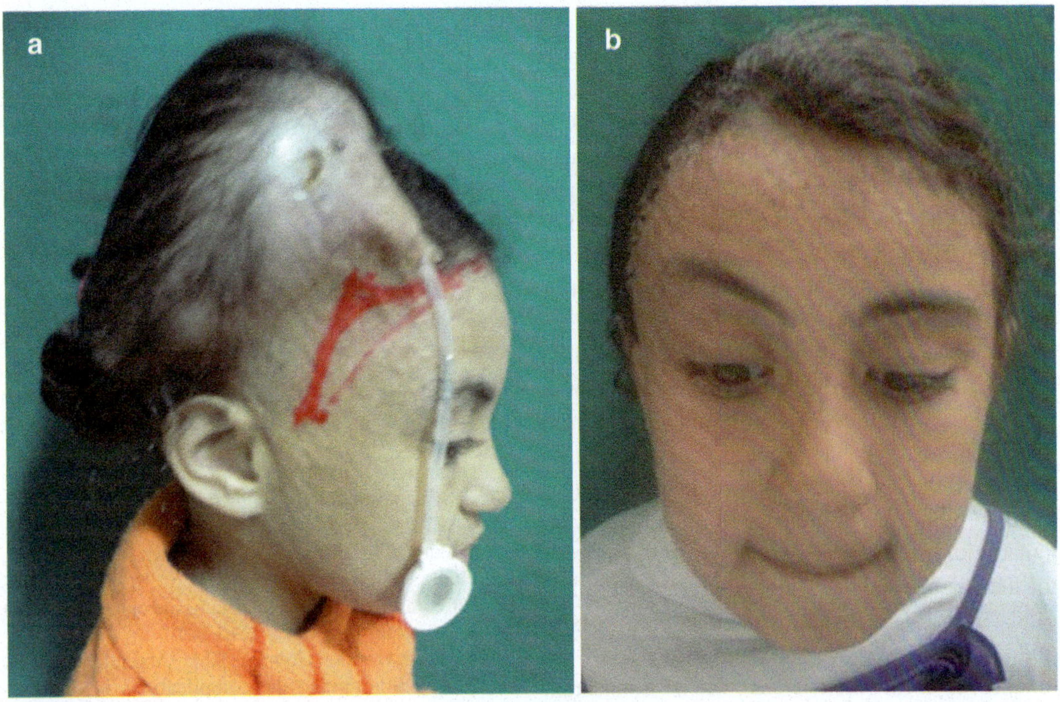

Fig. 8 Female child aged 6 years in Group A. (**a**) Complete expansion in 4 weeks without expander extrusion. (**b**) Postoperative

might not provide satisfactory results or may result in necrosis [16].

Pain/discomfort during the expansion process was the most common complication noted, especially in the later stages of expansion for Group B. No case of infection was noted in either group. In most cases, we used rectangular-, oval-, or crescent-shaped tissue expanders. A large series of 57 patients presented by Qing et al. [17] showed a complication rate of 14%. Similarly, the study by Saleh et al. [18] had a 21.5% complication rate with 8.25% infection and 5% expander extrusion. None of these complications were seen in Group A of the present study. Another study by Zellwegar et al. [19] showed a 22% complication rate, compared to a total complication rate of 0% in our Group A. Cunha et al. [20] reported a low complication rate (22.2%) in a series of over 300 expanders. Most complications involved implant exposure (51.4%) while only a few cases of perforation were reported (2.8%). This correlates with the incidence of expander exposure in our Group B (10/20 = 50%).

El Sadat et al. [21] have reported an innovation, using an endoscopic approach for tissue expander placement in the pediatric population in an attempt to reduce morbidity and complication rates. For the post-burn alopecia patients in this study, tissue expanders with galeotomies achieved better results than when the subgaleal plane was used without galeotomies. We believe that galeal tissue is important in protecting the integrity of hair follicles, preserving their circulation during the expansion procedure. As demonstrated, rapid expansion does not affect the integrity of hair follicles and does not promote pain. Supragaleal placement of the tissue expander induces excessive bleeding which may lead to more reactive tissue around the prosthesis and, when the vessels need to be cauterized, cause injury to the hair follicles, leading to local alopecia [22]. Larger and comparative studies must be done to modify the traditional procedure. The benefits of galeotomies increase if they are performed in a loose scalp region that is inherently more distensible [9].

The author believes that adding galeotomies to subgaleal tissue expander insertion may also lessen the risk of a widened, splayed scar due to the stretch-back phenomenon of scalp skin, which has been encountered in the second stage. However, wide-ranging multicenter research is needed to address this issue. The main hazard of galeotomies is the accidental transection of the abundant vasculature overlying the galea. It is important to remember that the galea is a thin layer, and in order to reduce the risk of bleeding, galeotomies should be performed under direct vision. The scalp receives its blood supply from the scalp margins, and thus, galeotomies that transect this plane, i.e. which are performed in a coronal plane, are at greater risk of causing vascular injury if the incision is too deep. As a result of the stiffness of the scalp's connective tissues, scalp arteries are unable to retract into spasm, unlike arteries at other sites, and, hence, they are unable to seal themselves when transected. Intraoperative bleeding can therefore be heavy if these vessels are severed. Similarly, postoperative hematoma is a potential hazard, so it is better to insert suction drain for at least 24 h.

Conclusions

Galeotomies are a reproducible and reliable method of increasing tissue distensibility through a reduction of the tensile properties of the scalp, without affecting the integrity of hair follicles.

References

1. DeFilippo RE, Atala A (2001) Stretch and growth: the molecular and physiologic influences of tissue expansion. Plast Reconstr Surg 109(7):2450–2461
2. Cherry GW, Austad E, Pasyk K, McClatchey K, Rohrich RJ (1983) Increased survival and vascularity of random pattern skin flaps elevated in controlled, expanded skin. Plast Reconstr Surg 72:680–687
3. Bauer BS, Vicari FA, Richard ME (1990) The role of tissue expansion in pediatric plastic surgery. Clin Plast Surg 17(1):101–113
4. Neumann C (1957) The expansion of an area of skin by progressive distension of a subcutaneous balloon. J Plast Surg 19(2):124–130
5. Manders EK (2000) Reconstruction using soft tissue expansion. In: Achauer BM, Erickson E, Guyuron B, Coleman JJ III, Russell RC, CVander Kolk CA (eds) Plastic surgery: indications, operations, and outcomes. Mosby, Philadelphia, pp 201–235
6. Epstein JS (2006) Scalp reconstruction: the role of tissue expansion. Hair Transpl Forum Intl 16:171–172
7. Leedy JE, Janis JE, Rohrich RJ (2005) Reconstruction of acquired scalp defects: an Algorithmic approach. Plast Reconstr Surg 116:54e–72e
8. Ahmad M, Mohmand MH (2013) Tissue expansion and hair restoration. J Pakistan Assoc Dermatol 23(4):423–427
9. Panje WR, Minor LB (1995) Reconstruction of the scalp. In: Baker SR, Swanson NA (eds) Local flaps in facial reconstruction. Mosby, St. Louis
10. Raposio E, Nordstrom REA (1997) Tension and flap advancement in the human scalp. Ann Plast Surg 39:20–23
11. Raposio E, Santi PL, Nordstrom REA (1998) Effects of galeotomies on scalp flaps. Ann Plast Surg 41:17–21
12. Friedman RM, Ingram AE, Rohrich RJ, Byrd HS, Hodges PL, Burns AJ, Hobar PC (1996) Risk factors for complications in pediatric tissue expansion. Plast Reconstr Surg 98:1242–1246
13. Elkafarawi HY, Goma'a RM, Aboueldahab AK (2013) Minimizing the complications in hair restoration by tissue expansion for pediatric post-cicatricial alopecia. Egypt J Plast Reconstr Surg 37(1):97–100
14. Bilkay U, Kerem H, Ozek C, Erdem O, Songur E (2004) Alopecia treatment with scalp expansion: some surgical fine points and a simple modification to improve the results. J Craniofac Surg 15:758–765
15. De Agustin JC, Morris SF, Zuker RM (1993) Tissue expansion in pediatric burn reconstruction. J Burn Care Rehabil 14:43–50
16. Marzola M (2010) Alopecia reduction. In: Unger WP, Shapiro R, Unger M, Unger R (eds) Hair transplantation, 5th edn. Informa Healthcare, London, pp 483–504
17. Qing Y, Cen Y, Liu Y (2006) Prevention and treatment of postoperative complication after skin soft tissue expansion for scar alopecia. Zhongguo Xiu Fu Chong Jian Wai Ke Za Zhi 20:1193–1195
18. Saleh Y, Hafezi F, Naghibzadeh B, Pegahmer M (2004) Scalp reconstruction using tissue expander. Egypt J Plast Reconstr Surg 28:71–75
19. Zellweger G, Kunzi W (1991) Tissue expanders in reconstruction of burn sequelae. Ann Plast Surg 26:380–388
20. Cunha MS, Nakamoto HA, Herson MR, Faes JC, Gemperli R, Ferreira MC (2002) Tissue expander complications in plastic surgery: a 10-year experience. Rev Hosp Clin Fac Med Sao Paulo 57:93–97
21. El Sadat AM (2010) Endoscopic approach for tissue expansion for different cosmetic lesions in pediatric age. Ann Pediatr Surg 6:27–33
22. Prakash V, Tendon R, Mantra RA (2006) Supragaleal placement of tissue expander for post-burn alopecia. J Plast Reconstr Aesthet Surg 59:1102–1104

Autologous Skin Cell Transplantation and Medical Needling for Repigmentation of Depigmented Burn Scars on UV-Protected and UV-Exposed Skin

Matthias Aust and Antigona Aliu

1 Introduction

In the following chapter, we are going to present medical needling as an ideal therapy for the treatment of scars and its combination with ReCell. Several clinical studies and scientific researches concerning the percutaneous collagen induction (PCI) do not only prove its efficiency on different indications but also its variety of benefits. Whereas medical needling itself does not influence the repigmentation of large hypopigmented scars, combining both methods does indeed create this effect [1], making use of autologic skin cells for especially those skin areas which have been treated by medical needling before implementing the idea of ReCell.

As the demand for less invasive but strongly effective cosmetic treatments is steadily growing, the establishment of innovative and successful methods is required from the development of plastic surgery. In the course of modern medicine, maximizing profit and providing successful results in the sense of the patient's satisfaction, PCI seems to be the ideal method compared to ablative treatments of several skin-related indications such as scars, wrinkles and skin laxity. As a new and very simple regenerative technique, it improves and rejuvenates the skin. Its success has been already detected in the treatment of different indications, particularly of severe, widespread burn scars. It neither requires expensive apparatus nor the need of complex instruments, setting a new trend in plastic and aesthetic medicine. According to that, this ideal intervention is aimed to achieve a natural regeneration of the skin and to improve its appearance as well as quality and function. It is proved that medical needling increases the quality of scars with comparatively low risk and stress for the patient with regard to important physiologic factors of the skin structure.

PCI is definitely marked by initiating the skin's own regenerative potential as its most important feature. It stimulates the synthesis of collagen and the expression of endogenous growth factors, which verify the association of PCI with scarless wound healing. Epidermal as well as dermal layers of the skin remain intact, and the improvement of the skin structure regarding its thickness and smoothness is apparent. In consideration of both, clinical and scientific data, PCI is proved to be a comparatively simple, fast and controlled method which can be safely repeated and also suited to regions where semi-ablative or ablative treatments reveal limited usage. Evaluated from the medical perspective, none of these would reach neither method nor results of PCI.

Moreover, the last-mentioned treatments covering non-invasive (e.g. silicone patches), minimal invasive (e.g. cortisone injections) or surgical options such as scar excision, tissue transfer, W- and

M. Aust (✉)
Department for Plastic and Reconstructive Surgery, Johanniter Hospital, Bonn, Germany
e-mail: aust_matthias@gmx.de

A. Aliu
Medical student, University of Düsseldorf, (Heinrich Heine Universität), Düsseldorf, Germany

Recent Clinical Techniques, Results, and Research in Wounds (2017)
DOI 10.1007/15695_2017_26, © Springer International Publishing AG
Published Online: 24 October 2017

Z-plasties or flaps, the quest has led to the application of many different topical therapies. Laser resurfacing, dermabrasion and deep chemical peels are all together defined by the same principal: they lighten the scar by destroying its structures and lead to an inflammatory response. As a result, the treated area is replaced by a thinner epidermis with flatter rete ridges and parallel-orientated scar collagen which is distinctive for pathological skin [2–4]. Furthermore, the skin is now more vulnerable to bacterial and viral infections.

Compared to that, medical needling is a minimal invasive non-ablative procedure which is capable of increasing the scar quality with regard to skin elasticity, moisture, erythema and functionality in terms of a dermal reorganization. This also includes an elevated incidence of physiological collagen and fibronectin as well as a decrease of transepidermal water loss due to an increase of macromolecules such as glycosaminoglycans [1, 5–7]. The stimulation of specific structure proteins and components of the extracellular matrix does also improve epidermal thickness. Thus, the skin is less vulnerable to extern stress-causing factors [8].

For patients with residuals of their cicatrical deformity and scars which remain a serious issue for the affected ones, medical needling suggests a controlled, simple and fast accessibility to aesthetic and functional results of their scars. This ideal treatment would overcome this shortcoming of numerous methods available for treatment of scars such as ablative methods by in fact not destroying epidermal structures and rather promoting the formation of a physiological skin collagen instead of scar collagen. Initiating the natural wound healing cascade and the expression of growth factors, this method can be associated with a scarless wound healing and regeneration of the skin.

2 How Does Medical Needling Exactly Work?

The core of medical needling is actually based on a simple idea of a repeated puncturing of the epidermis as well as the dermis in terms of inducing a physiological regeneration of the skin through activated messenger substances which are essential for the following procedure. Specific features of both skin layers are not only conserved in their functional structure but also promoted in a positive qualitative way. Both components of the skin remain intact and in their natural order, whereas the epidermis is marked by a throughout increased thickness. Concluding, this guarantees great stability and leads to a reduced vulnerability to damaging factors such as physical influences (UV radiation) [8]. Several studies confirm that also dark skin types are privileged by not facing any dyspigmentation, lack of pigmentation or even hypopigmentation, as soon as melanocytes within the basal layer are not impaired. Neither the amount of those pigment cells nor their mechanism of synthesizing melanin is affected. Moreover, the wound area is exactly limited to problematic regions which are treated in the first place. For this reason, there is a low risk for the development of viral or fungal infections enhancing a scarless and unproblematic wound healing (Figs. 1 and 2) [8].

Approximately 20 years ago, Camirand and Doucet got significant clinical improvement by treating hypertrophic scars with a tattoo gun [1]. Orentreich and Orentreich also reported about “dermal needling” as an alternative for treating scars and wrinkles. Based on this therapeutic approach, Fernandes developed the percutaneous collagen induction technique. In 1999 he entrenched this scientific discovery, by letting a roller equipped with needles produce thousands

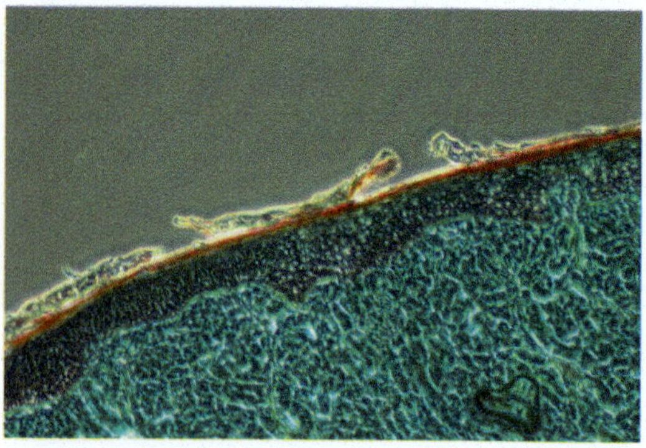

Fig. 1 Preoperative histology of a burn scar with a thin epidermis typical of scar tissue

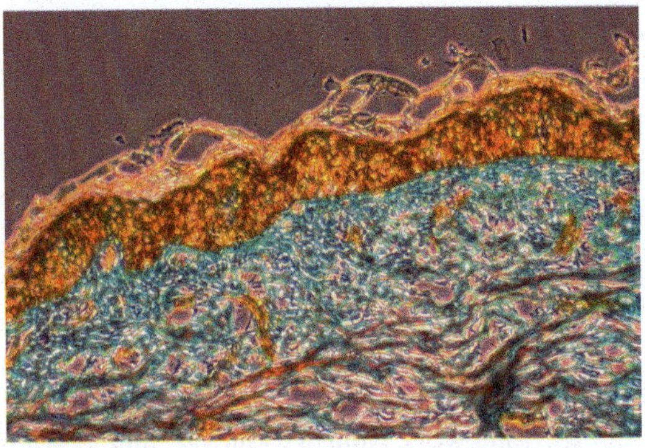

Fig. 2 One year postoperatively, the Van Gieson staining shows a normalization of the collagen-elastin matrix in the reticular dermis and an increase in collagen fibres. The orientation of the fibre bundles resembles that of healthy skin and an increase in vital epidermal skin cell layers are apparent

of neighbouring microwounds in the dermis and an intradermal bleeding [12]. Thanks to targeted research within the last 15 years, impressive scientific data is now available which underlines the efficacy and safety of medical needling.

3 Induction of the Wound Healing Cascade

3.1 Focus on Effects of Medical Needling on a Molecular Level

The intended trauma through the repetitive puncturing initiates the activation of the physiological wound healing cascade. Platelets and neutrophils secrete growth factors such as platelet-derived growth factor (PDGF), fibroblast growth factor (FGF), vascular endothelial growth factor (VEGF), tissue growth factor and transforming growth factor-α and transforming growth factor-ß (TGF-α, TGF-ß). An interactive cooperation of these factors initiates blood coagulation and the synthesis of dermal structures such as collagen, elastin and fibronectin by stimulating the migration and formation of fibroblasts and ceratinocytes.

Seen from a dermatological view especially growth and transforming factor-ß has a specific function regarding the wound healing cascade and its regulation based on a molecular level. Wound healing can be divided in three phases interacting through numerous growth factors and other essentials. The procedure of wound healing happens in an ideal time frame of 1 month distinguished in sequences of inflammation, proliferation and regeneration (Fig. 3).

Right after the injury, a natural and typical reaction of inflammation shows up in terms of activating immune cells and blood coagulation [11]. The following act of proliferation is marked by growth factors especially focused on TGF-ß due to its high importance in regulating processes. The activity of fibroblasts which are necessary for the regeneration of the extracellular matrix and the synthesis of collagen indicate a proper wound healing procedure as a result of the needling. Over the secondary phase of regeneration, an intact dermal skin barrier and a mechanically durable skin structure are evident.

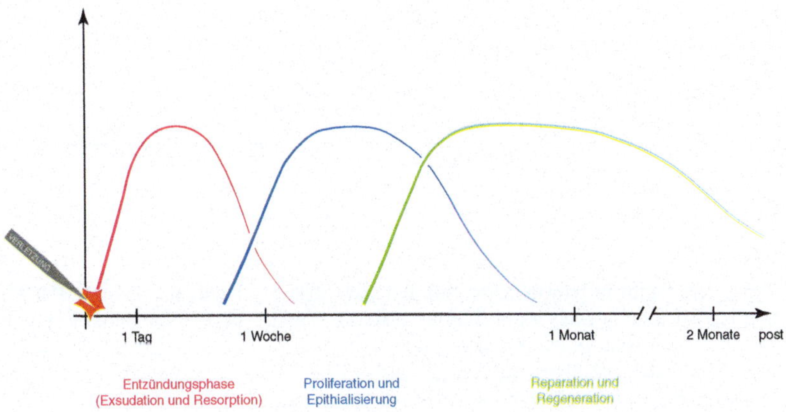

Fig. 3 Wound healing course

3.2 Scarless Wound Healing

In this context the relation of TGF and the induction of collagen type I represent a key role in repair and regeneration mechanisms. Collagen I is the physiological type of lattice-pattern collagen in healthy skin whereby collagen III with parallel-orientated fibrils is remarkable for scar collagen. Growth factors TGF-ß 1 and 2 are highly concentrated during the formation of scar collagen in cicatrice. Their level gets notably downregulated when it comes to scarless embryonal wound healing which is associated with the effectiveness of TGF-ß 3 [7, 13]. High levels of this specific growth factor do not only synthesize collagen I but also manage the conversion from collagen type III to the desired type I collagen (Fig. 4) [14].

3.3 Dermal Repairing

Furthermore, PCI modulates the gene expression of molecules, which are responsible for remodelling the extracellular matrix. This therapy approach can thus produce a quantitative and qualitative improvement in the appearance of the skin. Therefore, it stimulates the blood coagulation and the production of structure proteins including fibronectin and glycosaminoglycan molecules in correspondence of dermal remodelling. After reaching the wound region, these proteins promote the proliferation of ceratinocytes which changes physical and biological characteristics of the skin. The entire connective tissue framework appears thicker and denser. Other endogenous factors contribute towards improved skin elasticity, as the amount of elastin is significantly higher after the treatment with medical needling.

Not only for this reason, the activity of TGF-ß 3 remains constantly high regulated in the inflammation phase and also reaches high expression levels in the following phases of regeneration and proliferation [15]. In conclusion, medical needling influences the liberation of TGF as well as the production of type I collagen interacting within the procedure of dermal reorganization. The signal transduction pathway of TGF-ß 3 as one of the most important

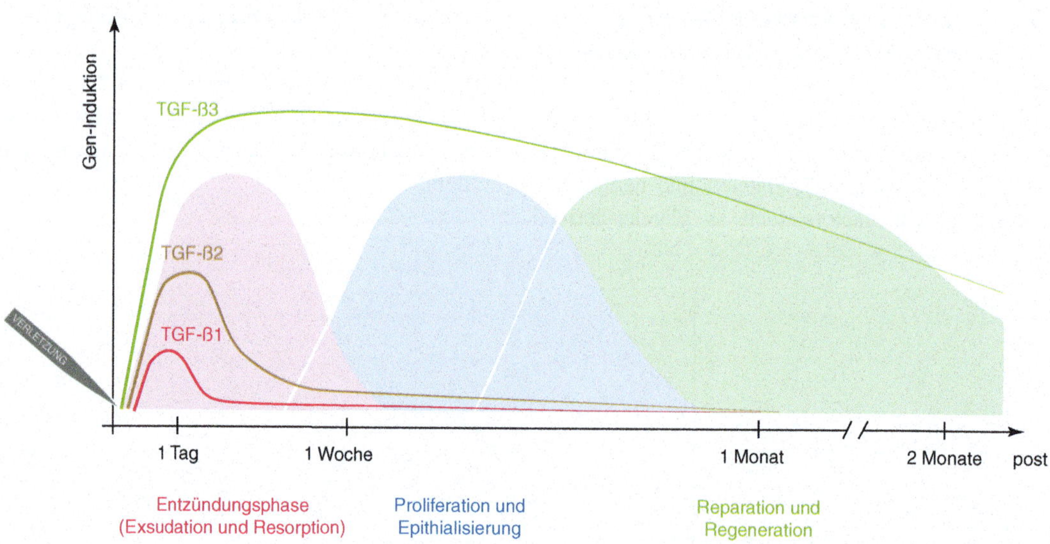

Fig. 4 Regulation of growth factor TGF-ß 3 and scarless healing. Microarray analyses of TGF-ß 1, TGF-ß 2 and TGF-ß 3 expression levels in treated and untreated animals show that the needling treatment stimulates TGF-ß 3 to a greater extent than TGF-ß 1 or TGF-ß 2. Moreover, the induction of TGF-ß 3 gene expression continues even beyond the initial wound healing phase, whereas the two other genes are downregulated during the second week post needling

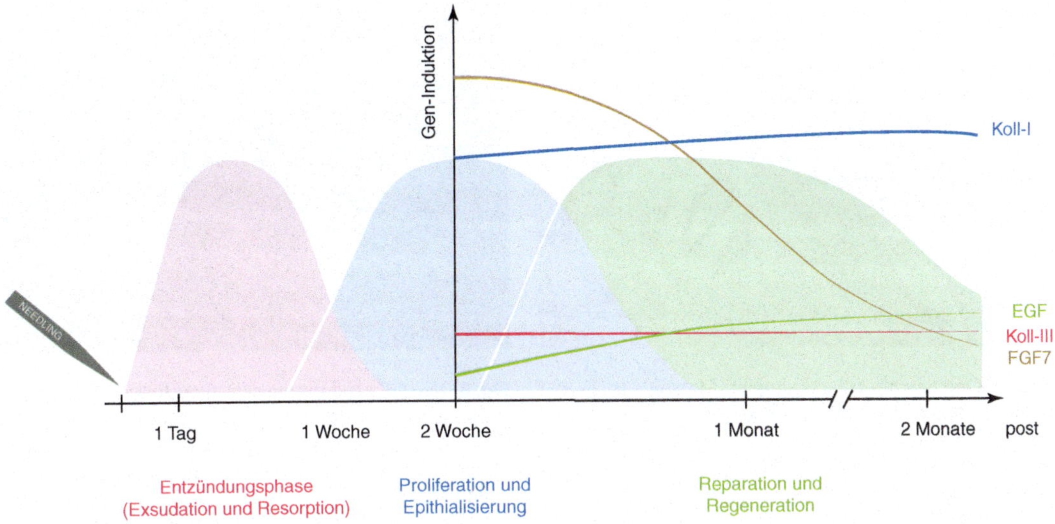

Fig. 5 Quantitative evidence: Remodelling through needling. Microarray analyses show that the expression of the genes associated with dermal remodelling has been increased in the treated animals compared to the untreated control group. Initially, collagen I is more induced than collagen III and remains elevated even after 2 months post needling

PCI-related factors allows an association with a scarless wound healing. Therefore, this method reaches results to a high extent of satisfaction (Fig. 5) [15].

3.4 Improved Perfusion

Another factor showing high appearance during the wound healing cascade after medical needling is VEGF. Its main function of creating new blood vessels is not only restricted to embryonic development but also shows activity after injury as the amount of VEGF rises significantly after treatment. A secretion of VEGF stimulates angiogenesis and vasculogenesis by forming blood vessels in the dermis in terms of normalizing and throughout supporting a better perfusion. It also helps regenerating characteristic pathological erythema of scars after burn injuries.

3.5 Increase in Dermal Thickness and Richness of Moisture

The regulation of the skin's water balance has high contingent potential of becoming a stress factor under adverse circumstances. In regard to this, medical needling proves a positive effect by preventing transepidermal water loss and maximizing the moisture of skin. Due to this fact, the higher secretion of glycosaminoglycans is integrated as an essential implication of medical needling. Instead of impairment, the skin's epidermal and dermal layers are not sustainably damaged. According to the differential diagnosis of the skin structure, the normal "lattice-work" collagen matrix is preserved, and a demonstrable increase in the vital thickness of the epidermis is apparent (Figs. 6 and 7) [13].

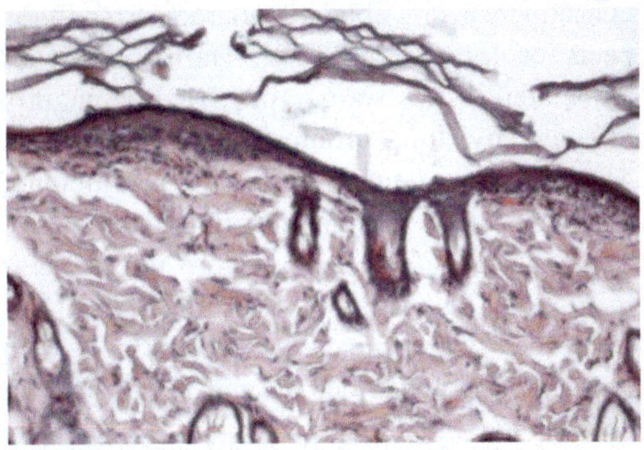

Fig. 6 Regenerative effects on the epidermis through needling

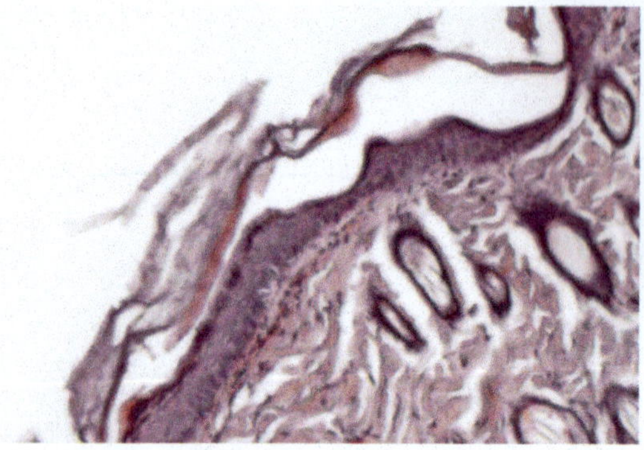

Fig. 7 One day after the treatment, Masson's trichrome staining shows no injuries in either the epidermis or dermis. The cell layers of the epidermis are completely intact, and no signs of ablation or cell damage are apparent untreated animal

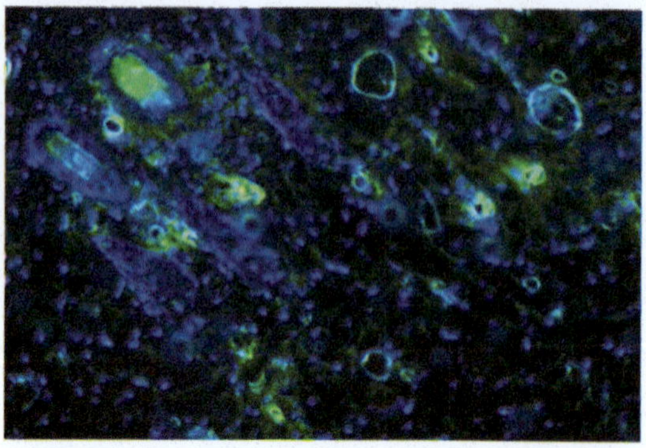

Fig. 8 Needling and dyspigmentation: Immunohistological staining, visualization of melanocytes in the epidermis. The number of melanocytic cell nuclei (blue dots) remains unchanged comparing untreated and treated conditions

3.6 No Dyspigmentation Through Needling

Post-inflammatory dyspigmentation is a usual consequence of ablative therapies such as peels or laser resurfacing. Dark skin types associated with skin type III are mainly affected by this problematic phenomenon. They already tend towards higher melanin synthesis under normal physiological conditions and therefore exhibit more intense pigmentation. Pale skin types I and II are less concerned which means that a treatment with those ablative methods is generally inadvisable in darker skin types. Medical needling does not change the amount of melanocytes but specifically modifies the expression levels of the melanocyte-stimulating hormone (MSH) and interleukin-10 (IL-10). MSH which influences the proliferation and activity of melanocytes is significantly downregulated within days after treatment. IL-10 as an anti-inflammatory cytokine is postoperatively upregulated. Medical needling does not hold the risk of dyspigmentation and support the hypothesis of a greater safety relative to ablative methods in terms of both, histological and molecular basis (Figs. 8 and 9) [13, 14].

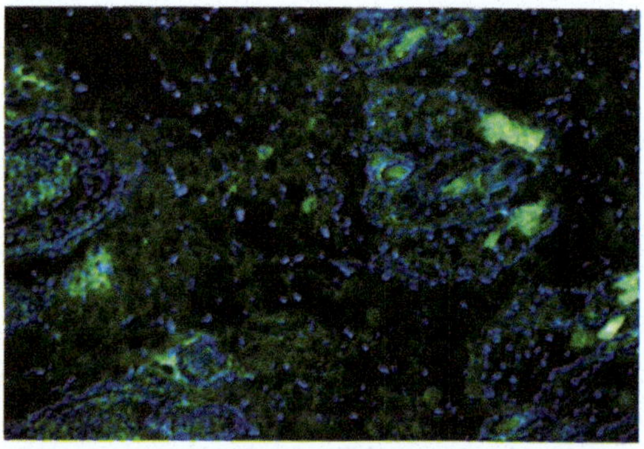

Fig. 9 A treatment-related proliferations or deficiency in the melanocyte count is not detectable in the histological section

4 Needling Techniques

4.1 Importance of Needle Length Selection

The procedure of PCI is generally based on a standardized principle towards the high variety of indications: The needling device is repeatedly rolled over the scar in three directions, longitudinally, diagonally and horizontally. The needles displace the skin cells temporarily and penetrate the dermis leading to thousands of microwounds and intradermal bleeding. Thus, repetitive puncturing evokes the posttraumatic inflammation cascade. Respecting the extent of the scar, this procedure can last 30 min or longer. Therefore, it is important to use the instrument with constant pressure and in a straight way to prevent shear forces.

Nevertheless, the needling treatment needs to be planned and prepared in advance. The procedure itself encompasses many features and has a decisive effect on the outcome. Preoperative preparation means selecting the appropriate length of needles depending on indication, pain management and expectation from the patient's site. Comparing input and outcome, maximizing the patient's profit is aimed to achieve.

In principle, needling can be classified into cosmetic, medical and surgical performances, which differ with regard to the intensity of the physiological effects and the postoperative regime they require [12]. The first-mentioned type of needling is performed as a purely cosmetic treatment with needles 0.1–0.5 mm in length. Generally, structural skin modifications based on a rather superficial level are apparent. This needle length is predominantly used to encourage the transepidermal transport and penetration of topically applied active substances. As the intradermal haemorrhage does not take place, there is no postinterventional reaction visible. Using the minimal length of needles does not require any anaesthesia and allows repeating the treatment after 1 day of recovering. The patient does not experience any downtime and gets back to his daily routine without any complications. All together, the cosmetic needling is used as a penetration enhancer for local externa (Fig. 10). Medical needling can finally be considered as a percutaneous collagen induction therapy when it comes to the usage of at least 1–2 mm needles. Needles of this length reach just beyond the basal membrane and lead to minimal petechial haemorrhages in the papillary dermis which already activate the TGF-ß signal cascade and a skin-regenerating effect. The used needle length is proportional to the provoked bleeding as it gets more intense by increasing the length of the needles. In this case, occurring intradermal lesions are so small that there is a minimal downtime without the appearance of oedema or bruises. Moreover, general anaesthetic can be replaced by effective topical anaesthetics as the process is nearly painless. However, the treated area is of a rosy complexion, and a resting time of at least 1 week is highly recommended (Figs. 11 and 12). From the perspective of clinical efficacy, surgical needling proves to be more intense and impressive in context of using 3 mm needles in length. Intensive intradermal haemorrhages due to lesions of extensive areas including dermis and the upper layer of the subcutis are usually carried out under general or regional anaesthesia and can also require a stay in hospital [15]. The painful operating act promotes reactions with more prolonged reddening, swelling and bruising. The potential of aesthetic correction as well as the correspondingly greater wound healing are on their highest level. Selecting a length of 3 mm, the patient accepts a protracted

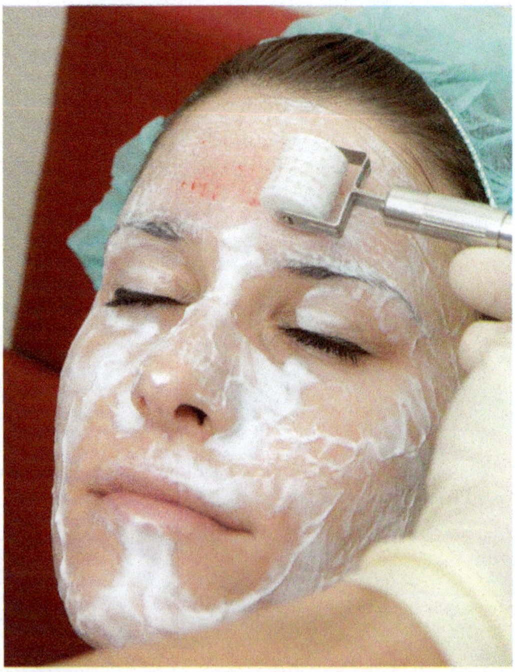

Fig. 10 Procedure of cosmetic needling with a needle length of 1 mm

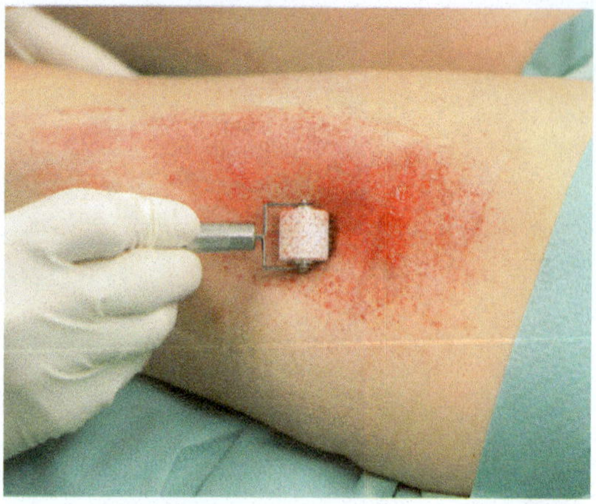

Fig. 11 Technique of surgical needling performed with a needle length of 3 mm

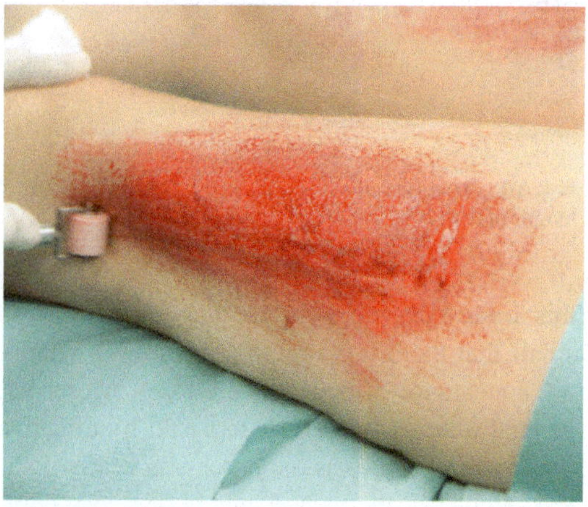

Fig. 12 Technique of surgical needling performed with a needle length of 3 mm with the aim of producing marked oedema and haematoma to induce therapeutically effective collagen production during the wound healing

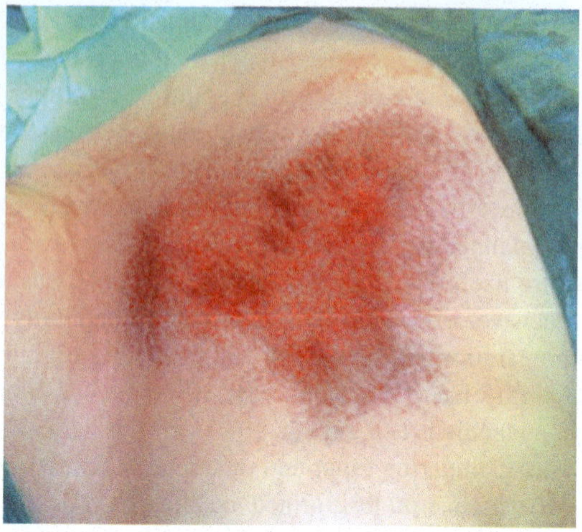

Fig. 13 A heavier bleeding caused by the 3-mm needling method

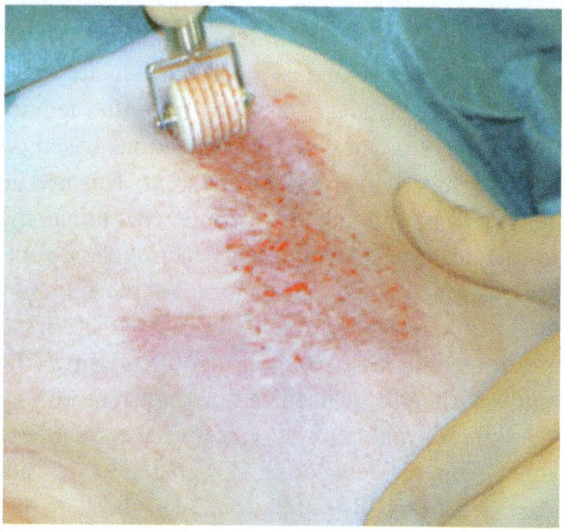

Fig. 14 Petechial haemorrhages produced by 1-mm needling

downtime and maximal results at the same time. Accordingly, longer recovery sections of weeks or months (maximal 3 months) should be taken into account (Figs. 13 and 14).

Thus, the selection of the needle length varies relative to the severity level of specific indications and finally to the patient's capacity of high effort. Moreover, important dependencies are revealed: The shorter the needles, the more often treatments need to be carried out in order to reach desired effects. The more pronounced pathology appears, the more preferred are longer needles. Summing up, the combination of the patient's expectations and the desired result decide upon the amount of therapies and the selection of the needle length considering three possible types.

5 Postinterventional Treatment Measures

5.1 Postoperative Wound Management

The urgent intention of optimizing and maximizing results implicates the right treatment of the skin in the course of pre- as well as postoperative measures. Especially the application of vitamin A and antioxidants such as vitamins E and C is of a necessary need and maximum success, respectively. Skin care measures combining the upper mentioned vitamins with a strongly recommended cleansing utilizing gentle washing lotion containing tea tree oil should be performed every 2 h as long as the needling canals are still opened. While skin irritation is persisting, direct exposure to sunlight should also be avoided [12]. A moisty wound healing in terms of applying vitamin-based creams, lotions and cleansing gels prevents a crust formation after the initial bleeding which could eventually harm results. A loss of serous fluid through the puncture holes in the immediate postinterventional period can lead to crusting which needs to be carefully averted by the removal of any surface serum. In consequence, preventing crusting can obviously eliminate the risk of bacterial superinfections. Further on, a secondary wound healing associated with cicatrization is definitely declined.

5.2 Managing Complications

As needling does not produce open wounds, the postoperative complication rate is rather low, and postinterventional monitoring is not necessary. However, local oedema can eventually develop related to the depth of the treatment and the size of the treated area. For this reason, it is suggestive to keep the patient in the clinic for a few hours after undergoing the operative act by surgical needling. Added to that, the patient may experience burning pain in the needled area following an extensive surgical needling under general anaesthesia. In the first hours postoperatively, pain should be managed with effective drugs [12].

The minimal intradermal haemorrhage right after the operating act seems to be the core reaction of medical needling, by motivating the endogenous potential for a natural and biological wound healing starting a few minutes after injury. The extent of the initial bleeding and the excretion of serous liquids can appear in a different intensity and mainly depend on the localization of the treated area as well as the needle length which has been selected on purpose. In consequence, facial skin regions show a higher bleeding propensity. These regions are more affected by swelling and bruising because skin tends to be thinner and therewith reacting more sensitive to operative interventions than skin of other regions. Eventually, PCI-related results are achieved by replacing scar typical collagen under the epidermis with normal collagen of healthy skin [2, 15, 16].

6 Indications

From a medical point of view, the method of percutaneous collagen induction shows a vast repertoire of effectiveness and success concerning different indications. First attractivity is especially characterized by the fact that medical needling is suitable for every type of skin and its accessibility to nearly every region of human body. Contemplating this dimension of PCI, limits are set far beyond anything which has been nowadays experienced with medical needling. The minimal invasive procedure combined with an appropriate skin care evokes sustainable results. Patients are able to ideally get back to routine 1 week after treatment which reduces psychological stress and other indirectly influenced parameters [18].

Realizing first results shortly after the first treatment, further improvements are increasingly visible in the course of months up to 2 years. Rejuvenation factors as a consequence of PCI achieve remarkable dimensions through a thicker, smoother and also tighter skin.

6.1 Age-Related Indications

PCI as an anti-ageing method promises a natural rejuvenation as well as regeneration of the skin structure by preserving characteristic cells of each layer and especially the basal membrane. Age-related indications such as wrinkles and lax skin are also suitable to be treated by medical needling. However, PCI does not affect the volume ratio or the muscle contraction of the mimic musculature. Intrinsic as well as chronological ageing factors reducing subcutaneous volume and muscle activity do not correlate with the effectiveness of

PCI. Whereas skin structure focused on the arrangement of collagen fibres benefit from a treatment with PCI, subdermal structures remain unaffected. Both, muscle contraction and the volume of the subcutis, fall into the spectrum of treatments with either botulinum toxin or hyaluronic acids. Subsequently, PCI ensures the maintenance of the flexibility and mobilization of facial factors as the mimic musculature remains unattached and thus intact. Further regions and surely extensive areas preferably undergo a treatment with medical needling representing a greater way to escape from more demanding and damaging surgical methods. These are usually interconnected with longer healing processes and postoperative complications which support the hypothesis that sustainable results and greater satisfaction can be reached by means of less effort as it becomes evident through medical needling. Additionally, postinterventional improvements are displayed also a few years after the treatment. It also clarifies the tight relationship between time, result and satisfaction focused on the patient's well-being.

6.2 Scars

6.2.1 Hypertrophic Scars

Outstanding results have already been described in the treatment of hypertrophic scars such as burn scars and are represented by the method of PCI. As burn scars remain a physical and psychological problem for the affected people, there was no other effective and reliable method of resolution found so far. The morphology and physiology of hypertrophic scars constitute a real challenge for other treatment approaches. A hypertrophy develops either during or after the wound healing cascade by an overproduction of the connective tissue fibres, mainly fibroblasts and ceratinocytes. The scar tissue is steadily growing in an uncontrolled and invasive way but however respects the original traumatic area which is not the case when it comes to the formation of proliferating scars such as keloids. In accordance with these circumstances, a surgical needling is unavoidable to achieve an intradermal bleeding and the collagen induction in the first place. Due to the constant proliferation of the cicatrization, the needles cannot penetrate as deeply as they should. Therefore, a horizontal needling from the outside to the inside of the scar is advisable [12]. Other methods such as skin transplantations or plasties are not as attractive as performing medical needling comparing income and outcome which results in a rather negative balance. The simple idea of needling in affecting healthy skin provided grounds for testing its effect on skin with impaired function. Several treatments have shown a positive response on medical needling. An improvement regarding the elasticity of the scarred region is evident, and the scar texture changes towards a slightly smaller and softer condition feeling more comfortable for the patients (Figs. 15 and 16) [12].

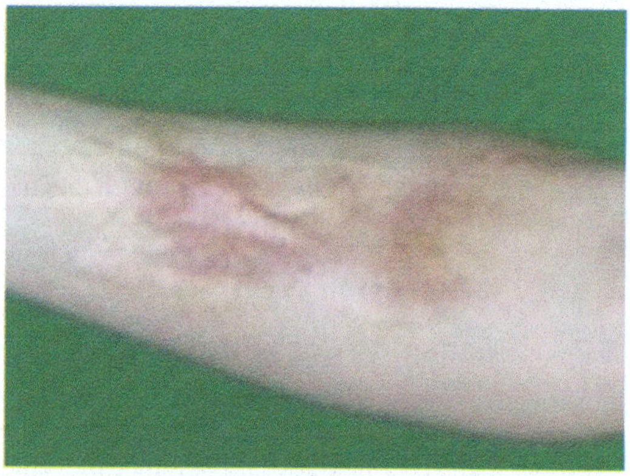

Fig. 15 Wide spread hypertrophic burn cars on the upper arm and forearm before needling

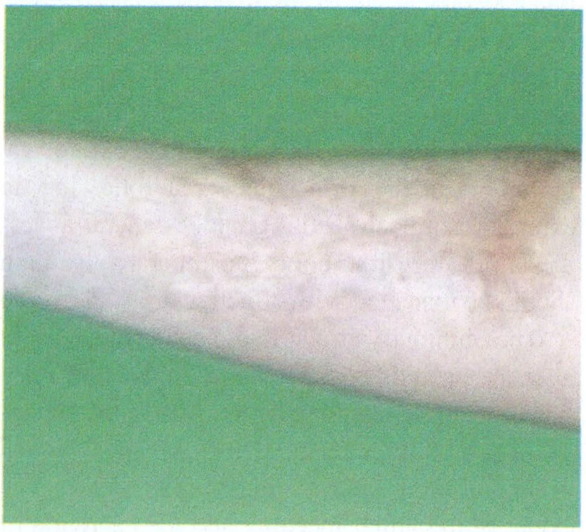

Fig. 16 Seven months postoperatively. Notable improvement of hypertrophic scars after 3-mm needling

6.2.2 Atrophic Scars

In contrast to hypertrophic scars, the appearance of atrophic scars, e.g. acne scars, may occur more often. An insufficient collagen synthesis during the wound healing cascade creates the characteristic sinking of an atrophic scar. Additionally, acne scars can be found sporadically and simultaneously in larger areas. Moreover, they are enclosed by healthy skin which makes accessibility towards the scar more difficult as long as healthy skin should remain in its physiological condition. The aim of needling therapy for those kinds of scars is to regenerate skin and build up the level of the scar through neocollagen induction in the dermal connective tissue, without damaging the healthy skin surrounding them. Ablative methods do exactly follow the reverse principle by reducing the level of the healthy skin to the level of the scar and inducing regenerative processes based on a large and uniformly flat wound surface [12]. These processes automatically implicate the danger of a renewed cicatrization as well as postoperative complications during the wound healing cascade. Physiological sequences within the ideal wound healing of certain time frame are guaranteed by medical needling and compatible with an improved appearance of the skin concerning different factors (Figs. 17 and 18).

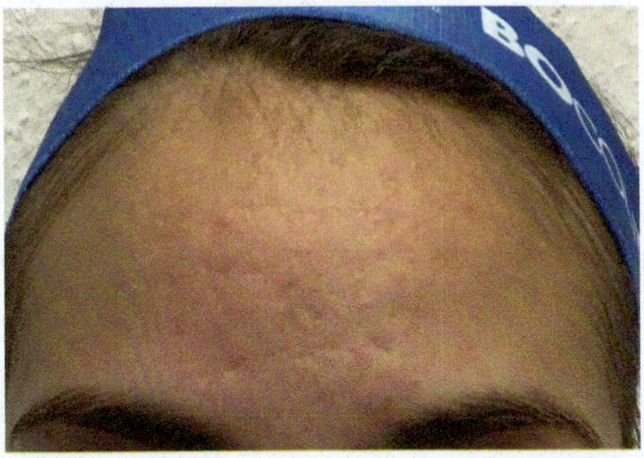

Fig. 17 Preoperative image of an acne scar on the patient's forehead

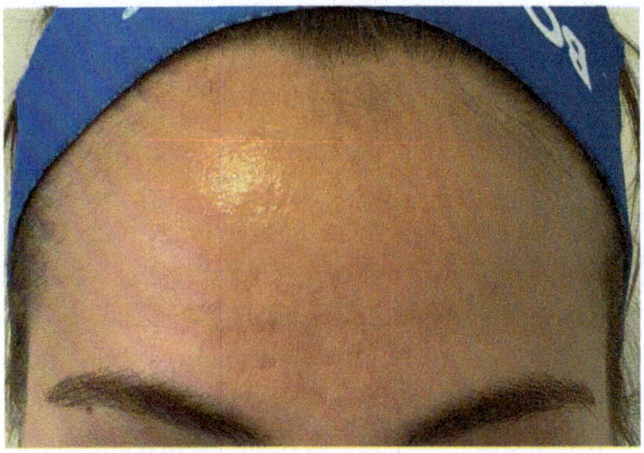

Fig. 18 The same patient 8 months postoperatively

6.2.3 The Combination of Medical Needling and Non-cultured Autologous Skin Cell Transplantation: Repigmentation of Hypopigmented Scars

As medical needling proves to be an ideal method for different types of skin damage represented by the variety of indications, special results could be achieved in the treatment of hypopigmented scars. In this case, a combination of medical needling and ReCell, meaning the repigmentation of hypopigmented skin, does exactly define an ideal and sustainable therapy from a medical perspective.

7 Need of Innovative Methods

Clinical studies as well as basic scientific research have shown that medical needling can significantly increase the quality of burn scars with comparatively low risk and stress for the patient. Making use of the skin's own regenerative potential, the needling technique influences skin elasticity, moisture, erythema and transepidermal water loss in many positive ways. Nevertheless, the repigmentation of large hypopigmented scars as they usually appear after burns does not succeed from the needling method itself. For this reason combining medical needling in order to improve the scar quality and ReCell in consideration of repigmentation, the goal for plastic and aesthetic medicine, has been set up immensely.

Following, numerous scientific studies of the past few years as well as current scientific data describe physical and biological effects in detail and entrench this combination as a promising therapy for hypopigmented scars.

As affected people do suffer from their burns and integrated disabilities, medical research and practice have become aware of handling serious physical and psychological problems such as burn scars [17–20]. Under given circumstances usual consequences integrate developmental, functional and aesthetic status which needs to be taken serious in advance of developing more efficient techniques [11, 17]. Attached patients are confronted with a different appearance and texture of their skin and many of them are supposed to deal with hypopigmentation after healing [21]. Mechanisms leading to dyspigmentation or rather reinforcing this phenomenon after treatment can be the death of melanocytes or a disruption of melanogenesis. Furthermore, ceratinocytes and fibroblasts are essential connective tissue cells which communicate and interact with melanocytes on paracrine networks with regard to influencing pigmentation and potentially leading to dyschromia [20]. Added to that, the scar tissue may provide a barrier for melanin transfer or melanocyte migration [22, 23].

The existence of numerous methods and approaches to treating hypopigmented skin such as split skin grafting [24, 25], laser treatment [26] and cultured skin cell transplantation [27] cannot be neglected, but their efficiency reasonably questioned. In recent years research has concentrated on involving a non-cultured autologous skin cell suspension (NCASCS), produced by the autologous cell-harvesting device. These are harvested intraoperatively and directly applied on the prepared wound area. This method is frequently used to repigment hypopigmented lesions of vitiligo and postburn scars by spraying the suspension of several intact skin cells onto the wound bed where they are able to penetrate deeper layers. Skin cells especially ceratinocytes are mainly located in the basal membrane where they start to proliferate and to continue growing as well as differentiating. Additional skin cells from the autologous skin cell suspension accelerate this process and support regeneration (Figs. 19 and 20).

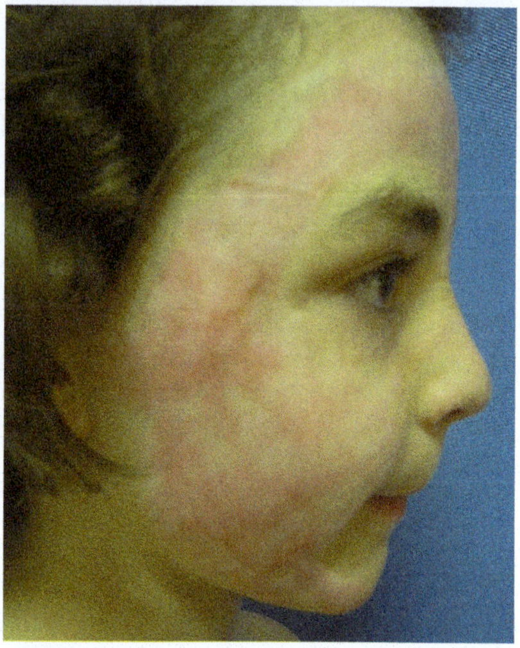

Fig. 19 Hypopigmented burn scar on the patient's face preoperatively

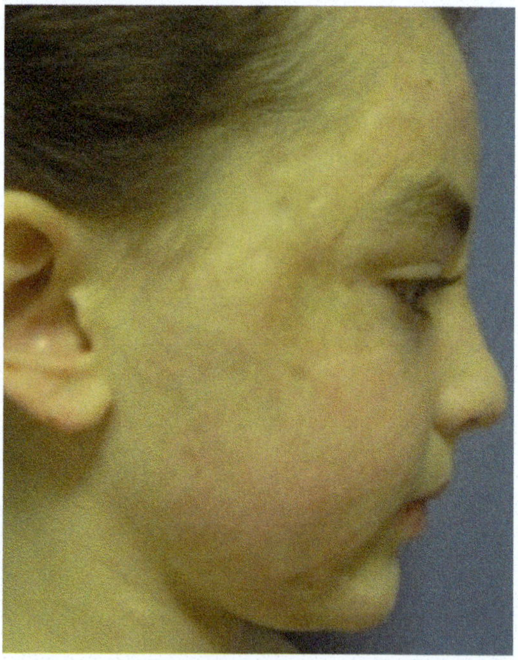

Fig. 20 After combined treatment with medical needling and NCASCS 12 months postoperatively

7.1 Medical Needling Preparing an Optimal Wound Bed for NCASCS

Optimal conditions concerning the preparation of the wound for a therapy with NCASCS are relevant for maximizing therapy results. Usually NCASCS is combined with ablative treatments such as dermabrasion or laser ablation [28–30]. The use of these interventions as already mentioned before involves many potential complications and implicates several risks of skin degradation. In this context, their purpose on reducing healthy skin to the scarred skin level does remove intact skin cells and structures such as the basement membrane which results in a thinner epidermis with flatter rete ridges [2–4, 20]. The subsequent inflammatory response, being the initial factor of the following wound healing cascade, stimulates fibroblasts to produce parallel-orientated scar collagen instead of physiological lattice-pattern collagen of healthy skin. As this is related to the expression of essential growth factors, the synthesis of type III collagen creating the characteristic scar texture is promoted. Additionally, the risk of dyspigmentation increases after these ablative treatments destroying epidermal as well as dermal structures [13, 14]. Producing larger wound areas and deeper lesions including structures of the basal membrane cause damage to melanocytes being revealed by their loss of function or eventually their destruction. For this reason, ablative treatments should be done with caution.

In order to overcome the shown deficits of ablative treatments by not harming the epidermis or eliminating important structures, medical needling has shown greatest response and offers accessibility for other skin-repairing treatments. The non-ablative and minimal invasive method of percutaneous collagen induction rather promotes the formation of physiological collagen and the expression of growth factors and decreases the risk of hypopigmentation [7, 16]. Several advantages concerning medical needling have been shown in detail before.

Fig. 21 Preoperative image of a hypopigmented scar on the patient's lower back

Fig. 22 Postoperative image of the same patient 1 year after treatment. Notable repigmentation through the combination of medical needling and NCASCS

A combination of both procedures can be performed after preparing a wound bed with medical needling as the first step. Afterwards, the autologous cell suspension is applied through a spray syringe on the wound. An interaction between already available and added skin cells through the suspension is directly linked to the induced processes. The transplantation of melanocytes shows direct interrelations to hyper- and hypopigmentation (Figs. 21 and 22).

7.2 Preparing NCASCS

First of all, a split skin sample of approximately 2 cm by 2 cm needs to be harvested from the patient. Uninvolved areas such as inner upper thigh or hairline which are also not directly exposed to the outside are suitable for this step. Then, the harvested skin sample is processed (Figs. 23 and 24) within the specific device functioning on the basis of four important components: an incubator well, a well for buffer solution, a work surface and a collection well for the final suspension [20].

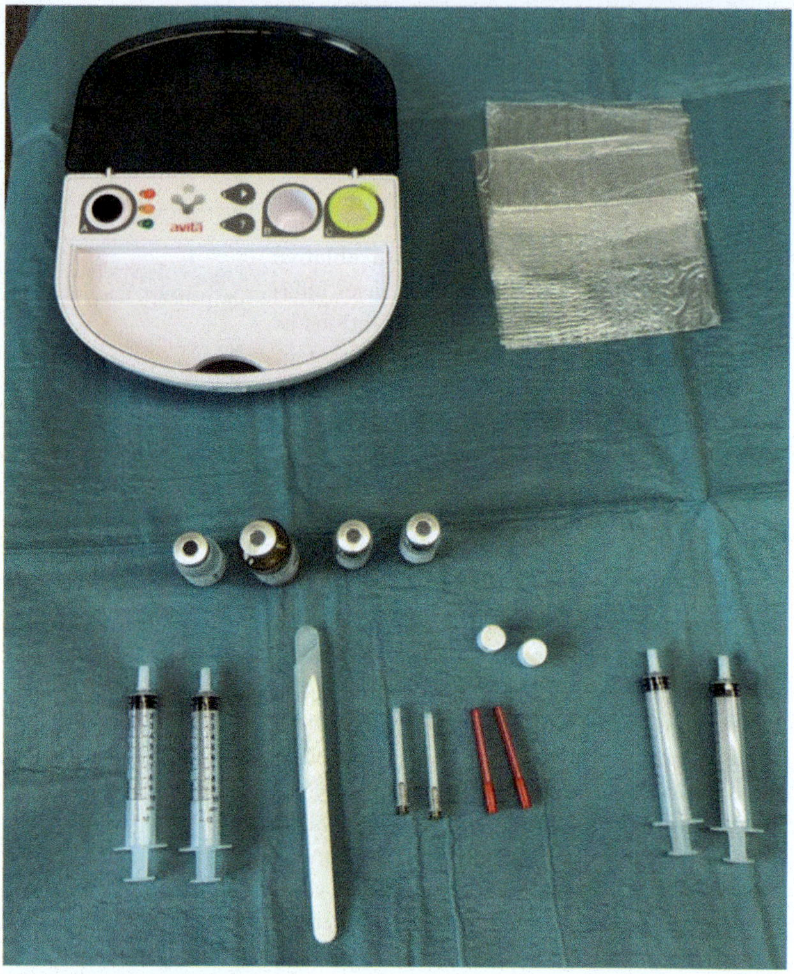

Fig. 23 Preparing NCASCS: Enzyme kit and other utensils

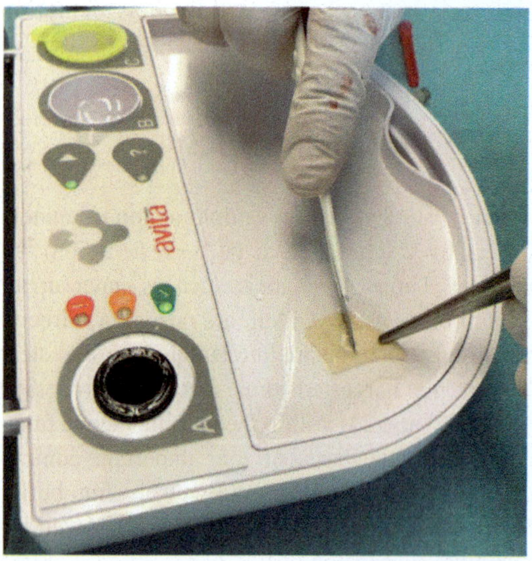

Fig. 24 Preparing NCASCS: Isolating skin cells from the harvested skin sample after processing

Enzymatic activity of the serine endopeptidase trypsin is used to isolate the skin cells from their extracellular matrix network for the next 20 min. After that, the skin sample is placed on the work surface where 4 mL of the buffer solution is added in order to inactivate the enzyme and therewith stop digestion. The skin is now in the condition for the mechanical process of disaggregation, so that the cells can be easily removed by scraping them from the prepared skin sample using a scalpel. The combined solution of both, buffer and cells, is then transferred into a collection well where a selection takes place through a sieve separating skin cells from skin appendages or other useless parts of the initial skin sample. The final solution is then collected using a syringe which is afterwards capped with a diffusor nozzle in order to not waste obtained material by accident. Before spraying the suspension onto the wound, its surface needs to be cleaned with wet compresses. After applying NCASCS, the wound is dressed with TelfaClear in order to fixate the skin cell suspension on the wound as long as the needling channels remain open. Only in this condition, transplanted skin cells are able to link through the parenchymal canals onto the basal membrane. For this reason, patients are instructed to keep the treated area immobile for at least 24 h after surgery until the needling channels do close [20].

8 Regulation of Melanogenesis Through Medical Needling and NCASCS

Medical needling seems to be a promising wound preparation for NCASCS considering several features and especially the synthesis of melanin. By producing a large number of microwounds for the percutaneous collagen induction, lesions never go deeper than 3 mm which depends on the selected needle length. Structures and cells located in deeper areas than the maximal needle length would reach are thus not directly affected. This also excludes the risk of destroying important structures. Instead of changing the amount of melanocytes, stimulating processes are observed by altered levels of the melanin-stimulating hormone (MSH) and interleukin-10 (IL-10) [7]. MSH influences the expression and activity of melanocytes which is downregulated 2 weeks postoperatively, where IL-10, an inflammatory cytokine, is upregulated postinterventionally. Based on these facts, medical needling minimizes the risk of inflammatory dyspigmentation [20].

In order to examinate the relation between the stimulation of melanogenesis and the actual quantity of melanin at the point of time after the application NCASCS, specific detection procedures combined with absorption spectroscopy have been executed. Outcomes are assessed objectively in terms of quantifying the presence of melanin. Based on the tissue's narrow wavelength light absorption, the light absorption of melanin can be measured. Knowing the defined wavelength for melanin, the amount of emitted light can be detected. After defining the quantity of emitted light, the quantity of light absorbed by the skin can be calculated. Accordingly, the result is proportional to the melanin content in the skin. These measurements of melanin are made in scar areas treated by medical needling itself and combined with NCASCS as well as in untreated and healthy skin. Remarkable results have shown up, as the melanin content in healthy and untreated skin is constant, whereas a significant increase in melanin in the skin treated by both, medical needling and NCASCS, is evident. Examinations by means of the physical behaviour of melanin prove the efficiency of combining both methods. The fact that higher levels of melanin are promoted offers the opportunity for repigmentation of hypopigmented scars.

8.1 Precautionary Measures Influencing Outcome

The highest priority after the combined treatment of medical needling and NCASCS is the temporary immobilization for at least 24 h after surgery which appeals the patient's discipline and cautiousness. As this seems quite long for a minimal invasive intervention, the idea of this instruction has splendidly to do with the desired melanocyte transfer through the puncture channels which could be compromised by an early mobilization of the treated area. Consequently, poorer outcome is expected. That is the reason why age-related concerns should not be neglected when it comes to the treatment of younger patients focusing on the lack of immobilization and thus a worsening of the surface area and death of cells over time [20, 24, 31]. The management of paediatric burn wounds and scars is therewith more challenging because of multiple factors. Ancillary physiological conditions of a young age include the immature vascularity silencing the petechial bleeding and the skin texture represented by a thinner epidermis and dermis.

Results can be harmed by different circumstances obtaining after the treatment or even before applying the cell suspension and during the procedure. The cell transfer can be negatively influenced by an invalid needling technique prior to the NCASCS application when the rolling device has not been hold in a straight line or used properly regarding pressure and direction of the rolling technique. Shear forces or the removal of the dressing means a loss or in the worst case the death of transferred cells [20]. However, the selection of the adequate needle length might also be a factor for the open probability of the puncture channels affecting the amount of cells being transferred.

Constraints within the preinterventional wound managing can also have a negative impact on the outcome as a hygienical wound preparation is neglected. In case of an insufficient cleaning, the needling channels can be blocked by serous fluid. Correlated to that, the potential for bacterial infections and a disturbed wound healing cascade is elevated.

9 Formalities and Guidelines

Both techniques of medical needling and NCASCS are approved and licenced therapies and used on a daily basis in terms of repigmentation of hypopigmentation. As all pre- and postoperative examinations are performed in vivo, ethical approval for invasive examinations has not been necessary. Several steps of the whole procedure such as anaesthesia, medical needling, harvesting a skin sample and skin cell transfer by creating NCASCS are performed in an operative theatre. As usual an informed consent form needs to be signed by the informed patient or the parents in case of patients younger than 18 years of age [20].

Conclusions

Objective as well subjective data taken from several studies on satisfaction and efficiency for both methods combined do indeed reveal a consistent picture insisting on subjective opinions and scientific researches. Overall ratings on repigmentation show a highly positive balance supported by standardized photo documentation used to confront extern observers with results. Based on this matter of fact as well as scientific and clinical data, it has been proven that the combination of medical needling and NCASCS makes the repigmentation of hypopigmented scars possible. This combination does not only demonstrate a safe performance but also a suitable implementation ensuring reliable results which reach new levels of satisfaction at the same time. Seen from this point of view and regarding the complexity of treating hypopigmented scars, an innovative and sustainable approach to the repigmentation of large hypopigmented scars is represented. Furthermore, it preserves the skin and thus provides a minimized risk of new scarring or dyspigmentation. These characteristic advantages are followed by an increased establishment of medical needling combined with NCASCS in the medical sphere of plastic and reconstructive medicine.

References

1. Açikel C, Ulkür E, Güler MM (2000) Treatment of burn scar depigmentation by carbon dioxide laser-assisted dermabrasion and thin skin grafting. Plast Reconstr Surg 105:1973–1978
2. Aust MC, Bahnte S, Fernandes D (2013) llustrated guide to percutaneous collagen induction: basics, indications, uses. Quintessence, London, pp 36–126
3. Aust MC, Fernandes D, Kolokythas P, Kaplan HM, Vogt PM (2008) Percutaneous collagen induction therapy: an alternative treatment for scars, wrinkels and skin laxity. Plast Reconstr Surg 121:1421–1429
4. Aust MC, Gohritz A, Redeker J, Knobloch K, Altintas AM, Herold C, Schwaiger N, Vogt PM (2010) Die Perkutane Kollageninduktion durch "Medical Needling". In: Plastische Chirurgie 1/2010, S. p. 39–46
5. Aust MC, Reimers K, Gohritz A et al (2010) Percutaneous collagen induction. Scarless skin rejuvenation: fact or fiction? Clin Exp Dermatol 35:437–439
6. Aust MC, Reimers K, Kaplan HM et al (2011) Percutaneous collagen induction—regeneration in place of cicatrisation? J Plast Reconstr Aesthet Surg 64:97–107
7. Aust MC, Reimers K, Repenning C et al (2008) Percutaneous collagen induction: minimally invasive skin rejuvenation without risk of hyperpigmentation—fact or fiction? Plast Reconstr Surg 122:1553–1563
8. Bandyopadhyay B, Fan J, Guan S et al (2006) A "traffic control" role forTGFbeta3: orchestrating dermal and epidermal cell motility during wound healing. J Cell Biol 172:1093–1105
9. Bernstein LJ, Kauvar AN, Grossman MC, Geronemus RG (1997) The short and long-term side effects of carbon dioxide laser resurfacing. Dermatol Surg 23:519–525

10. Berman B, Viera MH, Amini S, Huo R, Jones IS (2008) Prevention and management of hypertrophic scars and keloids after burns in children. J Craniofac Surg 19:989–1006
11. Busch KH, Bender R, Walezko N, Aziz H, Altintas MA, Aust MC (2016) Combination of medical needling and non-cultures autologous skin cell transplatation (renovacell) for repigmentation of hypopigmented burn scars in children and young people. Ann Burns Fire Disasters 29(2):116–122
12. Busch KH, Bender R, Walezko N, Altintas MA, Pech T, Rohn T, Aust MC (2015) Repigmentierung von hypopigmentierten Verbrennungsnarben durch die Kombination von Medical Needling und ReCell. In: derm 2/2015 S. p. 67–72
13. Cho S, Zheng Z, Park Y, Roh MR (2011) The 308-nm excimer laser: a promisingdevice for the treatment of childhood vitiligo. Photodermatol Photoimmunol Photomed 27:24–29
14. Davoodi P, Fernandez JM, O SJ (2008) Postburn sequelae in the pediatric patient: clinical presentations and treatment options. J Craniofac Surg 19:1047–1052
15. Fernandes D (2002) Percutaneous collagen induction: an alternative to laser resurfacing. Aesthet Surg 22:314–317
16. Ferguson MW, O'Kane S (2004) Scar-free healing: from embryonic mechanisms to adult therapeutic intervention. Philos Trans R Soc Lond B Biol Sci 359:839–850
17. Hultman CS, Friedstat JS, Edkins RE, Cairns BA, Meyer AA (2014) Laser resurfacing and remodeling of hypertrophic burn scars: the results of a large, prospective, before-after cohort study, with long-term follow-up. Ann Surg 260:519–529. discussion 529–32
18. Hultman CS, Edkins RE, Wu C, Calvert CT, Cairns BA (2013) Prospective, before-after cohort study to assess the efficacy of laser therapy on hypertrophic burn scars. Ann Plast Surg 70:521–526
19. Kahn AM, Cohen MJ (1996) Treatment for depigmentation following burn injuries. Burns 22:552–554
20. Laws RA, Finley EM, McCollough ML, Grabski WJ (1998) Alabaster skin after carbon dioxide laser resurfacing with histologic correlation. Dermatol Surg 24:633–636
21. McGwin G, Cross JM, Ford JW, Rue LW (2003) Long-term trends in mortality according to age among adult burn patients. J Burn Care Rehabil 24:21–25
22. Onur Erol O, Atabay K (1990) The treatment of burn scar hypopigmentation and surface irregularity by dermabrasion and thin skin grafting. Plast Reconstr Surg 85:754–758
23. Peck MD (2011) Epidemiology of burns throughout the world. Part I: Distributionand risk factors. Burns 37:1087–1100
24. Rashaan ZM, Krijnen P, Klamer RRM et al (2014) Nonsilver treatment vs. silver sulfadiazine in treatment of partial-thickness burn wounds in children: a systematic review and meta-analysis. Wound Repair Regen 22:473–482
25. Rawlins JM, Lam WL, Karoo RO, Naylor IL, Sharpe DT (2006) Quantifying collagen type in mature burn scars: a novel approach using histology and digital image analysis. J Burn Care Res 27:60–65
26. Ross EV, Naseef GS, McKinlay JR et al (2000) Comparison of carbon dioxide laser, erbium: YAG laser, dermabrasion, and dermatome: a study of thermal damage, wound contraction, and wound healing in a live pig model: implications for skin resurfacing. J Am Acad Dermatol 42:92–105
27. Roy D (2005) Ablative facial resurfacing. Dermatol Clin 23:549–559. viii
28. Spies M, Herndon DN, Rosenblatt JI, Sanford AP, Wolf SE (2003) Prediction of mortality from catastrophic burns in children. Lancet 361:989–994
29. Thomas JR, Somenek M (2012) Scar revision review. Arch Facial Plast Surg 14:162–174
30. Waibel J, Beer K (2008) Fractional laser resurfacing for thermal burns. J Drugs Dermatol 7:59–61
31. Zhang D, Hong W, Fu L, Wei X, Xu A (2014) A randomized controlled study of the effects of different modalities of narrow-band ultraviolet B therapy on the outcome of cultured autologous melanocytes transplantation in treating vitiligo. Dermatol Surg 40:420–426

A Novel Chitosan-Based Gel for Burn Wounds

Soheila S. Kordestani

1 Introduction

1.1 What Is Burn Wound?

Burns are one of the most common injuries in both children and adults [1, 2]. Although the mortality rate from burns has declined in the past decade; however, it is still high in some countries. When more than 70% of the body surface is affected by burn wounds, it may be fatal [3]. The classification of burns is according to the depth of the injury. Epidermis and partial dermis damage is classified as first-degree burns [4]. When the dermis is damaged in large scale, it is considered as second-degree burns. This type of burn causes the skin to blister and becomes extremely red and sore. When the entire skin and hypodermis are damaged, it is classified as third-degree burns. In fourth-degree burns, the skin, hypodermis, and even bones are largely damaged.

1.2 Importance of Healing Burn Wound

1.2.1 Inflammation

Inflammation is vital to initiate the process of burn wound healing, and inflammatory mediators such as cytokines, kinins, lipids, etc. provide immune signals to recruit leukocytes and macrophages that initiate the proliferative phase [3]. Meanwhile aberrant inflammatory pathways have been linked to hypertrophic scarring, and anti-inflammatory treatments could potentially aggravate symptoms and delay wound healing [4]. In the proliferative phase wound, reepithelialization is activated via keratinocyte and fibroblast [4]. Significant edema that is initiated by several factors including vasodilation, extravascular osmotic activity, and increased microvascular permeability often accompanies inflammation [5].

Treatment of inflammation in large burns is difficult. Early excision and grafting have become the gold standard for treatment of full and deep partial-thickness burns [5], in part because early excision helps reduce the risk of infection and scarring [5].

1.2.2 Infection

The skin functions as a barrier to the external environment to maintain fluid homeostasis and body temperature while providing sensory information along with metabolic and immunological support. Damage to this barrier following a burn disrupts the innate immune system and increases susceptibility to bacterial infection [4]. Burn wound infection was defined in a rat model with *Pseudomonas aeruginosa* [4, 5], in which the following progression was observed: burn wound colonization, invasion into subjacent tissue

S.S. Kordestani, Ph.D.
Department of Biomedical Engineering, Amirkabir University of Technology, Tehran, Iran

ChitoTech Inc Company, Tehran, Iran
e-mail: ss.kordestani@chitotech.com

Recent Clinical Techniques, Results, and Research in Wounds (2017)
DOI 10.1007/15695_2017_27, © Springer International Publishing AG
Published Online: 31 October 2017

within 5 days, destruction of granulation tissue, visceral hematogenous lesions, and leukopenia, hypothermia, and death.

Burn patients are at high risk for infection [6], especially drug-resistant infection [5], which often results in significantly longer hospital stays, delayed wound healing, higher costs, and higher mortality [5, 6]. Infection can lead to the development of a pronounced immune response, accompanied by sepsis or septic shock, which results in hypotension and impaired perfusion of end organs, including the skin—all processes that delay wound healing. Furthermore, the leading causes of death following a severe burn are sepsis and multiorgan failure [4–6], so prevention and management of infection are a primary concern in the treatment of burn patients.

Application of chitosan-based gel (ChitoHeal® gel) is for burn wound healing. Chitosan is a polysaccharide comprising copolymers of glucosamine and *N*-acetylglucosamine. It is derived by partial deacetylation of chitin from crustacean shells [7, 8]. Chitosan gel also acts as an ideal wound dressing. It is biocompatible, biodegradable, hemostatic, and antibacterial, and more importantly it accelerates wound healing [9]. A previous study showed that chitosan-treated wounds were epithelized when compared with wounds of the control group after the treatment [10].

Animal models have been used to investigate burn wound pathology, local therapy [11], the influence of systemic drug application on the burn wound, and the effect of burn trauma on the entire organism [12]. Guinea pigs [13–15], Sprague-Dawley rats [16–21], Wistar rats [22], Long-Evans rats [23], and gold hamsters [24] have been used in burn research. A further commonly used animal in burn experiments is the pig [25–27]. The hairless porcine skin is very similar to human skin. However, pigs pose practical problems as research subjects. They need more housing space and are more expensive to maintain than smaller animals.

Rabbits were chosen in the following study mainly for two reasons. Firstly, New Zealand white rabbits have been shown appropriate for burn studies [28–30]. Secondly, rabbits are large enough to obtain adequate blood samples for several days without impairing their general condition. Furthermore they are easy in terms of handling and housing and cost less than laboratory pigs. The structural configuration of the skin layers in rabbits is similar to human skin [31]. In humans and other mammals, there are regional differences in the thickness of skin layers as well as in the distribution of hair follicles and sweat and sebaceous glands. The skin of rabbits is more elastic than human skin. However, this difference does not interfere with the usefulness of this model to study the phenomenon of burn depth.

The present studies describe the efficacy of chitosan-based ChitoHeal® gel on accelerating the rate of burn wound healing in animal model.

2 Technique

Experimental design and treatment of animals were approved by the Animal Care Committee of Islamic Azad University, Science and Research Branch. The animals were kept under veterinary supervision and given adequate food.

2.1 Animals

Following the guidelines and recommendations of the Animal Research Board of the American University of Beirut, eight New Zealand rabbits with a weight range of 1.8–2.0 kg were used in this study, designed to continue for 30 days after the experimental burns were inflicted.

The animals' backs were shaved with a standard electric shaver 3 days before the experimental burn. Just before inflicting the burn, the area was depilated with a commercial depilatory cream to obtain smooth and hairless skin. The animals were kept under standard laboratory conditions with veterinary supervision and no restrictions on water and food.

2.2 Anesthesia

The animals were anesthetized by intramuscular injection of 3 mg/kg ketamine and 5 mg/kg xylazine 2% (Chanazine). Booster injections of up to half of the initial dose were administered as needed, in order to ensure that the rabbits were pain-free during the procedure and subsequent application of the dressing.

2.3 Burn Injury

A round aluminum stamp, described by Knabl et al. [32], measuring 4 cm in diameter and 81 g in weight was heated to 80 °C. It was then applied for 14 s with no extra pressure on the skin to produce a superficial, partial-thickness burn (SPT). In each animal, one SPT burn was produced on the vertebral and paravertebral area 10 cm from the tail and 14 cm from the last cervical vertebrae (Fig. 1).

2.4 Treatment

The animals were divided into two groups. Group 1 was the control group, in which the burn wounds were covered by sterile gauze dressing. Group 2 received a daily application of a chitosan-based gel covered with sterile gauze dressing. The chitosan-based gel was applied with a thickness of about 1 mm. Both treatment and control group wounds were then covered by a wraparound bandage.

2.5 Change of Dressing

The dressings were changed daily, after sedating the rabbits with an intramuscular injection of 0.4 mL/kg of 2% xylazine, for the 30-day treatment period. Before the application of a new dressing, the wounds were cleansed with saline solution for both groups.

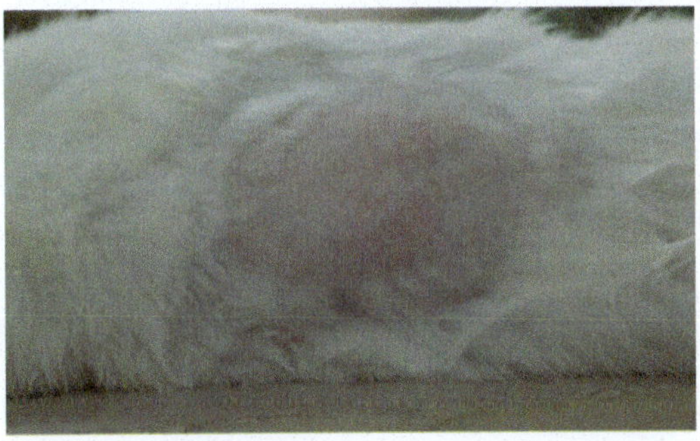

Fig. 1 Burn infliction area

2.6 Burn Tissue Assessment

Punch biopsies were taken from the center of the burn areas along with small bits of normal skin from around the wounds on days 10, 20, and 30 from both groups. The biopsied tissues were cut into two halves: one was fixed in 10% formalin for routine microscopy staining and the other half was fixed in 2.5% glutaraldehyde for analysis by scanning electron microscope (SEM) and transmission electron microscopy (TEM), respectively.

The specimens for light microscopy were processed according to standard methods and stained with hematoxylin and eosin. The harvested specimens were fixed in 10% formalin for 24 h. After conventional ethanol gradient dehydration, the tissues were embedded in paraffin and sectioned at 5 mm for hematoxylin and eosin staining.

2.7 Other Assessments

Morphological, histological, and molecular parameters were used to evaluate the efficacy of chitosan-based gel on SPT burns in the treatment group, compared with a gauze dressing used in the control group.

Immediately after the burn was inflicted on the rabbits, the burned tissue was biopsied. The biopsied tissue was fixed in 10% formalin. After light microscopy assessment, the pathologist confirmed an SPT burn. Based on the TEM protocol, the cell nucleus was stained with uranyl acetate, and the cell cytoplasm was stained with lead citrate.

Body mass index (BMI) was calculated using the Lee formula:

$$\text{BMI} = \text{BW}1/3(\text{g})/\text{nasoanal length}(\text{cm})$$

2.8 Results

Morphological, histological, and molecular parameters were used to evaluate the efficacy of ChitoHeal® gel on superficial partial-thickness burns in treatment group compared to a gauze dressing used in the control group.

2.8.1 Macroscopic Assessments

Lee index (body mass index)

Body mass index was calculated using the Lee formula (1):

$$\text{BMI} = \text{BW}1/3(\text{g})/\text{nasoanal length}(\text{cm}) \quad (1)$$

On day 10, the Lee index noticeably declined in both groups. The decline in this index, resulting from trauma-based weight loss, was expected. In time, the Lee index improved in all groups, due to the progression of wound healing and reduction of stress (Figs. 2 and 3).

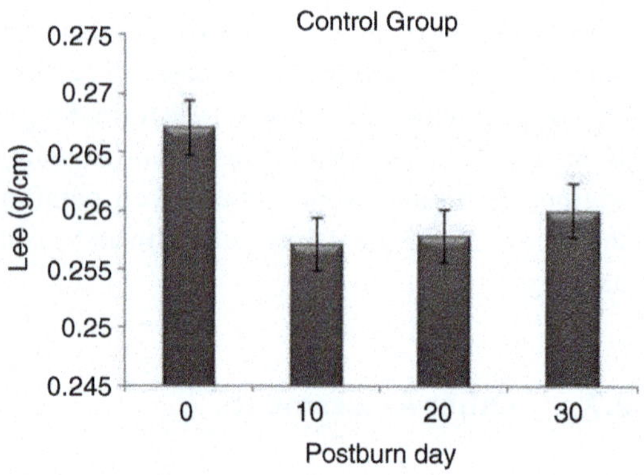

Fig. 2 Lee index for control group

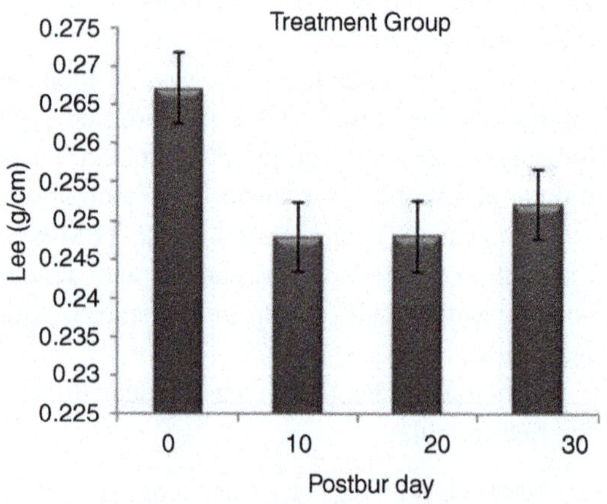

Fig. 3 Lee index for treatment group

2.8.2 Wound Edge Migration Rate Assessment

The area and periphery of the wounds were calculated using digital photographs and the Auto CAD program. Wound edge migration rate was calculated using Gilman's modified Eq. (2):

$$\text{WEMR}(\text{mm}/\text{day}) = \{(Ab - Aa)/([Pa + Pb]/2)\}/(b - a) \quad (2)$$

In this equation, A represents area, P represents periphery, and a and b represent the start and end days of observations.

The area and periphery of wounds treated with ChitoHeal® gel were smaller than the wound area and periphery in the control group (Figs. 4 and 5).

Wound edge migration in the treatment group was noticeably higher than that in the control group as shown in Fig. 6. In the proliferation phase in wound, which occurs after synthesis and deposition of intra cellular matrix, the division, differentiation, and migration of epithelial cells begin. As ChitoHeal® gel accelerated wound closure, it seems it has induced all stages

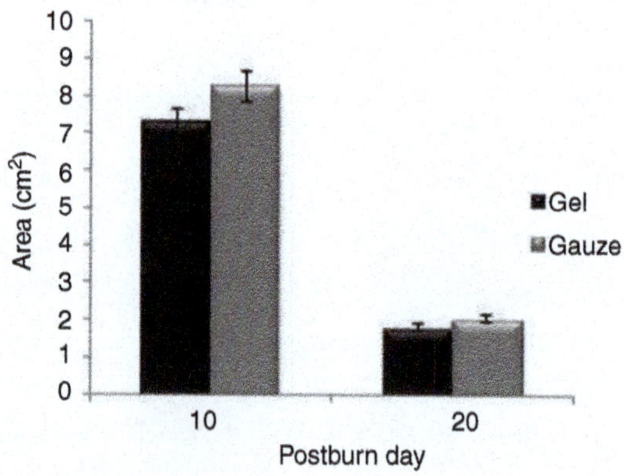

Fig. 4 Wound area—post-burn day

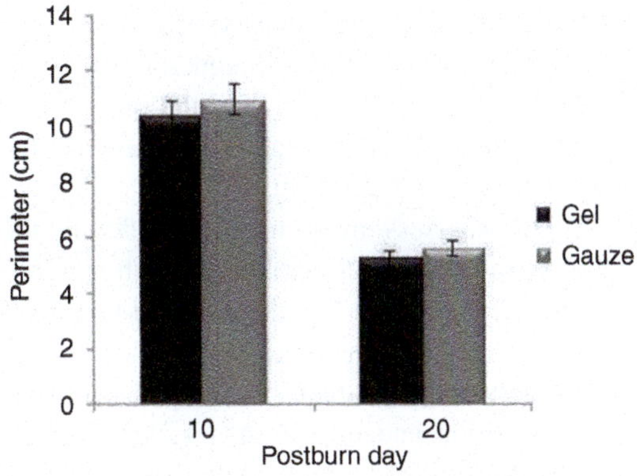

Fig. 5 Wound periphery—post-burn day

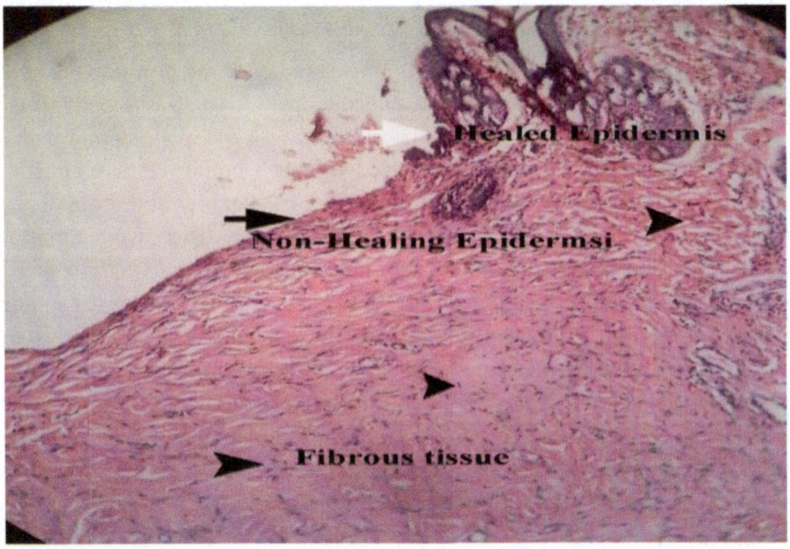

Fig. 6 Treated specimen, day 10

of the proliferation phase, especially cell migration, due to the moist environment which it provides, allowing the cells to move more easily and farther.

2.8.3 Clinical Assessment

On days 2 and 5, the scabs on the wounds in the treatment group were thicker than those in the control group. The necrotic tissue, however, was completely adhered to the wound, and its underside was soft and flexible. This indicated the rapid healing process, since the faster the damaged tissue degrades, the more quickly the wound bed clears, and healing enters the next phase. The softness of the scab in the treatment group in comparison with that of the control group may well be associated with the application of the chitosan-based gel dressing.

2.8.4 Histopathology

In the light microscopy assessment of normal skin, intact epidermis and dermis were distinguished. Melanocytes were irregularly present among keratinocytes. Since rabbit skin is more flexible than human skin, a large number of elastin fibers were observed.

On day 10, no reepithelialization was observed. The epidermis was present only in necrotic and ulcer forms. In the dermis, both fibrous and granular tissues were observed, a sign of the progression and matrix deposition processes. Hemostasis and inflammation precede epidermal cell proliferation, and the presence of inflammatory cells and coagulation phase residue was considered normal (Fig. 6).

There was less inflammation (33%) in the treated group on day 10 compared with the control group, suggesting that the chitosan-based gel decreased the inflammatory reaction. Less inflammation results in less collagen synthesis and deposition and, therefore, less scar formation. In the control group on day 10, granulation was observed. The epidermis was not reconstructed, ulceration was noticeable, and inflammation continued.

On day 20, in the treated group, proliferation of epidermal cells was observed. Reepithelialization was completed, and the epidermis was healed and had a near normal appearance. Furthermore, all wounds showed almost complete epidermis reconstruction, while 50% of the control group specimens showed ulcers and poor or partial reconstruction of the epidermis. The acceleration of healing in the treatment group was confirmed microscopically. In the group, 67% of wounds healed; however, there was no trace of hair follicles. In the control group, 50% of wounds healed (Fig. 7). The epidermis in the control group appeared to be partially reconstructed; however, ulceration was observed. The epidermis thickness seemed to be thin, and inflammatory cells were present in the dermis. The formation of wound bed, before epidermis formation in the expected healing direction, from depth to surface, was observed (Fig. 7).

In the treated group, by day 30, the epidermis was thoroughly reconstructed and was a normal thickness. There was no melanocyte overgrowth, indicating the absence of hyperpigmentation and the restoration of normal color of the skin. In some cases, swelling in keratinocytes was observed; that was due to their moisture absorption as a result of the moist wound healing environment provided by chitosan-based gel. Inflammation had mostly disappeared. Epidermis growth and the number of keratinocytes appeared to be normal (Fig. 8). In the control group, by day 30, the epidermis was reconstructed. There was papillary growth in the wound bed, which could be associated with hyper-keratinocytes expression.

There were numerous active melanocytes, and melanin was dispersed in the stratum spinosum of the epidermis and dermis. A number of keratinocytes appeared swollen. The epidermis displayed a higher than normal thickness in the control group, comparing the light microscopy images to that of the treatment group. This indicated an abnormal healing in the control group (Fig. 8).

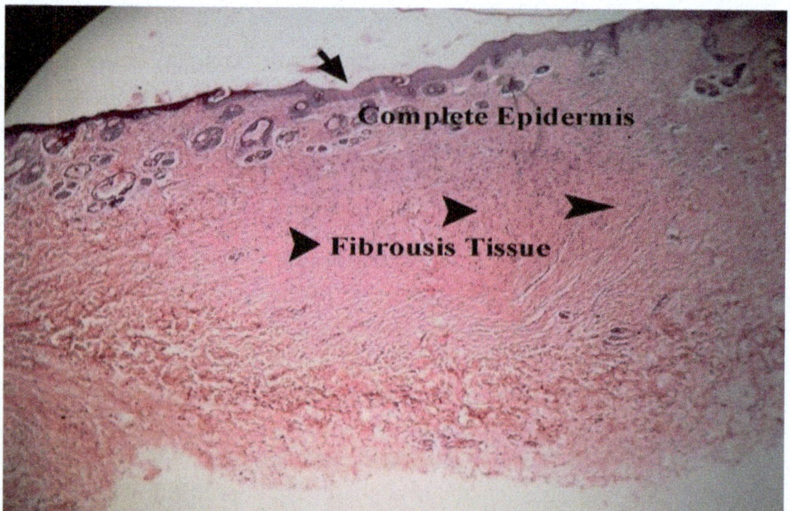

Fig. 7 Treated specimen, day 20

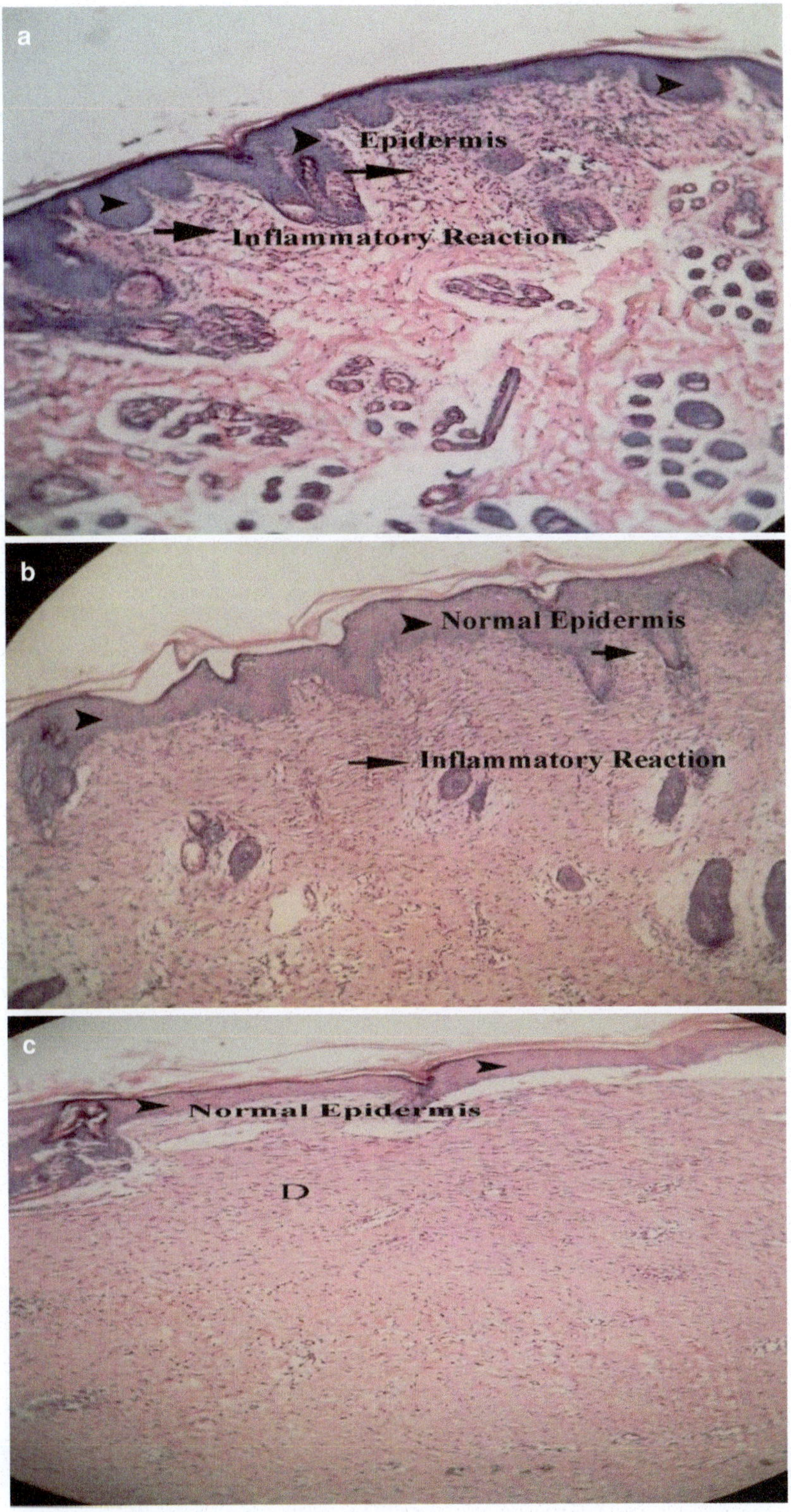

Fig. 8 (**a–c**) Treated specimen, day 30. (**d–f**) Control specimen, day 30

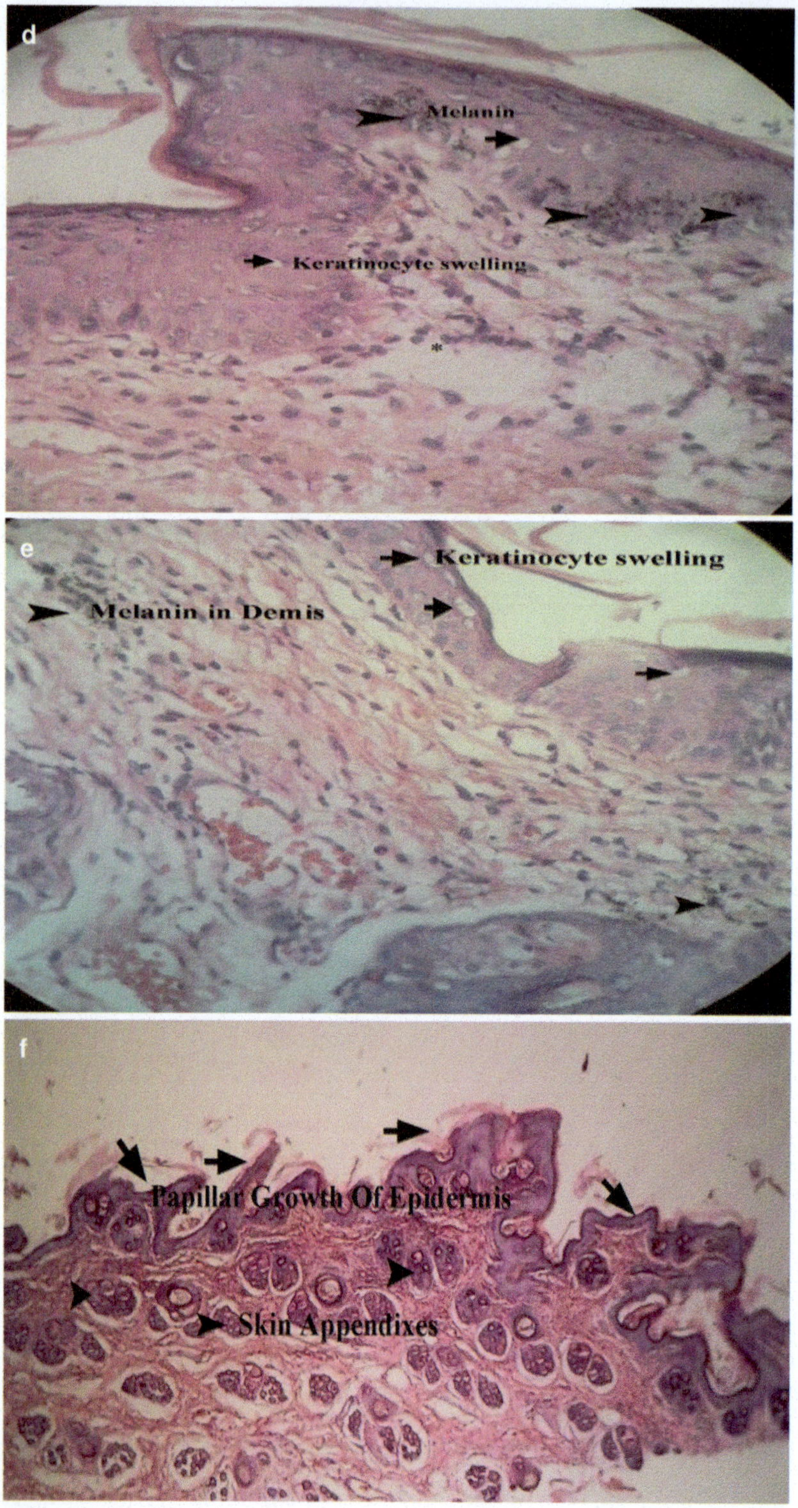

Fig. 8 (continued)

2.8.5 Microscopic Assessment

Scanning Electron Microscopy

Melanocyte Investigation

On the tenth day of healing, it was noticed that fibrous tissue was present in both treatment and control groups. Fibroblasts were the main cells present, and the inflammatory phase was almost over. In SEM images of both the control and treatment groups on day 10, small immature cells together with tissue granules were noticeable, indicating the start of the cell proliferation and tissue granulation phases. In the control group, the presence of blood and inflammatory cells was more noticeable, indicating a longer inflammatory phase in the control group (Fig. 9).

On day 20 the wounds were mostly healed in the treatment group. As the epidermis was reconstructed, keratin fibers were detectable. In the dermis of treatment group, some immature granules were present, showing the accelerated reepithelialization and formation of epidermis. The epidermis in the treatment group was more intensified before the dermis was completely mature. In the control group, less keratin was noticed (Fig. 10).

On day 30, keratin, representing the reconstructed epidermis, and contracted mature granular tissue, representing the reconstructed

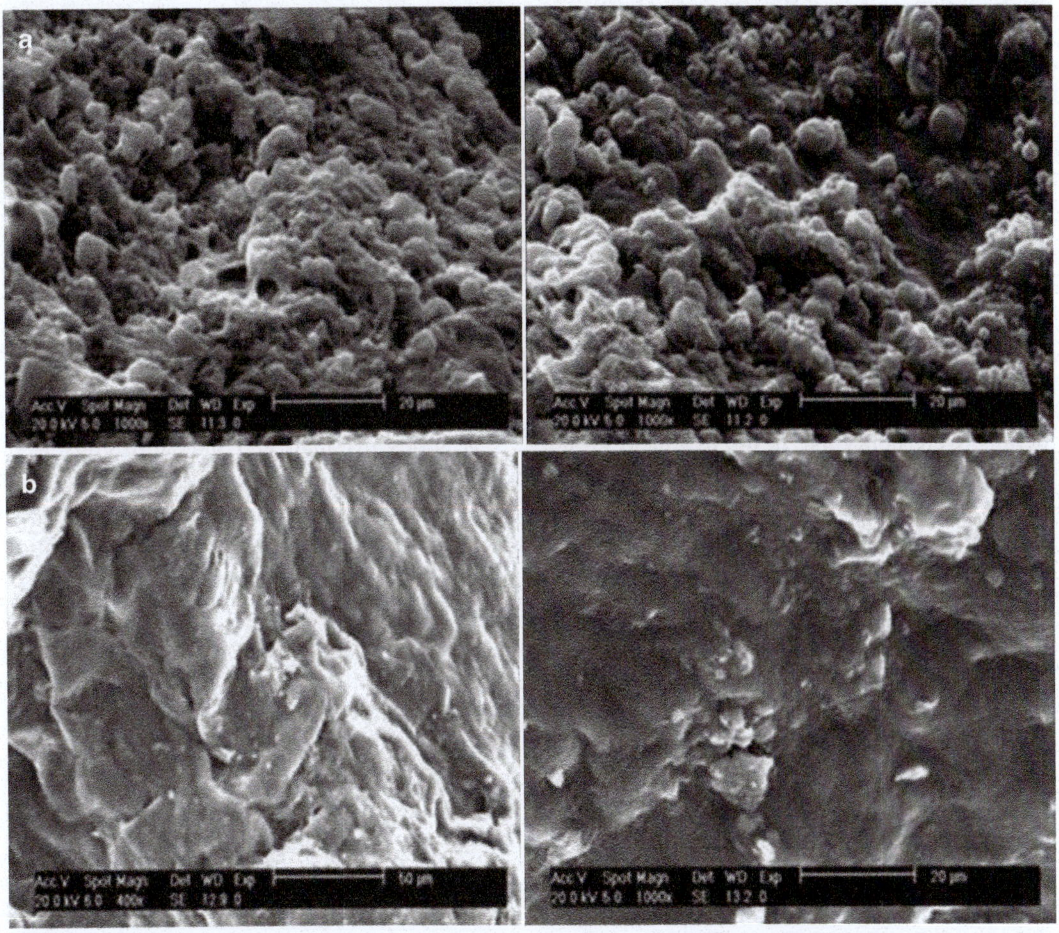

Fig. 9 (**a**) SEM images of control group day 10. (**b**) SEM images of treatment group day 10

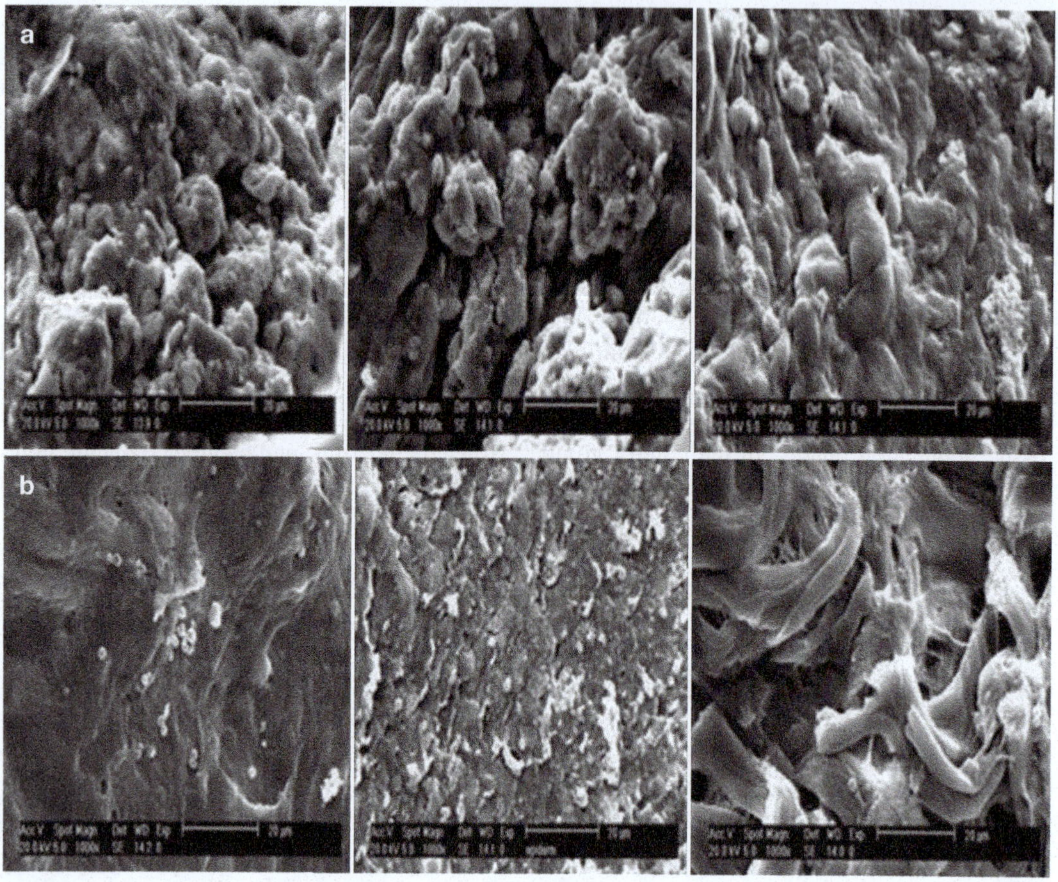

Fig. 10 (**a**) SEM images of control group day 20. (**b**) SEM images of treatment group day 20

dermis, were noticeable in the treatment group. Red blood cells indicated effective angiogenesis. In the control group, tissue granules were still visible. There were little keratins as compared to the treatment group, indicating poor epidermis reconstruction (Fig. 11).

Keratinocyte Investigation

The scanning electron microscope was used for observation of the morphology of the cells. A control and a treated sample SEM pictures are presented from the tenth, the twentieth, and the thirtieth days in Figs. 12, 13, and 14.

In general, on the tenth day of repair, wounds were in the process of contraction. Matrix and fibrous tissue were produced. Therefore, fibroblast and protein strings were observed for the most part.

A series of small and immature cells were observed in the SEM pictures of the control and experimental samples from the tenth day indicating cell division and production of granulation tissue. These cells were observed in pictures of both samples. There were greater presence of blood and inflammatory cells in control samples than treated cells indicating longer inflammation stage in control sample in comparison to the treated sample.

Repair of superficial burn wounds were almost completed by the 20th day. As indicated by the microscopic and histopathology results, repair was in the treated samples, and epidermis and dermis layers were noticed in the treated group.

However, in control samples, fewer keratin fibers were observed. In other words, these

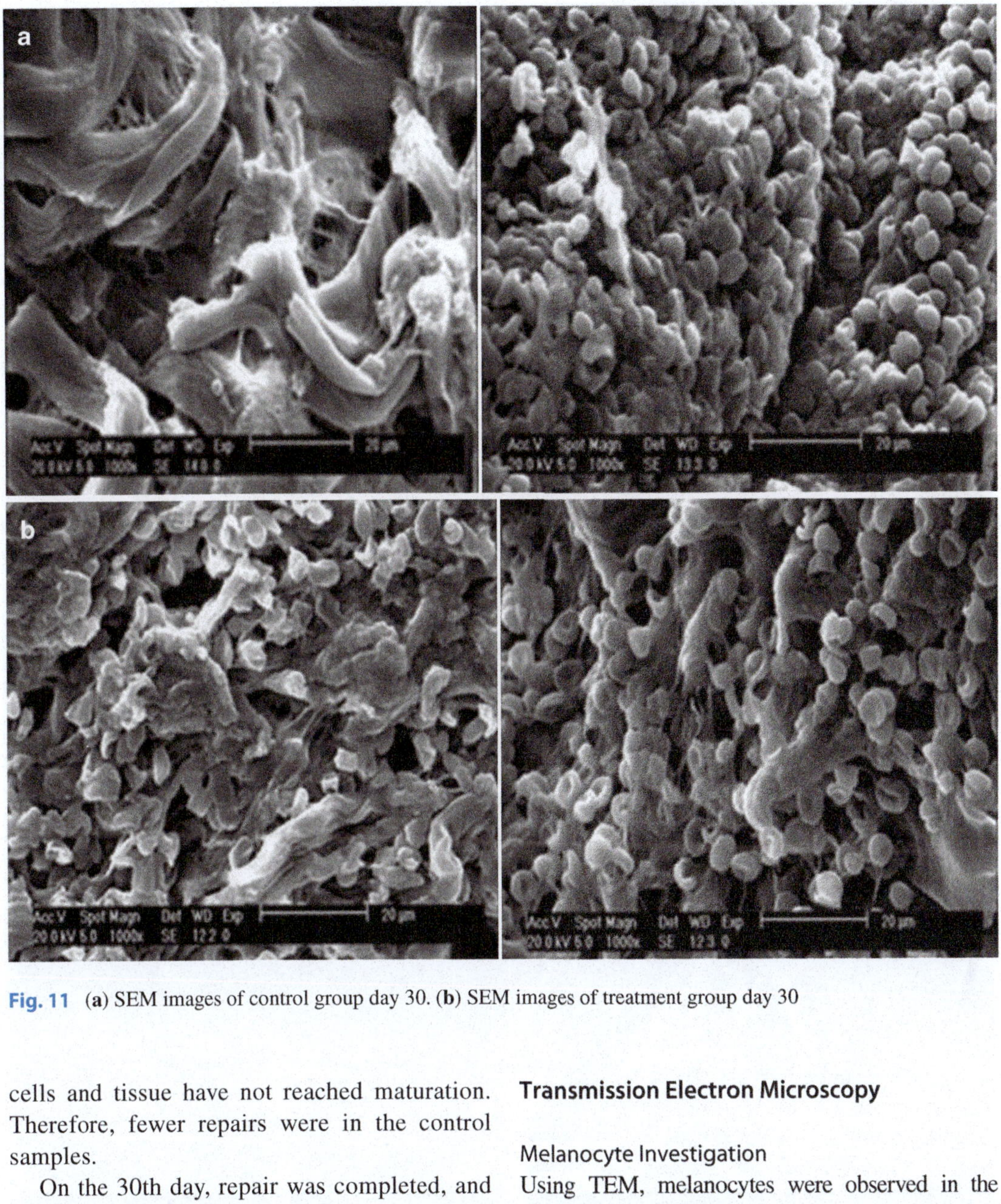

Fig. 11 (**a**) SEM images of control group day 30. (**b**) SEM images of treatment group day 30

cells and tissue have not reached maturation. Therefore, fewer repairs were in the control samples.

On the 30th day, repair was completed, and wounds were completely closed, and epidermal and dermal layers looked normal especially in the treated group. Due to slower rate of repair in the control group, the epidermis layer appeared thinner with lower density. The dermis did not show any signs of the repair of blood capillaries. Blood flow seems normal and lower in the treated samples since repair process is ending.

Transmission Electron Microscopy

Melanocyte Investigation

Using TEM, melanocytes were observed in the treatment group (Fig. 14). As a result of reepithelialization, melanocytes were present among the keratinocytes. The morphology of the melanocytes was normal, implying that, in appropriate wound healing, epidermal melanocytes are reconstructed.

Keratinocyte Investigation

As illustrated in Fig. 15, keratinocytes were present next to melanocyte cells. These pictures

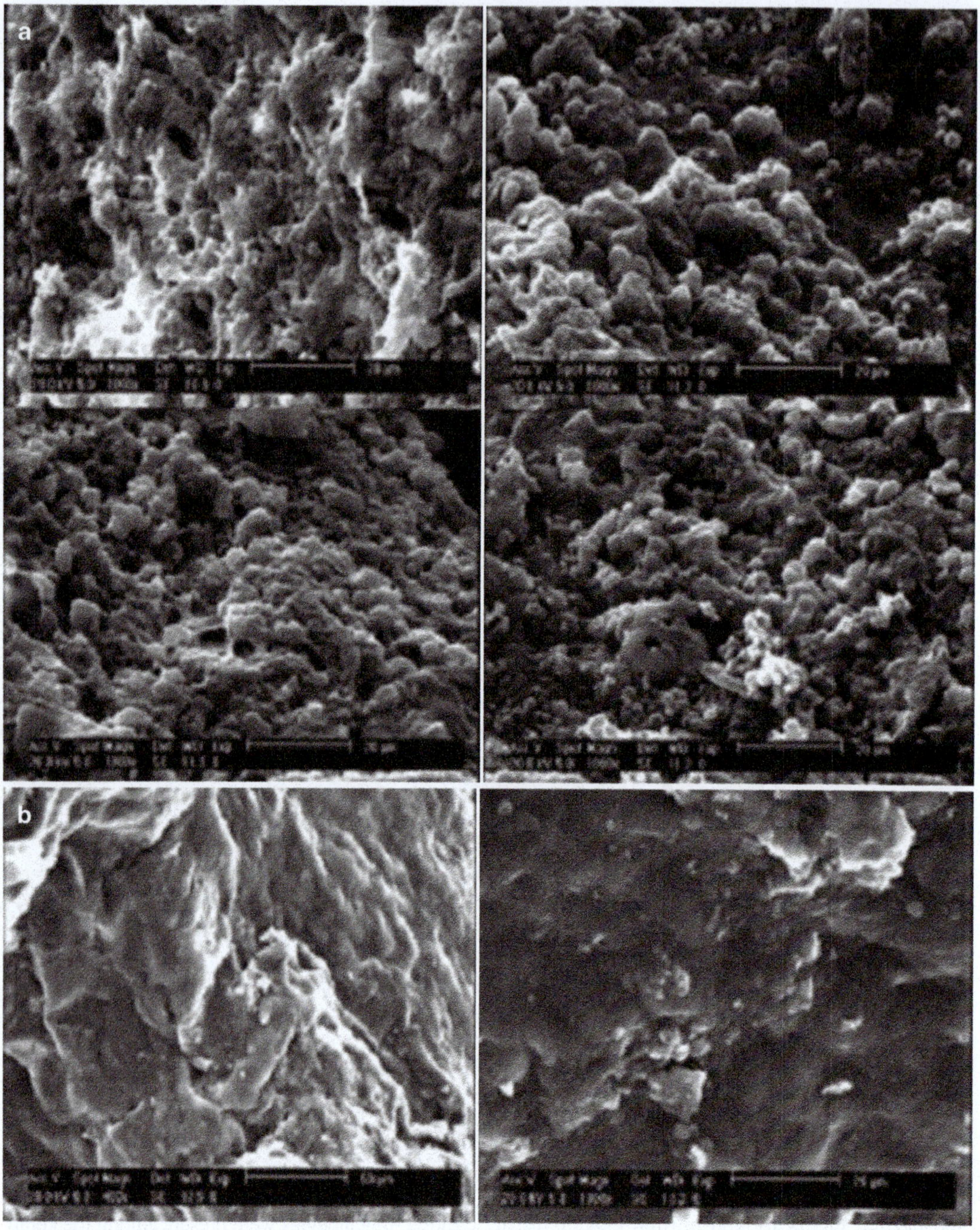

Fig. 12 (**a**) SEM images of control group day 10. (**b**) SEM images of treatment group day 10

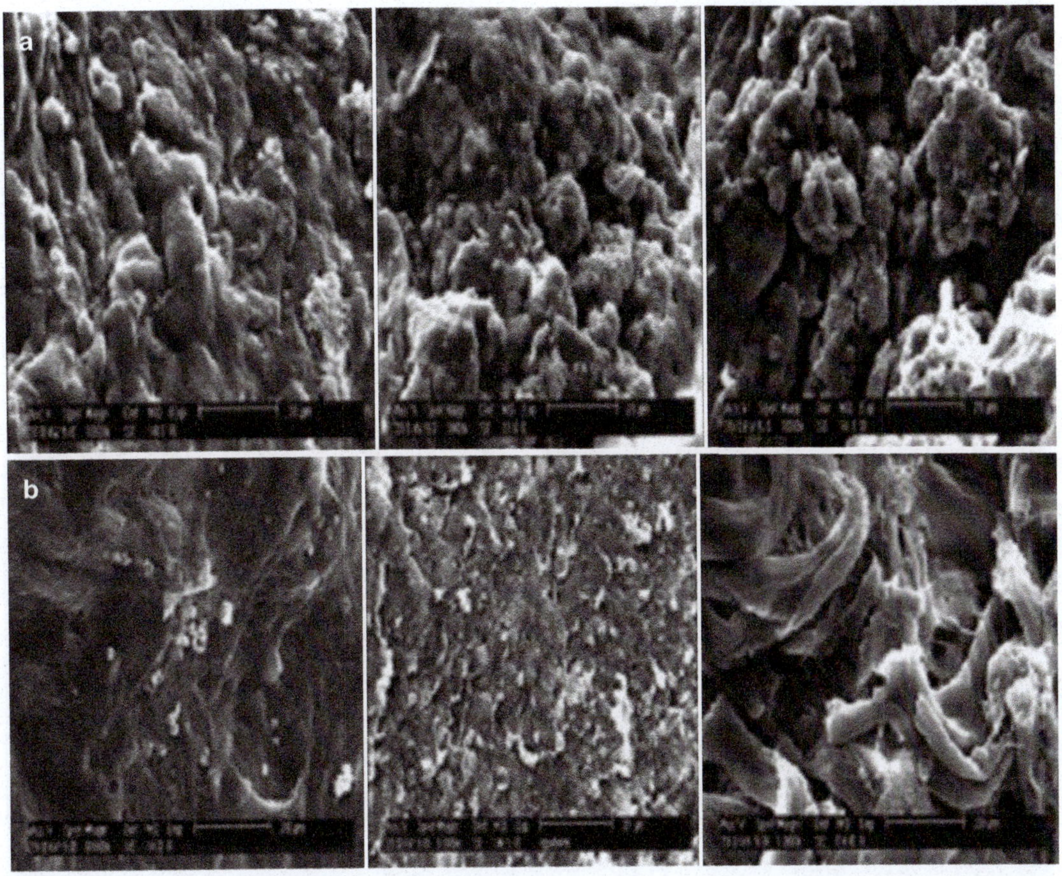

Fig. 13 (**a**) SEM images of control group day 20. (**b**) SEM images of treatment group day 20. (**c**) SEM images of control group day 30. (**d**) SEM images of treatment group day 30

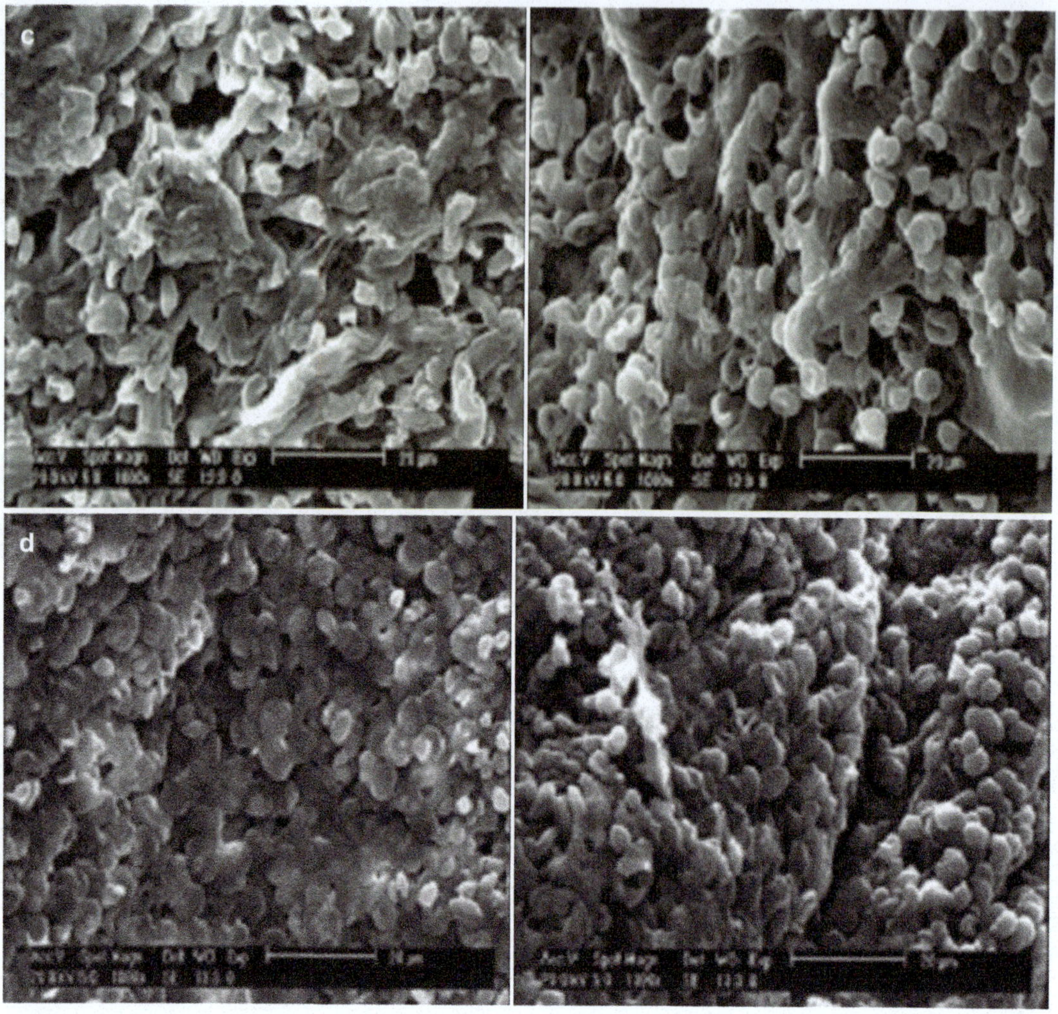

Fig. 13 (continued)

showed keratinocyte layers producing epidermis cells. Considering rate of healing in treated group, it appears that ChitoHeal® gel has caused the acceleration of reepithelialization and production of normal epidermis containing keratinocyte cells. As evident from the images, morphology, shape, and composition of these cells appear normal.

These fibers indicate epidermal repair and presence of active and normal keratinocytes in repaired tissues.

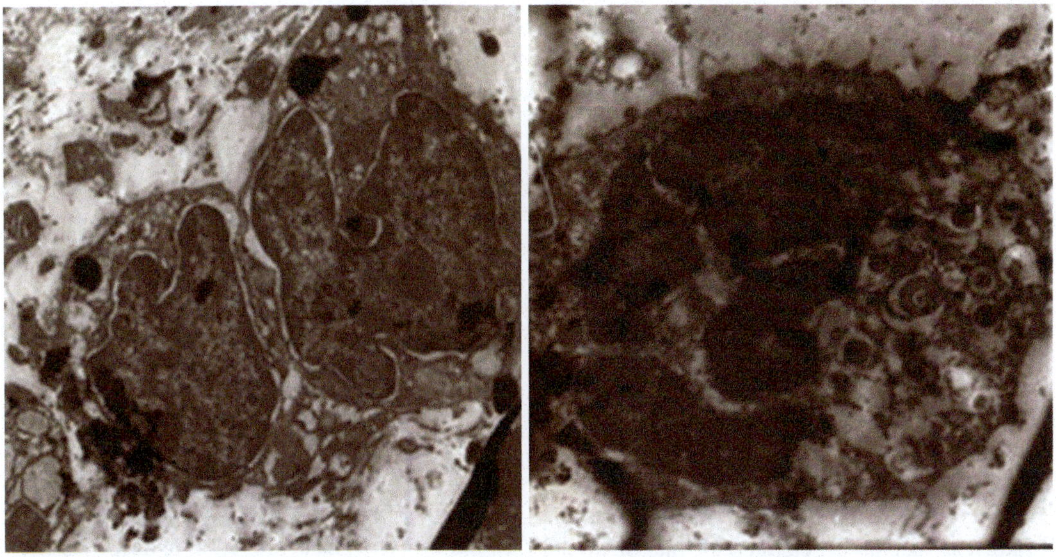

Fig. 14 TEM images of melanocyte cytoplasm in treatment group day 30

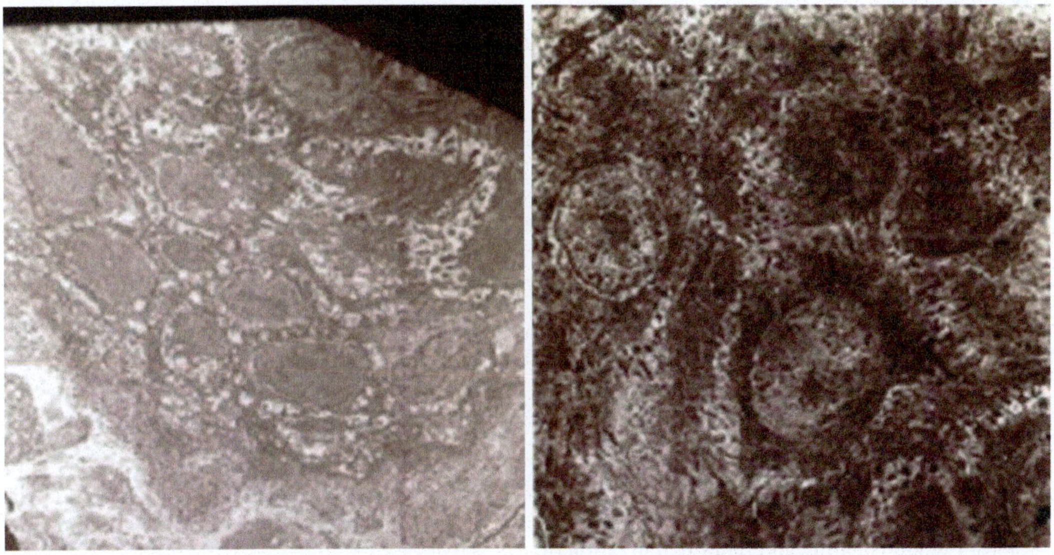

Fig. 15 TEM images of keratinocyte next to melanocyte cells in treatment group day 30

3 Discussion

The mammalian epidermis is a stratified, multilayered epithelium, consisting of the interfollicular epidermis and associated appendages, which extend into the dermis and include hair follicles, sebaceous glands, and sweat glands [5]. The epidermis is made almost entirely of keratinocytes (95%). Other cell types found include melanocytes, Langerhans cells (dendritic cells), and Merkel cells (sensory receptors). The epidermis is a dynamic epithelium that is constantly renewed throughout life. Its turnover is estimated at about 60 days in humans. The aim of this study was to investigate about keratinocyte and melanocyte cells behavior and morphology after wound healing using ChitoHeal® gel in comparison with traditional methods.

The use of ChitoHeal® gel, which is based on chitosan, has improved the rate of wound healing in burn wounds. In fact the application of bioactive dressings consisting of different biomaterials, natural or synthetic, is becoming more widespread in modern wound care treatment [19, 20] as it has been demonstrated by Archana et al. [33]. Application of chitosan and chitosan blend dressing is effective in accelerating burn wounds healing [21].

Results in animals' burn wounds in treatment group compared to control group indicate that ChitoHeal® gel has accelerated the rate of wound healing, the formation and deposition of fibrous matrix, as well as the proliferation and migration of epithelial cells toward the center of the wound. Since epithelial cells proliferate from the wound edges toward its center, as wound heals, its dimensions decrease. Thus, a faster wound closure, with recovering epithelial, shows a satisfactory rapid healing.

The results of the present study demonstrated that the application of ChitoHeal® gel in treatment group has accelerated the rate of wound healing process as compared to the control group where traditional gauze dressings were used.

Conclusions

The outcome of the present study is likely to be important for the development of novel strategies for wound healing, since it sheds light on the potential of the therapeutic regimens. Faster wound healing and reepithelialization of burn wound could result in the reduction of collagen deposition hence preventing severe scar formation.

References

1. Department of Health, Education, and Welfare (1982) Reports of the epidemiology and surveillance of injuries. Atlanta: Centers for Disease Control. (DHEW publication no. (HSM) 73–10001)
2. Brigham PA, McLoughlin E (1996) Burn incidence and medical care use in the United States: estimate, trends, and data sources. J Burn Care Rehabil 17:95–107
3. O'Connor NE, Mulliken JB, Banks-Schlegel S, Kehinde O, Green H (1981) Grafting of burns with cultured epithelium prepared from autologous epidermal cells. Lancet 317:75–78
4. Rowan MP, Cancio LC, Elster EA, Burmeister DM, Rose LF, Natesan S, Chan RK, Christy RJ, Chung KK (2015) Burn wound healing and treatment: review and advancements. Crit Care 19:243
5. Barret JP, Herndon DN (2003) Effects of burn wound excision on bacterial colonization and invasion. Plast Reconstr Surg 111:744–750
6. Braun KM, Prowse DM (2006) Distinct epidermal stem cell compartments are maintained by independent niche microenvironments. Stem Cell Rev 2(3):221–231
7. Illum L (1998) Chitosan and its use as a pharmaceutical excipient. Pharm Res 15(9):1326–1331
8. Ishihara M, Ono K, Sato M, Nakanishi K, Saito Y, Yura H, Matsui T, Hattori H, Fujita M, Kikuchi M, Kurita A (2001) Acceleration of wound contraction and healing with a photocrosslinkable chitosan hydrogel. Wound Repair Regen 9(6):513–521
9. Ishihara M, Nakanishi K, Ono K, Sato M, Kikuchi M, Saito Y, Yura H, Matsui T, Hattori H, Uenoyama M, Kurita A (2002) Photocrosslinkable chitosan as a dressing for wound occlusion and accelerator in healing process. Biomaterials 23:833–840
10. Alemdaroğlu C, Değim Z, Celebi N, Zor F, Oztürk S, Erdoğan D (2006) An investigation on burn wound healing in rats with chitosan gel formulation containing epidermal growth factor. Burns 32:319–327
11. Honardar S, Kordestani SS, Daliri M, Nayeb Habib F (2016) The effect of chitosan-based gel on second degree burn wounds. J Wound Care 25(8):488–494
12. Aulick LH, Bace WB, Johnson AA, Wilmore DW, Mason AD (1981) A large animal model of burn. Hypermetabolism J Surg Res 31:281–287
13. Sevitt S (1949) Local blood-flow changes in experimental burns. J Pathol 61:427–442
14. Robson MC, Kucan JO, Paik KI, Eriksson E (1978) Prevention of dermal ischemia after thermal injury. Arch Surg 113(5):621
15. Raine TJ, Heggers JP, Robson MC, London MD, Johns L (1981) Cooling the burn wound to maintain microcirculation. J Trauma 21(5):394–397
16. Arturson G, Jakobsson OP (1985) Edema measurements in a standard burn model. Burns 12:1–7
17. Wang HJ, Chen TM, Yang TS, Wang DS, Lin SZ (1995) Regional skin blood -flow in deep burn wounds: a preliminary report. Burns 21(2):340–343
18. Langlade A, Carr DB, Serrie A, Silbert BS, Szyfelbein SK, Lipkowski AW (1994) Enhanced potency of intravenous, but not intrathecal, morphine and morphine-6-glucuronide after burn trauma. Life Sci 54(22):1699–1709

19. Chance WT, Nelson JL, Foley-Nelson T, Kim MW, Fischer FE (1989) The relationship of burn-induced hypermetabolism to central and peripheral catecholamines. J Trauma 29(3):306–312
20. Caldwell FT, Graves DB, Wallace BH (1994) The response in heat production, plasma catecholamines and body temperature of burned rats to hypothalamic temperature displacement. J Burn Care Rehabil 15(4):315–321
21. Berthiaume F, Ezzell RM, Toner M, Yarmush ML, Tompkins RG (1994) Transport of fluorescent dextrans across the rat ileum after cutaneous thermal injury. Crit Care Med 22(3):455–464
22. Kistler D, Hafemann B, Schmidt K (1988) A model to reproduce predictable full-thickness burns in an experimental animal. Burns 14(4):297–302
23. Mulligan MS, Til GO, Smith WC, Anderson DC, Miyasaka M, Tamatani T, Todd RF, Issekutz TB, Ward PA (1994) Role of leukocyte adhesion molecules in lung and dermal vascular injury after thermal trauma of skin. Am J Pathol 144(5):1008–1015
24. DaCosta R, Aggarwal SJ, Diller KR, Baxter CR (1992) The effects of epinephrine, ibuprofen and tetrachlorodecaoxide on cutaneous microcirculation in thermally injured hamsters. J Burn Care Rehabil 13(4):396–402
25. Brans TA, Durtieux RP, Hoekstra MJ, Kreis RW, du Pont JS (1994) Histopathological evaluation of scalds and contact burns in the pig model. Burns 20(1):48–51
26. Behounkova-Houskova E, Moserova J (1978) Histology of healing of deep dermal burns in pigs. Scand J Plast Reconstr Surg 13:57–60
27. Breuing K, Eriksson E, Liu P, Miller DR (1992) Healing of partial thickness porcine skin wounds in a liquid environment. J Surg Res 52:50–58
28. Oluwasanmi J, Chvapil M (1976) A comparative study of four materials in local burn care in rabbit model. J Trauma 16(5):348–353
29. Mileski WM, Borgstrom D, Lightfoot E, Rothlein R, Faanes R, Lipsky P, Baxter C (1992) Inhibition of leukocyte-endothelial adherence following thermal injury. J Surg Res 52:334–339
30. Bucky LP, Vedder NB, Hong HZ, Ehrlich HP, Winn RK, Harlan JM, May JW Jr (1994) Reduction of burn injury by inhibiting CD18-mediated leukocyte adherence in rabbits. Plast Reconstr Surg 93(7):1473–1480
31. Militzer K (1982) Vergleichende morphologie der haut und der haare von maus, ratte, hamster, meerschweinchen und kaninchen (Teil 1). In: Militzer K (ed) Haut- und Hautanhangsorgane kleiner Laboratoriumssa Èugetiere. Verlag Paul Parey, Berlin/Hamburg, pp 25–28. 108–9
32. Knabl JS, Bayer GS, Bauer WA, Schwendenwein I, Dado PF, Kucher C, Horvat R, Turkof E, Schossmann B, Meissl G (1999) Controlled partial skin thickness burns: an animal model for studies of burn wound progression. Burns 25(3):229–235
33. Archana D, Dutta J, Dutta PK (2013) Evaluation of chitosan nano dressing for wound healing: characterization, in vitro and in vivo studies. Int J Biol Macromol 57:193–203

Treatment of Partial-Thickness Scalds by Skin Xenografts

Peter Bukovčan and Ján Koller

1 Introduction

Burns are primarily damaging the skin and nearby structures. Secondarily, they are able to endanger all the systems in the human body. From this point of view, the management of burns represents a part of the medicine, where multidisciplinary approach is needed. Nevertheless, the basic and inevitable prerequisite of successful treatment of burns represents a treatment of the burn wound, where the skin substitutes are still holding an irreplaceable position.

Burn wound is like an opened door. Through this opened door, not invited guests are coming (causing bacterial contamination/colonization/infection). On the contrary, inhabitants which wished to stay (body heat, wound fluid, electrolytes, proteins) are leaving. The more the door is opened (the larger extent of burn and depth are) and the longer the time period of opening is (length of time delay between injury and wound cover/closure), the greater negative impact they are likely to have. Except the burn depth, burn extent, and time delay of the treatment, many other factors can influence the speed and quality of wound closure (burn etiology and localization, age, associated illnesses/injuries), so it is not always easy to close the door (perform wound coverage/closure) securely and in time.

The main requirement in the management of partial-thickness burn wounds is an economical, easy-to-apply, readily available dressing or method of coverage that would provide pain relief, protect the wound from infection, induce healing, prevent heat and fluid loss, and provide other beneficial activities while waiting for spontaneous epithelialization.

According to epidemiological studies [1–3], scald injuries are the most frequent cause of burns afflicting lower age groups of the patients (<15 years of age). Scald injuries are an important public health issue and cause considerable morbidity. Mainly the partial-thickness scald burns are creating one of the frequent indications for the utilization of biological skin substitute—porcine skin xenograft at the authors' workplace. In regard to the high incidence of this type of injury—43% of the whole amount of burned patients admitted in the years 1989–1993 in Bratislava [4], their reasonable and efficacious treatment is of great importance. To prove the beneficial effects of skin xenograft as biological skin substitute, the retrospective study had been created and performed [5].

By describing the preparation method of skin xenografts, wound management protocol, clinical results of the retrospective study, their comparison with other methods of wound coverage used at other clinical workplaces, and discussion, it would be possible for the reader to gain comprehensive approach to the wound management of partial-thickness burns.

P. Bukovčan, M.D., Ph.D. (✉)
J. Koller, M.D., Ph.D.
Department of Burns and Reconstructive Surgery of Comenius University, Universital Hospital Ružinov, Bratislava, Slovak Republic
e-mail: bukovcanmed@gmail.com

Recent Clinical Techniques, Results, and Research in Wounds (2017)
DOI 10.1007/15695_2017_28, © Springer International Publishing AG
Published Online: 24 October 2017

2 Technique

The retrospective study was performed in 109 patients with fresh superficial and deeper partial-thickness burns, who were hospitalized at the Teaching Department of Burns and Reconstructive Surgery of the University Hospital Bratislava, Ruzinov Hospital, Slovakia, in the years 2005–2007. The study was approved by the Ethics Committee of the Ruzinov Hospital.

2.1 Xenograft Preparation Method

Skin xenografts (SXG) have been used as biological skin substitutes at the Department of Burns and Reconstructive Surgery since 1987. They have been prepared for clinical use in the Central Tissue Bank (CTB), a part of the Teaching Department of Burns and Reconstructive Surgery Bratislava, Slovakia, where SXG preparation method has been performed according to the original method of Moserová (1974) [6] with some minor modifications. Porcine skin removed from veterinary-certified slaughtered pigs, stored at the temperature of 4 °C, has been transported from the slaughterhouse to CTB. Within 24 h after the slaughter, under sterile conditions, the retrieval of the dermoepidermal grafts has been done by electrical dermatome (Fig. 1). After the washing of grafts retrieved in a solution of chloramine, lavage in antibiotic solution, and lavage in cryoprotective agent (Fig. 2), four small samples (0.5 × 0.5 cm each) have been taken from each graft for the bacteriological control. After then, each graft has been put on the sterile gauze with the dermal side up, folded up to create four layers at maximum (Fig. 3), and sealed in the sterile plastic bag. Prepared SXG have been placed into the deep-freezer appliance and stored at the temperature of −80 °C. After obtaining negative results of the sterility tests according to Czech-Slovak Pharmacopoeia, 4th Ed., the SXG could have been released for the clinical use.

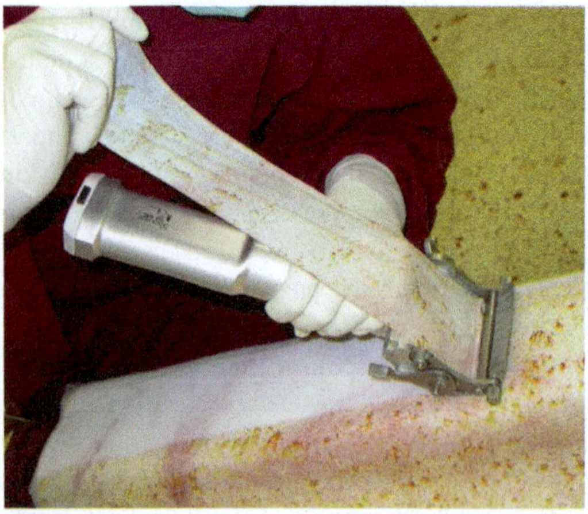

Fig. 1 Pig skin xenograft retrieval

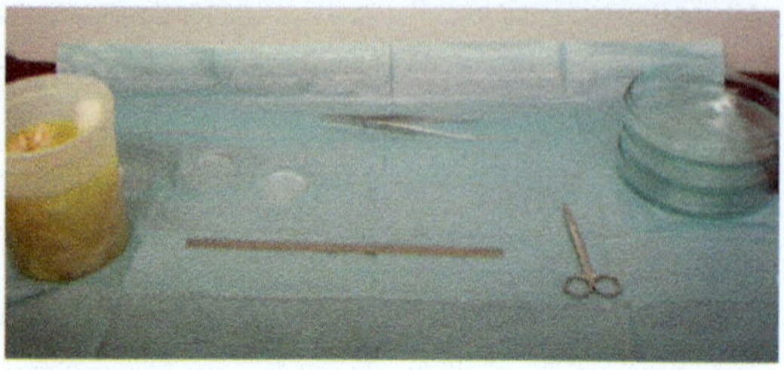

Fig. 2 Skin xenografts are lavaged in antibiotic solution and in cryoprotective agent

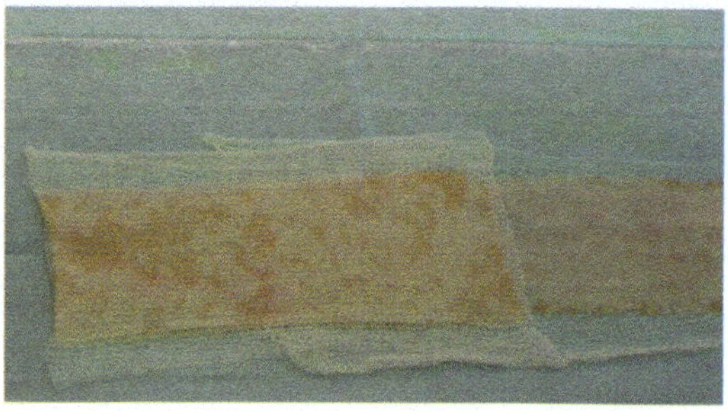

Fig. 3 Skin xenografts are placed on the sterile gauze with the dermal side up, folded up to create four layers at maximum

2.2 Wound Management Protocol

During the admission of the patient, initial assessment of the depth and extent of burns has been performed. For estimation of an extent of burns, body surface area of burns (BSAB), the Lund-Browder chart has been used. The depth of the burn has been expressed in degrees. When indicated for the xenograft coverage, after the disinfection of the wounds with Betadine, all patients underwent complete debridement of the nonviable epidermis using blunt debridement (gauze) under systemic analgesia, by children with greater extent of burns under general anesthesia. After obtaining the clean surface of the wound with the dermis exposed (Fig. 4), the cryopreserved porcine xenografts (defrosted rapidly in saline immediately before the usage) were applied (Fig. 5). Treated areas were then covered by tulle dressing impregnated with Vaseline, gauze with silver sulfadiazine, dry gauze layers, and elastic bandage. In the case of placement of xenografts over the joints of the limbs mainly by children, Kramer

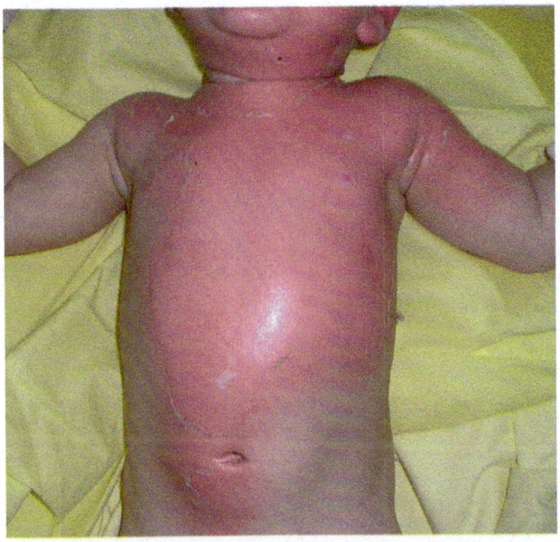

Fig. 4 IIa-degree scald burn by a 13-month-old child

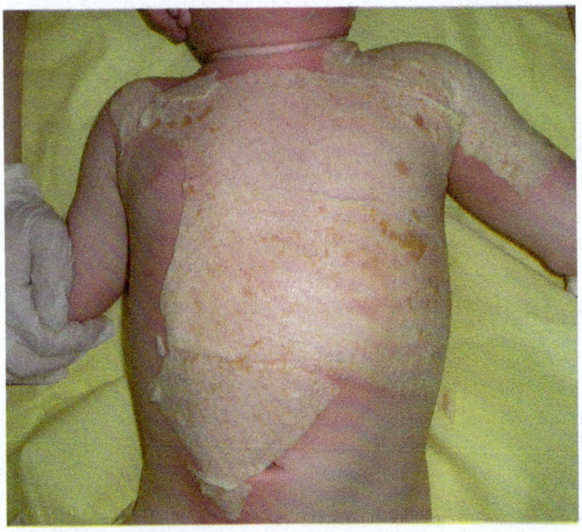

Fig. 5 The same child after immediate coverage by skin xenografts

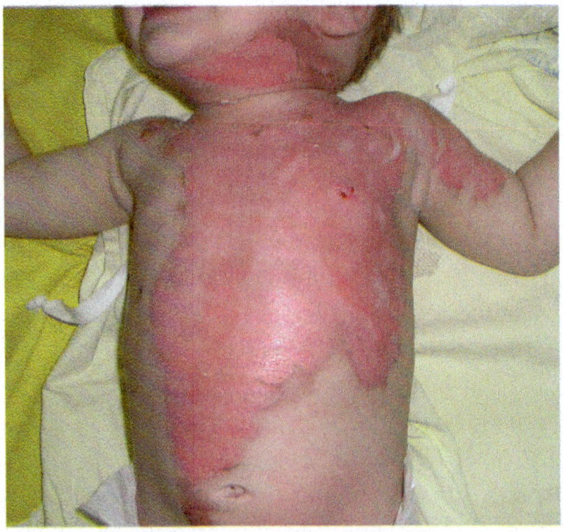

Fig. 6 Separation of the xenografts by means of transepithelial elimination 8th day post-injury

splints were used. Systemic antibiotic prophylaxis was provided by intravenous administration of penicillin in standard doses in cases with negative history of penicillin allergy. Wound cultures were taken by initial treatment and also regularly during the hospital stay. If the wound dressings were not displaced and if no complications occurred, the dressing changes were performed every 48 h. The xenografts were left to adhere to the wound surface till their separation by means of transepithelial elimination (Fig. 6). The residual defects (if present) were treated by application of topical antimicrobial agents within a scope of the methods for the wound healing during the hospital stay or on an outpatient basis.

Inclusion Criteria

The inclusion criteria were as follows:

1. Patients were hospitalized during the 3-year period (from the beginning of 2005 to the end of 2007).
2. All patients sustained partial-thickness (superficial and deep dermal) scald burns.
3. All patients were admitted and treated within the first 24 h after injury.
4. All patients were indicated for wound coverage by biological skin substitutes.
5. Patients of every age, extent of burn, and associated illness were included.

Evaluation Criteria

1. Total number of patients healed within 14 days postburn and their mean healing time
2. Mean healing time of all patients included to the study (total healing time)
3. Mean discharge time to outpatient management
4. Total number of patients whose treatment required operation—wound closure by skin autografts

Total healing time was defined as the time necessary to reach 95% of reepithelialization by each patient. Hospital discharge was enabled to all patients, an outpatient management of whom could have been done safely and comfortably.

3 Results

One hundred nine patients were included in the study. From these patients 59 were males (54%) and 50 females (46%). The male/female ratio was by adults 1.16:1 and 1.2:1 by children. The mean age of the patients was 7.6 years (min., 6 months; max., 80 years). The majority of 109 patients were children (96 cases). The mean BSAB was 13% (min., 3%; max, 43%). By all patients the burns were caused by hot liquids (water, tea, coffee, soup). The numbers of patients, sex, mean age, mean BSAB, minimal and maximal values (min.-max.), and standard deviations (S.D.) are shown in Table 1.

According to BSAB the patients were divided into three groups:

1. Within 10% (48 patients with mean extent 7.6%)
2. 11–20% (45 patients with mean extent 13.4%)
3. More than 20% (16 patients with mean extent 29.4%)

The results are displayed in Table 2.

Healing was within 14 days. Among 109 patients 78 (71%) patients healed within 14 days with a mean time 9.6 days (S.D.: 3.2). One sample *t*-test which compared mean healing times achieved

Table 1 Patients included in the study

			Sex			
			Male (59)		Female (50)	
		№ patients (109)	Men (7)	Boys (52)	Women (6)	Girls (44)
Age (years)	Mean	**7.6**	44.3	2.5	42.1	3.1
	S.D.	**15.3**	20.7	2.5	26.0	2.8
	(min.–max.)	**(0.5–80)**	(21–75)	(0.5–12)	(18–80)	(0.5–11)
BSAB (%)	Mean	**13**	16.5	12.6	14.3	13.3
	S.D.	**8.2**	11.7	6.6	14.7	8.4
	(min.–max.)	**(3–43)**	(3–32)	(3–40)	(3–43)	(4–42)

Table 2 Results of the study

	Patients	Healing within 14 days				Total healing time		Discharge time		Operations	
BSAB (%)	№	№	%	Mean time (days)	S.D.	Mean time (days)	S.D.	Mean (days)	S.D.	№	%
<10	48	38	81	9.3	3.0	13.6	11.1	7.7	6.0	0	0
10–20	45	36	80	9.4	3.2	13.4	10.2	9.1	4.7	1	2.1
>20	16	4	25	12	4.3	24.6	12.7	18.61	8.0	3	18.7
All extents	109	78	71	9.6	3.2	15.1	11.6	9.96	6.7	4	3.6
		$p = 0.0001 < 0.05$				$p = 0.3 > 0.05$					

within 14 days with the value of 14 days proved the significant difference ($p = 0.0001 < 0.05$) by the level of significance 0.05. In the group with extents larger than 20%, the lowest amount of patients healed within 14 days.

This fact shows the correlation between the larger extents of burns and increased healing times in this group. Healing within 14 days serves for expression of the healing dynamics and as a parameter for comparison with another studies focused on the alternative treatment options.

3.1 Total Healing Time

Also in this category, the values in groups with extents up to 10% and from 10 to 20% were almost identical and within 14 days. In the group with extents more than 20%, the mean value of total healing time was 24.6 days which is in accordance to the increased value of mean healing time within 14 days in this group. For all the 109 cases, the mean total healing time was 15.1 days (S.D.: 11.6) with no significant difference between mean total healing times and the value of 14 days ($p = 0.3 > 0.05$).

3.2 Discharge Time

As the treatment of residual defects could have been done in many cases on the outpatient basis, the mean values of discharge time in each group were lower than mean values of total healing time. Among 109 patients altogether, the mean discharge time was up to 10 days.

3.3 Operations

In four cases, it was necessary to perform tangential excision of the deep parts of the wounds and their coverage with split-thickness skin autografts or the coverage of residual defects of larger extent, the spontaneous healing of which would require much more time. In the group with extents up to 10%, there were no operations. In the group with extents from 10 to 20%, one case of a 7-year-old girl with BSAB 13.5% was treated by operation. Because of the wound deepening of BSAB 3.5%, the tangential excision and temporary coverage with porcine skin xenografts had been performed on day 10 postburn. Skin xenografts had been replaced by split-thickness skin autografts on the second stage. The wound cultures at the day of admission were sterile, on day 4 postburn sterile—after multiplication *Staphylococcus aureus*. From 16 patients in the group with BSAB above 20%, three cases were operated, which represented 18.7% from this group. In two cases (one girl and one boy with the same age of 2 years and with BSAB 22% and 23%, respectively), the tangential excision and coverage with split-thickness skin autografts of BSAB 6 and 6.5%, respectively, had been performed. In one case (girl 2 years old, BSAB:21.5%), it was necessary to cover the residual defects, which represented BSAB 2% with split-thickness autografts.

Among 109 patients, 4 patients underwent surgery, which represented 3.6%. The mean surface operated was 4.5% TBSA (total body surface area).

4 Discussion

The authors compare the results of the retrospective study with cryopreserved skin xenografts with the results obtained at other workplaces, where another types of skin substitutes in this indication have been used.

A retrospective study of the treatment of scalds by glycerolized skin allografts had been performed by Brans [7]. In the period of 4 years, 45 patients with mean age of 23 months and mean BSAB 10.2% (from 3% to 23%) had been treated during the first 24 h postburn. From all patients 21 patients (47%) healed within 14 days. Better outcome of patients from the study of the treatment of scalds by skin xenografts (71%) could be only partially explained by the lower mean age of patients treated by skin allografts. The decisive could be the difference in the viability of these skin substitutes.

A prospective randomized study had been performed by Leicht [8], based on the comparison of the treatment of scalds by lyophilized allografts (LA) with the treatment by open technique. From 50 patients with scalds, 25 with the mean age 1.4 years and mean BSAB 8.35% received LA within the first 24 h postburn. From these 25 patients, 15 of them (60%) healed within 14 days. Better results achieved in the study with xenografts (71% healed within 14 days) could be explained by the higher mean age (7.6 years) but also by the similar reason mentioned previously, for as much as lyophilized skin allografts do not retain the viability in comparison with cryopreserved skin xenografts.

The results of another studies showed the necessity of the presence of bioactive surface to accelerate the reepithelialization through the contact orientation and stimulation of cell proliferation [9, 10]. From this point of view and with regard to the results achieved, the partially retained bioactivity of skin xenografts seems to be more advantageous. Partially retained bioactivity of cryopreserved skin xenografts (CXE) was observed also by Liangpeng Ge [11], where CXE has been shown to maintain a level of skin metabolism equal to 77% of the fresh sample when measured immediately after thawing (the viability value of fresh skin samples before cryopreservation was defined as 100%). The average viabilities of thawed skin samples were 77.01% (quick freezing) and 66.37% (slow freezing), respectively, measured by 3-(4,5)-dimethylthiazol-2,5-diphenyl tetrazolium bromide (MTT) salt assay immediately after thawing.

It is also possible to preserve skin allografts by deep freezing which partially retains their viability. However, utilization of them is recommended in such cases, where integration of the dermal component as a part of permanent wound closure is desired [12], because the glycerol-preserved or lyophilized allograft provides no viable coverage material and lacks the beneficial effect of integration and vascularization of viable allogeneic grafts [13].

Transmissions of human diseases via allografts, particularly infections with viruses such as HIV, CMV, and hepatitis, are a risk [14–16]. Although the disease transmissions through allografts are shown to be low [17], utilization of them should be reserved for wound closure in excised full-thickness burns of large extent with limited donor sites, where the benefit of wound closure (when combined with skin autografts) of large full-thickness burns would balance the possible (although very low) risk of disease transmission.

In cryopreserved skin xenografts, zoonotic infections above all porcine endogenous retroviruses (PERV) are a potential threat, but, to date, no evidence of pig-human PERV transfer has been observed [18]. Moreover, the actual risk for PERV infection, replication, and pathogenic outcome in human recipients of xenotransplantation products is still undefined [19]. Also in authors' clinical practice, for almost 30 years of using of cryopreserved skin xenografts, such complication has never been observed.

A prospective, randomized trial of 32 patients with partial skin thickness burns, mostly scalds (25 from 32), is reported by Healy [20] comparing E-Z Derm® (silver-impregnated porcine xenograft) with Jelonet® (petroleum jelly-impregnated widely meshed gauze) as a burn dressing. The bacterial colonization rate, need for surgical treatment, time for spontaneous healing, analgesic requirements, and frequency of dressing changes were assessed in each group. No statistically significant differences were found between the two groups, for any of these factors. Surgical treatment was required in 7 of the 16 E-Z Derm-treated patients, compared with 8 of the Jelonet group (mean body surface area burned 2.3% and 1.8%, respectively). Of the burns which healed spontaneously, the mean time to healing was 12.9 days for the E-Z Derm-treated group and 12.5 days for the Jelonet-treated group. Although the number of patients included in our study and the mean body surface area were higher (109 patients, 13 ± 8%), the mean healing time was comparable (15.1 days). Moreover, the number of patients who required surgical treatment in our study was significantly lower (4 patients from 109 vs. 7 patients from 16 in E-Z Derm group). In E-Z Derm, the collagen is chemically cross-linked with an aldehyde group, which makes it more resistant to bacterial collagenous degradation and reduces antigenicity, one of the early concerns about xenografts [21] but adherence is reduced [22], which could explain the differences between study results.

In prospective study performed by Zajicek and colleagues [23], 43 pediatric patients with superficial scald burns treated with Xe-Derma® (dry sterile biological cover derived from a cellular pig dermis) were compared with 43patients treated with Askina THINSite® (hydrocolloid dressing). No significant difference in the epithelialization time, percentage of conversion from superficial to deep dermal burns, and percentage of infectious complications was detected between the two groups. Xe-Derma® showed better adherence to the wound with no need to change in comparison to Askina THINSite®, where in 40% of patients (17 out of 43) had to be changed. In the Xe-Derma group and also in the Askina THINSite group, a part of the area covered with them converted in 16 and 18 patients, respectively. In converted areas, Flammazine® or autografting (the number of patients with autograft procedure not specified) was used for further treatment. According to the results of authors' retrospective study with cryopreserved skin xenografts, only 4 (3 of them with BSAB >20%) from 109 patients needed autograft procedure (mean surface operated 4.5% TBSA). Lower count of wound conversions can be explained by partially retained bioactivity of cryopreserved skin xenografts.

For the coverage of partial-thickness burns also, amnion obtained from the placentas of selected donors is being used. In 2007 Singh [24] compared the burn wound healing rate between the radiation-sterilized amniotic membranes and glycerol-preserved amniotic membranes. Fifty patients with partial-thickness burns (41 of them with scalds, the rest caused by flame) up to the 70% of BSAB were selected in the study. The wounds of each patient had been divided on halves, first half treated by glycerol-preserved and the second one by irradiated membrane, respectively. There were no significant differences in the rate of healing between the gamma-irradiated amniotic membranes and glycerol-preserved membranes indicating no adverse effect of the gamma irradiation on the efficacy of the membranes. According to the authors, in all the patients, membranes are desiccated and separated in 10–14 days time leaving behind epithelialized surface. Exact results of the healing were not stated.

The usage of allogeneic cultivated keratinocytes as a temporary wound coverage is advantageous mainly by IIb-degree burns, where the capability of keratinocytes to promote epithelialization by releasing the growth factors and mediators of the wound healing is combined with the ability of epithelialization from the adnexal structures of the viable parts of the dermis. On this approach "the Viennese concept" is based, published by Rab [25] in 2005:

1. Early tangential excision of partial- and full-thickness scalds (days 4–7 after trauma).
2. Coverage of the partial-thickness burns by cryopreserved allogeneic cultivated keratinocytes.
3. In scalded areas which have to be excised to the subcutaneous tissue, the coverage of autologous split skin grafts is still the method of choice.

The authors compared 22 scalded children with the wounds tangentially excised and covered with cultivated allogeneic keratinocytes on days 4–7 after trauma with 14 children who underwent the same procedure on days 4–7 after trauma covered with split skin autografts. They observed significantly lower volume of the blood transfusion and significantly better long-term results pertaining the hypertrophic scar formation in the group of patients covered by cultivated allogeneic keratinocytes. In compliance with the results achieved, according to the authors, the higher costs resulting from the usage of keratinocytes are justified. "The Viennese concept" is promising mainly by the management of scalds in the period after first 24 h after trauma, when the usage of temporary skin substitutes is more risky because of possible infectious complications which can in many cases disable their application.

Lower incidence of hypertrophic scars in the group of patients covered with cultivated allogeneic keratinocytes as a long-term result corresponds with the finding of Ghaffari [26], who observed significantly lower amount of collagen produced by dermal fibroblasts during their cultivation with keratinocytes. This fact he explains by the presence of keratinocyte-derived collagen-inhibitory factors (KD-CIFs) with the molecular weight 30–50 kDa, which are regulating type I collagen expression and synthesis in dermal fibroblasts.

There is a reason to suppose that this regulation acts also by other types of biological skin substitutes with preserved viability of keratinocytes when used.

During cutaneous wound healing, keratinocyte proliferation and migration are critical for reepithelialization. In addition the epidermis secretes growth factors, cytokines, proteases, and matricellular proteins into the wound microenvironment that modify the extracellular matrix and stimulate other wound cells that control the inflammatory response, promote angiogenesis, and facilitate tissue contraction and remodeling. Wound keratinocytes express at least seven different integrins—the major cell adhesion receptors for the extracellular matrix—that collectively control essential cell-autonomous functions to ensure proper reepithelialization, including migration, proliferation, survival, and basement membrane assembly. Moreover, it has become evident in recent years that some integrins can regulate paracrine signals from wound epidermis that stimulate other wound cells involved in angiogenesis, contraction, and inflammation. Importantly, it is likely that abnormal integrin expression or function in the epidermis contributes to wound pathologies such as over-exuberant healing (e.g., hypertrophic scar formation) or diminished healing (e.g., chronic wounds). Many challenges arise from the complex roles that multiple integrins play in wound epidermis, which may be regulated through extracellular matrix remodeling that determines ligand availability [27]. Future research should be focused on understanding of different integrin functions coordination in wound epidermis to determine how best to target them clinically to achieve maximum therapeutic benefit.

Besides biological skin substitutes also another types of skin substitutes of different origin and constitution are used for coverage of partial-thickness burns. In 1998 Ou [28] published a retrospective study of the treatment of scalds by Biobrane. In the period of 2.5 years, 106 patients with scalds with an average BSAB 12.5% had been treated within 24 h postburn. By 24 from these patients, the coverage was aborted because of the low adherence, 14 of them healed spontaneously. By 10 remaining patients, it was necessary to perform the coverage with split skin autografts. The cases of low adherence and accumulation of exudate below Biobrane were by the authors explained by the presence of devitalized upper dermis. Therefore they emphasized accurate initial diagnosis of the depth of burns because, according to them, best results can be obtained only on superficial partial-thickness burns. Patients operated represented 9.4% of all the patients from the study, in the study with cryopreserved skin xenografts 3.6%. Neither the healing within 14 days nor total healing time was stated. The mean time of separation of the skin substitute was 11.1 days (from 3 to 18 days).

In the period immediately after an injury, during initial treatment, it is sometimes difficult to make an exact differentiation of IIa- and IIb-degree burns. Therefore, as more suitable appears the usage of such types of skin substitutes, the adherence of which should not be influenced by this depth range.

On partial-thickness face burns, a biosynthetic skin substitute Transcyte has been used to comply with the changing irregular surfaces of the face. In a comparative study [29], the usage of Transcyte was compared with open technique (bacitracin ointment). The authors observed significantly shorter healing time, shorter time for the wound care, and lower pain in the group treated with biosynthetic skin substitute.

At present, there is still research for the permanent skin substitute the quality of which would be the closest to the ideal skin substitute [30]:

1. Inexpensive
2. Long shelf life
3. Used off the shelf
4. Nonantigenic
5. Durable

6. Flexible
7. Prevents water loss
8. Bacterial barrier
9. Drapes well
10. Easy to secure
11. Grows with child
12. Applied in one operation
13. Does not become hypertrophic
14. Does not yet exist

Also from these ideal properties, the concepts of the characteristics of a good wound dressing by which all burns should be covered in a primary care are more or less coming out [31]:

Considered Essential
1. Maintain moist wound environment
2. Contours easily
3. Non-adherent but retains close contact with the wound
4. Easy to apply and remove
5. Painless on application and removal
6. Cost-effective
7. Protects against infection

Considered Desirable
1. Lasts for 10 days (one application)
2. Minimal dressing changes
3. Waterproof to allow for washing and bathing

Conclusions

From the bioactive properties of cryopreserved skin xenografts, it follows:

1. Their adherence to the fresh wound surface decreases the leakage of electrolytes and salts (little or no exudate under the xenografts); good adherence also reduces the risk of secondary wound contamination.
2. Increased speed of epithelialization by growth factors, which they contain.
3. Faster wound healing is reducing the wound fibroplasia by which the final quality of scars is improved.
4. Unless the total healing time exceeds 14 days, the risk of scar hypertrophy is minimal.

Early application of cryopreserved skin xenografts on all IIa- and IIb-degree scalds can overwhelm the problem with their exact differentiation. Moreover, it decreases the risk of secondary wound deepening which would demand excision and coverage with split skin grafts. From clinical knowledge and experiences obtained from the usage of cryopreserved skin xenografts in given indication, the following results:

1. The treatment algorithm for indication and application of cryopreserved skin xenografts is at authors' clinical workplace on highly professional level.
2. The best effect of the application of skin xenografts is achieved when applied within the first 24 h after trauma, which reduces the risk of secondary infection.
3. According to authors' experiences, the wound surfaces covered with xenografts are during the dressing changes less painful; the consumption of analgetics is also lower.
4. The costs associated with the processing and storage of cryopreserved skin xenografts are 0.2€ per cm^2, which is significantly less amount than that needed for the purchase of synthetic or biosynthetic skin substitutes.
5. According to the results of the author's study, treatment of superficial scald burns with cryopreserved skin xenografts particularly in children proved to be an effective, safe, and reliable method.

The retrospective study proved the clinical efficiency of utilization of cryopreserved skin xenograft for the treatment of partial-thickness scald burns. This method with its treatment effect is fully comparable with the other ones, which are using biological or another type of skin substitutes in given indication, realized at other clinical workplaces.

Appropriate choice of skin substitute should always depend on careful consideration of the characteristics, indications for use, clinical experiences, results of clinical research, and also price of each available skin substitute. Only by this approach, it is possible to achieve the main goal—early wound closure of the best quality.

References

1. Ahuja RB, Bhattacharya S (2002) An analysis of 11,196 burn admissions and evaluation of conservative management techniques. Burns 28:555–561
2. Pruitt BA, Wolf SE, Mason AD (2007) Epidemiological, demographic, and outcome characteristics of burn injury. In: Herndon DN (ed) Total burn care. Elsevier, Philadelphia, pp 14–32
3. Forjuoh SN (2006) Burns in low- and middle-income countries: a review of available literature on descriptive epidemiology, risk factors, treatment, and prevention. Burns 32:529–537
4. Koller J, Orság M, Ondriašová E, Gräffinger I, Bukovcan P (1994) Analysis of 1119 Burn injuries treated at the bratislava burn department during a five-year period. Acta Chir Plast 36(3):67–70
5. Bukovcan P, Koller J (2010) Treatment of partial-thickness scalds by skin xenografts – retrospective study of 109 cases in the three- years period. Acta Chir Plast 52(1):7–12
6. Moserová J, Běhounková E, Vrabec R, Svátek V (1974) Methods of collection and storage of porcine dermoepidermal grafts. Rozhl Chir 53(3):190–194
7. Brans TA, Hoekstra MJ, Vloemans AFPM, Kreis RW (1994) Long-term results of treatment of scalds in children with glycerol-preserved allografts. Burns 20:10–13
8. Leicht P, Muchardt O, Jensen M, Alsbjörn BA, Sørensen B (1989) Allograft vs. exposure in the treatment of scalds – a randomized controlled clinical study. Burns 15:1–3
9. Brown R, Smith KD, Angus McGrouther D (1997) Strategies for cell engineering in tissue repair. Wound Rep Reg 5:212–221
10. Git M, Toda K, Grinell F (1990) Activation of human keratinocyte migration on type 1 collagen and fibronectin. J Cell Sci 96:197–205
11. Ge L, Sun L, Chen J, Mao X, Kong Y, Xiong F, Wuc J, Wei H (2010) The viability change of pigskin in vitro. Burns 36:533–553
12. Brož L, Vogtová D, Königová R (1999) Experience with banked skin in the Prague burn centre. Acta Chir Plast 41:54–58
13. Atiyech BS, Hayek SN, Gunn SW (2005) New technologies for burn wound closure and healing – Review of the literature. Burns 31:94456
14. Pirnay JP, Vandenvelde C, Duinslaeger L, Reper P, Vanderkelen A (1997) HIV transmission by transplantation of allograft skin: a review of the literature. Burns 23(1):1–5
15. Kealey GP (1997) Disease transmissions by means of allograft. J Burn Care Rehabil 18:S10–S11
16. Hermans MHE (2014) Porcine xenografts vs. (cryopreserved) allografts in the management of partial thickness burns: Is there a clinical difference? Burns 40:408–415
17. Csonge L, Pellet S, Szenes A, Istvan J (1995) Antibiotics in the preservation of allograft and xenograft skin. Burns 21(2):102–105
18. Boneva RS, Folks TM (2004) Xenotransplantation and risks of zoonotic infections. Ann Med 36(7):50
19. Wilson CA (2008) Porcine endogenous retroviruses and xenotransplantation. Cell Mol Life Sci 65(21):3399–3412
20. Healy CMJ, Boorman JG (1989) Comparison of E-Z Derm and Jelonet dressings for partial thickness burns. Burns 15(1):52–54
21. Ersek RA, Gadaria U, Surak G, Denton DR (1986) A new wound dressing that solves the retention and storage problems: a clinical history. Contemp Surg 28(3):72–79
22. Chiu T, Pang P, Ying SY, Burd A (2004) Porcine skin: friend or foe? Burns 30:739–741
23. Zajicek R, Matouskova E, Broz L, Kubok R, Waldauf P, Königova R (2011) New biological temporary skin cover Xe-Derma® in the treatment of superficial scald burns in children. Burns 37:333–337
24. Singh R, Purohit S, Chacharkar MP, Bhandari PS, Bath AS (2007) Microbiological safety and clinical efficacy of radiation sterilized amniotic membranes for treatment of second-degree burns. Burns 33:505–510
25. Rab M, Koller R, Ruzicka M, Burda G, Kamolz LP, Bierochs B, Meissl G, Frey M (2005) Should dermal scald burns in children be covered with autologous skin grafts or with allogeneic cultivated keratinocytes?—"The Viennese concept". Burns 31:578–586
26. Ghaffari A, Kilani RT, Ghahary A (2009) Keratinocyte-conditioned media regulate collagen expression in dermal fibroblasts. J Invest Dermatol 129(2):340–347
27. DiPersio CM, Zheng R, Kenney J, Van De Water L (2016) Integrin-mediated regulation of epidermal wound functions. Cell Tissue Res 365:467–482
28. Ou LF, Lee SY, ChenYC YRS, Tang YW (1998) Use of biobrane in pediatric scald burns – experience in 106 children. Burns 24:49–53
29. Demling RH, DeSanti L (1999) Management of partial thickness facial burns (comparison of topical antibiotics and bio-engineered skin substitutes). Burns 25:256–261
30. Tompkins RG, Burke JF (1992) Burn wound closure using permanent skin replacement materials. World J Surg 16:47–52
31. Alsbjörn B, Gilbert P, Hartmann B, Kaźmiersky M, Monstrey S, Palao R, Roberto MA (2007) Van TrierA, VoinchetV. Guidelines for the management of partial-thickness burns in a general hospital or community setting – Recommendations of a European working party. Burns 33:155–160

The Meek Technique in the Treatment of Burns

Paul I. Heidekrueger, Peter Niclas Broer, and Milomir Ninkovic

1 Introduction

To overcome the problem of extensive full thickness third-degree burns, the Meek technique was devised by Meek in 1963 [1]. This involved using a Meek-Wall microdermatome producing widely expanded postage stamp autografts, in which prefolded gauzes were used to gain a regular distribution of the autografts [2]. The technique, with an expansion rate of 1:9, was cumbersome and not frequently used. Tanner et al. (1964) [3] devised meshed skin grafts that improved the treatment of severe full thickness burns that replaced the Meek technique. Kreis et al. (1993) [4] modified the Meek technique by using a different device for cutting the grafts and employed aluminum foil backing to help the expansion of the skin grafts. The mean epithelialization rate was 90% (range 70–100%) within 5 weeks. The Meek technique utilizes small pieces of autograft and has proved to be a practical alternative to mesh grafts when donor sites are limited.

The authors describe their use of the Meek technique in a fair number of cases.

2 Technique

The authors reviewed 148 skin grafting surgeries from 2006 to 2015. The mean percentage body surface burned was 65% (range 50–87%), and full thickness injury occurred in 52% (range 40–81%) (Table 1).

Patients with associated inhalation injury were intubated on admission. Wounds were dressed with Flamazine (Smith & Nephew, Canada) that contained 1% silver sulfadiazine. Fluid resuscitation followed the Parkland formula (Table 2) [5]. For example, a person weighing 75 kg with burns to 20% of his or her body surface area would require $4 \times 75 \times 20 = 6000$ mL of fluid replacement within 24 h. The first half of this amount is delivered within 8 h from the burn incident, and the remaining fluid is delivered in the next 16 h [6]. The burn percentage in adults can be estimated by applying the Wallace rule of nines (see total body surface area): 9% for each arm, 18% for each leg, 18% for the front of the torso, 18% for the back of the torso, 9% for the head, and 1% for the perineum [7].

Surgery was performed on the 3rd to 5th postburn day after stabilization with fluids and electrolytes [8]. The Weck knife and the Humby

P.I. Heidekrueger, M.D. (✉)
Department of Plastic, Reconstructive, Hand, and Burn Surgery, StKM-Klinikum Bogenhausen, Academic Teaching Hospital Technical University Munich, Munich, Germany

Center of Plastic, Aesthetic, Hand and Reconstructive Surgery, University of Regensburg, Regensburg, Germany
e-mail: paul@heidekrueger.net

P.N. Broer • M. Ninkovic
Department of Plastic, Reconstructive, Hand, and Burn Surgery, StKM-Klinikum Bogenhausen, Academic Teaching Hospital Technical University Munich, Munich, Germany

Recent Clinical Techniques, Results, and Research in Wounds (2017)
DOI 10.1007/15695_2017_29, © Springer International Publishing AG
Published Online: 24 October 2017

Table 1 Patient demographics and outcomes

Pat. No.	% 3rd degree	Cause	No. of operations	Outcome
1	43	Flame	2	Survived
2	54	Flame	3	Survived
3	46	Flame	2	Survived
4	67	Inhalation injury	1	Died
5	50	Flame	2	Survived
6	62	Flame	3	Survived
7	72	Flame	3	Survived
8	40	Flame	2	Survived
9	44	Electrical	2	Survived
10	47	Flame	2	Survived
11	41	Inhalation injury	3	Survived
12	46	Flame	2	Died
13	42	Flame	2	Survived
14	47	Flame	2	Survived
15	50	Chemical	2	Survived
16	48	Flame	2	Survived
17	63	Flame	3	Survived
18	74	Flame	2	Died
19	49	Flame	2	Survived
20	41	Flame	2	Survived
21	46	Flame	2	Survived
22	69	Flame	3	Survived
23	45	Inhalation injury	2	Survived
24	74	Inhalation injury	2	Died
25	64	Inhalation injury	3	Survived
26	41	Chemical	2	Survived
27	42	Flame	2	Survived
28	48	Inhalation injury	2	Survived
29	61	Flame	3	Survived
30	43	Flame	2	Survived
31	48	Flame	2	Survived
32	62	Flame	3	Survived
33	59	Inhalation injury	3	Survived
34	42	Flame	2	Survived
35	49	Flame	2	Survived
36	73	Inhalation injury	3	Survived
37	43	Flame	2	Survived
38	50	Flame	2	Survived
39	48	Flame	2	Survived
40	43	Flame	2	Survived
41	40	Electrical	2	Survived
42	49	Flame	2	Survived
43	78	Flame	1	Died
44	46	Flame	2	Survived
45	42	Flame	2	Survived
46	48	Flame	2	Survived
47	77	Flame	3	Survived
48	47	Flame	2	Survived
49	40	Flame	2	Survived
50	55	Inhalation injury	3	Survived
51	64	Inhalation injury	4	Survived
52	46	Flame	2	Survived
53	42	Flame	2	Survived
54	48	Flame	2	Survived
55	41	Flame	2	Survived
56	81	Inhalation injury	1	Died
57	48	Flame	2	Survived
58	41	Flame	2	Survived
59	44	Flame	2	Survived
60	57	Flame	3	Survived
61	73	Inhalation injury	1	Died
62	69	Electrical	3	Survived
63	41	Flame	2	Survived
64	49	Chemical	2	Survived
65	40	Chemical	2	Survived
66	62	Flame	2	Survived
67	64	Inhalation injury	3	Survived

Modified from Almodumeegh A, Heidekrueger PI, Ninkovic M, Rubenbauer J, Hadjipanayi E, Broer PN. The MEEK technique: 10-year experience at a tertiary burn centre. Int Wound J. 2016 In publication

Table 2 Parkland formula

The Parkland formula is mathematically expressed as:
$V = 4 \times m\ (A \times 100)$
V = volume (mL)
m = Mass (kg)
$A \times 100$ = percent of body burned (2° plus 3°)

http://kallus.com/er/calculations/parkland.htm. Accessed 3 Aug 17

knife were used to debride until punctuate bleeding occurred and the layer was grossly judged to be viable. When indicated, the entire skin down to the fascia was removed and the Meek technique was employed to close the wound. Epigard alloplastic material was used to temporarily cover debrided wounds when portions of the debrided areas were not able to be covered immediately.

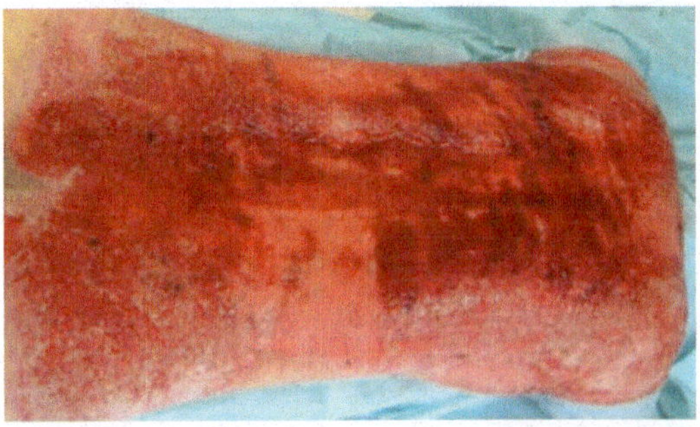

Fig. 1 Tangential excision of full thickness burn of the whole back. Modified from Almodumeegh A, Heidekrueger PI, Ninkovic M, Rubenbauer J, Hadjipanayi E, Broer PN. The MEEK technique: 10-year experience at a tertiary burn centre. Int Wound J. 2016 In publication

This procedure was repeated every 2–5 days, providing the patient's condition allowed for surgical intervention.

The wounds are excised down to the healthy layers and hemostasis secured (Fig. 1). The extent of skin expansion required was determined by the size of the wound and the size of the available skin for grafting. The harvested autograft skin is placed on 42 × 42 mm dampened cork with the dermis side down and trimmed to the required size (Fig. 2). Then it is placed on the carrier block and passed through a modified Meek-Wall dermatome, which contains 13 parallel blades, spaced 3 mm apart that cut the graft but not the cork (Fig. 3). After the first pass, the cork plate is rotated to 90° and passed through the dermatome once more thus cutting the graft in to 14 × 14 square islands measuring 3 × 3 mm.

The cork, with the cut graft in place, is removed. The epidermal side of the graft is sprayed with an adhesive dressing spray (Leukospray, Beiersdorf GmbH, Germany). After about 2–5 min, the sticky surface of the graft is brought into contact with the prefolded

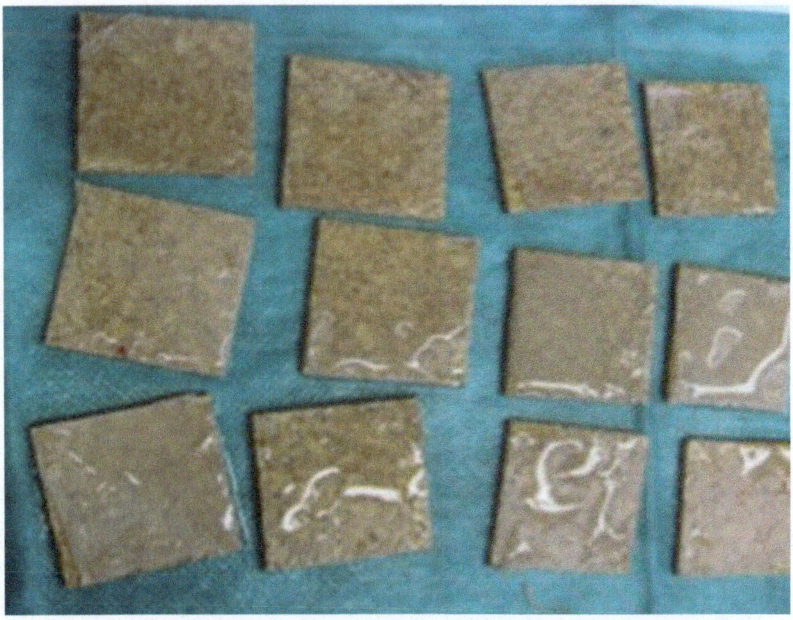

Fig. 2 After harvesting the split-thickness skin grafts in a normal fashion, the grafts are manually cut in pieces and stretched over the 42 × 42 mm moistened cork plate with the inner layer facing downward for final cutting. Modified from Almodumeegh A, Heidekrueger PI, Ninkovic M, Rubenbauer J, Hadjipanayi E, Broer PN. The MEEK technique: 10-year experience at a tertiary burn centre. Int Wound J. 2016 In publication

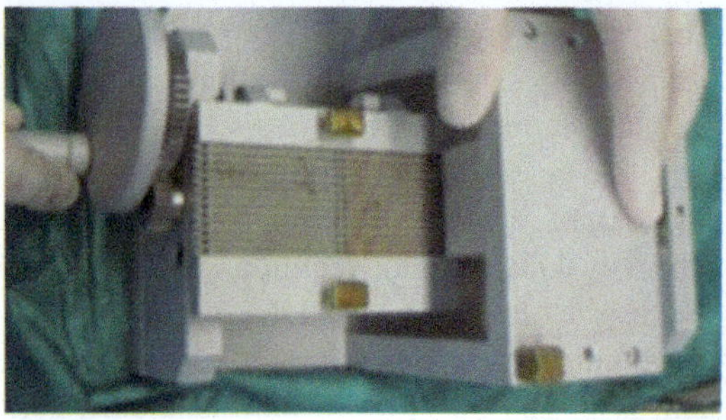

Fig. 3 Meshing of the graft is achieved using the modified Meek-Wall dermatome. Modified from Almodumeegh A, Heidekrueger PI, Ninkovic M, Rubenbauer J, Hadjipanayi E, Broer PN. The MEEK technique: 10-year experience at a tertiary burn centre. Int Wound J. 2016 In publication

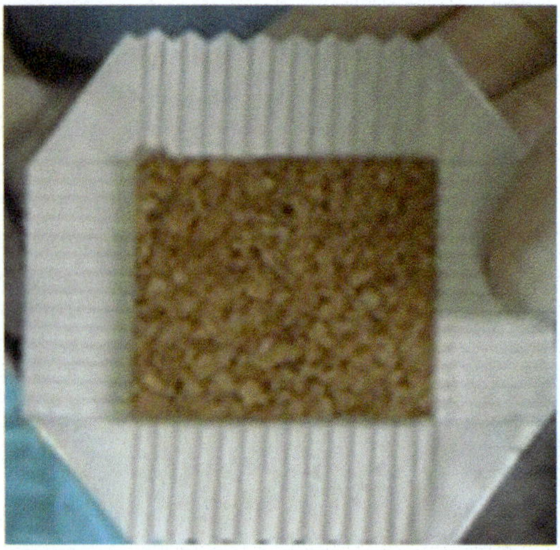

Fig. 4 The cork is removed once the minced grafts are transferred to prefolded polyamide gauze backed with aluminum foil. Modified from Almodumeegh A, Heidekrueger PI, Ninkovic M, Rubenbauer J, Hadjipanayi E, Broer PN. The MEEK technique: 10-year experience at a tertiary burn centre. Int Wound J. 2016 In publication

(pleated) gauze (Fig. 4), and the pleats are pulled out on all the four sides to provide uniform expansion of the islands (Fig. 5), with ratios varying from 1:3 to 1:9. The gauze is pulled steadily in all directions until it was completely smooth and flattened.

The graft is applied to the wound bed and the gauze tacked down with surgical staples (Fig. 6). The grafted wound is covered with Jelonet gauze (Smith & Nephew, Canada) impregnated with Lavasept-Gel (B. Braun Melsungen AG, Germany) containing polihexanide antimicrobial. The operative sites in the trunk and extremities are additionally dressed with Jelonet and wrapped with elastic bandages. After 3–5 days

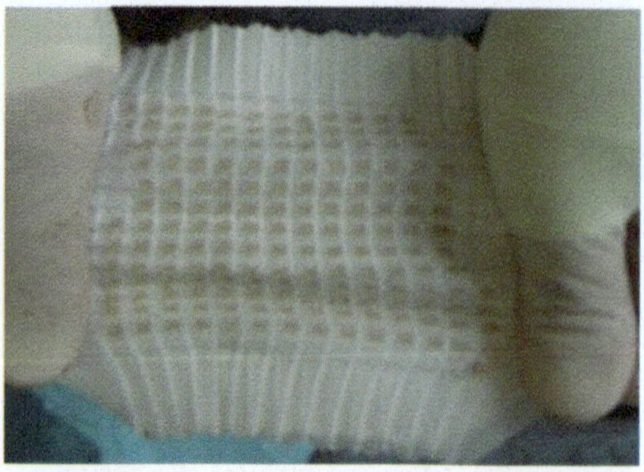

Fig. 5 The gauze is pulled steadily and firmly in all directions until it is completely smooth and flattened. Modified from Almodumeegh A, Heidekrueger PI, Ninkovic M, Rubenbauer J, Hadjipanayi E, Broer PN. The MEEK technique: 10-year experience at a tertiary burn centre. Int Wound J. 2016;14(4):601–5

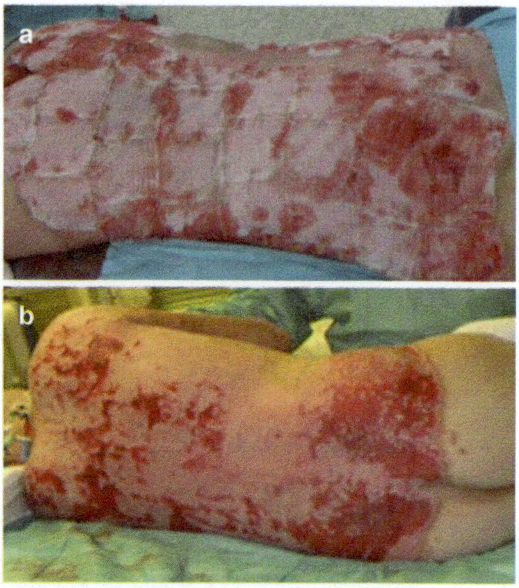

Fig. 6 (**a**) The skin graft is applied onto the wound bed, and the edges of gauze are tacked down with surgical staples. (**b**) The appearance of the grafted wound at the 10th day after the procedure. The viability of the graft was assessed as satisfactory. Modified from Almodumeegh A, Heidekrueger PI, Ninkovic M, Rubenbauer J, Hadjipanayi E, Broer PN. The MEEK technique: 10-year experience at a tertiary burn centre. Int Wound J. 2016;14(4):601–5

the dressing are changed every 2 days. Staples are removed after 7–10 days. One percent silver sulfadiazine cream is used to cover the wound if it showed signs of local infection.

The mean area graft per procedure was 20% (range 15–25%). The viability of the graft as assessed on the 7–10th day was generally in the range of 60–90% (Fig. 6). The average number of operations required was 1–3 (Table 1). When the initial graft application failed, infection or hematoma was most commonly responsible. Although blood replacement was prescribed as needed at surgery, transfusions seldom exceeded two units per session. Functional and aesthetic outcomes of wounds treated with Meek grafts were satisfactory in most instances.

Infection was noted in five patients. There were seven deaths, four dying from respiratory failure due to severe inhalation injury and three dying from septic shock.

3 Discussion

Meshed split-thickness skin grafting has been an accepted method of treatment for severely burned patients at most burn centers [8–10]. However, especially in large area burns, lack of autograft skin may become a limiting factor. In order to prevent wound infection and septicemia, remaining areas of eschar should be excised even if they cannot be covered with autografts immediately [11, 12]. Our experience utilizing the Meek technique in large burn areas suggests that it provides a reliable method to achieve wound healing with expanded autografts. The main advantage is that the Meek technique allows a greater expansion ratio as compared to mesh grafts [12]. The small autografts can be easily applied in contrast to the oftentimes challenging handling of higher expansion (1:6 or 1:9) mesh grafts [4, 13].

Infection, as noted in five of our cases, can be a common cause for graft failure. Similar to others, we found that the thickness of skin grafts used for wound coverage does not seem to affect the incidence of infection. Indeed, small postage stamp skin grafts appear to be more resistant to invasion by microorganisms, and we also observed that spacing and distribution of the micrografts allowed for faster and more uniform epithelialization [12–14].

In our experience, the cosmetic result following the Meek graft technique is comparable with that of widely expanded mesh grafts. A major downside of the micrografting technique is the fact that it is expensive and needs more staff in the operating room to be carried out [14].

Conclusions

When faced with large surface area burns and limited donor sites, the Meek technique is a satisfactory method to cover large wounds. While labor extensive, paying attention to the outlined principles allows achieving good functional and aesthetic results in this challenging patient population.

References

1. Meek CP (1958) Successful microdermagrafting using the Meek wall microdermatome. Ann J Surg 96:557–558
2. Meek CP (1963) Extensive severe burn treated with enzymatic debridement and micro dermagrafting: case report. Am Surg 29(1):61–64
3. Tanner JC, Vandeput JF, Olley JF (1964) The Mesh skin graft. Plast Reconstr Surg 34:287–292
4. Kreis RW, Mackie DP, Vloemans AW, Hermans RP, Hockstram MJ (1993) Widely expanded postage stamp skin grafts using a modified Meek technique in combination with an allograft overlay. Burns 19(2):142–145
5. Parkland formula. http://www.josephsunny.com/medsoft/parkland.html. Accessed 3 July 2017
6. Williams C (2008) Fluid resuscitation in burn patients 1: using formulas. Nurs Times 104(14):28–29
7. Explore Burns Mdcalc, Fluid Requirements, and more! https://www.pinterest/pin/440649144772194432/. Accessed 3 July 2017
8. Alexander JW, Macmillan BG, Law E, Kittur DS (1981) Treatment of severe burns with widely meshed skin autografts and meshed allograft overlay. J Trauma 21:433
9. Gang RK, Arturson G, Hakelius L (1981) The effect of split skin allografts on wound epithelialization from autologous patch grafts. Scand J Plast Reconstr Surg 15:1–4
10. Minanov O, Peterson HD (1997) Burn injury. In: Georgiade GS, Riefkohl R, Scott Levin L (eds) Plastic

maxillofacial and reconstructive surgery, 3rd edn. Williams & Wilkins, Baltimore, p 203
11. Macmillan BG (1958) Early excision of more than 25% of body surface in the extensively burned patients. Arch Surg 77:369
12. Raff T, Hartman B, Wagner H, German G (1996) Experience with modified Meek technique. Burns 38(4):142–146
13. Kreis RW, Mackie DP, Hermans RP, Vloemans AR (1994) Expansion technique for skin grafts: comparison between mesh and meek island (Sandwich) grafts. Burns 20(1):539–542
14. Zermani RGC, Zarabini A, Trivisonno A (1997) Micrografting in the treatment of severely burned patients. Burns 23:604–607

Acute Respiratory Distress Syndrome in the Burn Patient

Robert Cartotto

1 Introduction and Historical Background

It may seem unusual to include a chapter on the acute respiratory distress syndrome (ARDS) in a textbook on wounds. However, patients with burn wounds are clearly at risk of developing this life-threatening complication. While ARDS is most typically seen in patients following major burn injuries, we know that it sometimes occurs even in patients that have relatively small burn wounds. The development of ARDS after a thermal injury is not overly surprising since many of the known risk factors for ARDS, in addition to the burn wound itself, such as smoke inhalation, pneumonia, sepsis, and blood transfusion all commonly occur with burns. As is the case among critically ill patients without burns, ARDS contributes significantly to heightened morbidity and mortality following burn injury.

The first published report of what we now refer to as ARDS appeared in 1967 [1]. In that report Ashbaugh et al. described a syndrome which featured severe respiratory distress, hypoxemia, stiff non-compliant lungs, and the presence of extensive bilateral infiltrates on the chest radiograph. The twelve adult patients in that report suffered from various insults such as multiple trauma, pancreatitis, and pulmonary infections. While none had sustained burns or smoke inhalation, the same syndrome was almost certainly being recognized around the same time in patients that had suffered burn injuries. Dr. Pruitt, in 1970 [2], along with Nash et al., in 1974 [3], reported the autopsy findings of burned adults that had died from pulmonary complications. Extensive diffuse interstitial lung edema and alveolar hyaline membranes—now widely recognized as pathognomonic features of ARDS [4]—were clearly described.

Among critically ill but unburned patients, there was an evolution during the late 1980s and early 1990s of stricter diagnostic criteria and definitions for ARDS, such as a lung injury severity score [5] and the American-European Consensus criteria [6]. This was followed over the ensuing two decades by a massive output of research on ARDS in the critically ill. Most recently, newer diagnostic criteria for ARDS—referred to as the Berlin definition—have been adopted. In parallel but at a slower and delayed pace, the ARDS was also being increasingly recognized and more accurately diagnosed among the burn injured [7–11]. However, relative to the extensive body of research that includes several landmark randomized controlled trials in non-burn patients with ARDS, there has been very little published on ARDS in burn patients. Thus, it must be stated at the outset that almost all our understanding of

R. Cartotto, M.D.
Ross Tilley Burn Centre, Sunnybrook Health Sciences Centre Professor of Surgery, University of Toronto, Toronto, ON, Canada
e-mail: Robert.cartotto@sunnybrook.ca

Recent Clinical Techniques, Results, and Research in Wounds (2017)
DOI 10.1007/15695_2017_30, © Springer International Publishing AG
Published Online: 24 October 2017

ARDS in burn patients comes from translation of research conducted in the non-burn population.

While most of this translation is entirely appropriate, burn patients are a unique subpopulation of the critically ill, and important differences do arise. This chapter will review the epidemiology, pathogenesis, clinical features, and management of ARDS in the burn patient. Important distinctions and areas of controversy that arise because of the unique nature of the burn injury will be emphasized.

2 Pathogenesis

ARDS can be triggered by a wide variety of primary disease processes, which may be classified as pulmonary (i.e., originating in the lung) and extrapulmonary (i.e., originating outside the lung). Pulmonary causes most commonly include pneumonia and gastric aspiration and less commonly lung contusion, near-drowning, and smoke inhalation. The most frequent extrapulmonary causes are sepsis and severe trauma with shock and less frequently multiple blood product transfusions, drug overdose, and pancreatitis [4, 12]. While burns are usually not identified as a specific predisposing condition for ARDS, many of the risk factors such as pneumonia, smoke inhalation, sepsis, shock, and blood product transfusion may occur, often in combination, following thermal trauma. We also make the assumption that the burn wound itself is a rich source of inflammatory mediators which can likely injure the lung secondarily, leading to ARDS. It is not entirely clear how these diverse predisposing conditions ultimately lead to the final pathological and clinical picture of ARDS. What is important is that the insult induces a set of common pathological changes in the lung, regardless of the cause.

The primary change is a breakdown of the pulmonary microvascular endothelial lining and the alveolar epithelial surface—together referred to as the alveolar-capillary barrier. Injury to the alveolar-capillary barrier appears to be mediated by activated neutrophils and a complex bombardment of cytokines and inflammatory mediators including interleukin (IL)-8, tumor necrosis factor α, and various oxygen-free radicals and proteases. These pro-inflammatory mediators probably play a role not only in the initiation of the injury but also in amplification of the local inflammatory process. The net result of the alveolar-capillary disruption is that the interstitial and alveolar spaces are flooded with protein-rich fluid, neutrophils, fibrin, and fibroblasts. Protein-laden hyaline membranes are deposited on the denuded alveolar basement membranes. Normal transport of fluid out of the alveolar space is compromised by injury to the type I epithelial cells that normally predominantly line each alveolus, while injury to the smaller population of type II epithelial cells results in loss of surfactant production, and importantly, disruption of the ability of these cells to differentiate into type I cells which is an important part of the repair process after injury [4]. Following this acute inflammatory phase which can last up to 5–7 days, the lungs of some patients begin to show resolution of the process with resorption and mobilization of the fluid, reduction of inflammation, and repair of the alveolar epithelial lining by the type II cells. Such patients show rapid clinical recovery. Other patients' lungs progress to a fibroproliferative phase in which mesenchymal cells, neovascularization, and procollagen are deposited in the alveolar space. This development of fibrosing alveolitis is a poor prognostic sign and is associated with an increased risk of death [13]. Resolution of this phase is prolonged but again involves mobilization of fluid and protein and restoration of the normal alveolar lining of type I cells through proliferation and differentiation of the type II cells [4].

3 Defining ARDS

Following Ashbaugh et al.'s [1] description of ARDS, the American-European Consensus Conference (AECC) developed clinical diagnostic criteria for the definition of ARDS in 1994 [6]. This AECC definition of ARDS included acute hypoxemia with an arterial partial pressure of oxygen to fraction of inspired oxygen ratio

(PaO_2:FiO_2 ratio) ≤200 mmHg, bilateral infiltrates on chest radiograph, and no clinical evidence of left atrial hypertension or a pulmonary artery wedge pressure (PAWP) measured by the Swan-Ganz catheter of ≤18 mmHg. The AECC definition also identified a condition called acute lung injury (ALI) which had the same features of ARDS but which had milder hypoxemia with a PaO_2:FiO_2 ratio ≤ 300 mmHg. The AECC definition was highly important because it provided a common set of definitions that allowed researchers to study the epidemiology and clinical care of patients over nearly two decades. Several landmark randomized clinical trials including the famous ARDS Network low tidal volume ventilation (ARMA) trial [14] occurred, in part, because uniform definitions could be used to identify and recruit subjects.

However, in 2011, a panel of experts convened in Berlin to address deficiencies of the AECC definition and to develop an updated set of diagnostic criteria [15]. The main concerns with the AECC definitions included an unspecified timing of ARDS onset, misinterpretation of PaO_2:FiO_2 ratio and classification of ALI vs. ARDS, low reliability of the chest radiograph interpretation, inconsistent consideration of positive end-expiratory pressure (PEEP) levels, and the use of the PAWP in the definition.

A revised definition (the Berlin definition) was developed and validated and is shown in Table 1. The key features are (1) elimination of the term ALI and stratification of all ARDS as mild, moderate, and severe based on PaO_2:FiO_2 ratios of 200 to ≤300, 100 to ≤200, and ≤100, respectively, on at least 5 cm H_2O of PEEP, (2) clarified definitions of bilateral infiltrates on chest radiograph and origin of edema, and (3) specification of acute onset within 1 week of a known clinical insult. One of the most important components of the Berlin definition of ARDS is the emphasis on training to improve chest radiograph interpretation and diagnosis of hydrostatic pulmonary edema using a series of clinical vignettes and sample radiographs included in the supplement to the publication (Fig. 1, Table 1) [15].

The Berlin ARDS definition has now been applied to intubated and mechanically ventilated civilian and military burn patients [10, 11, 16–18]. One problem that arises in application of the Berlin ARDS definition to burn patients is the requirement to eliminate "fluid overload" as a possible origin of the pulmonary edema. Most patients with major burns have received substantial amounts of resuscitation fluid by 48–72 h post-injury and have considerable generalized

Table 1 The Berlin definition of ARDS, adapted from Ranieri et al. [15]

Timing	Within 1 week of known clinical insult or worsening respiratory symptoms
Chest radiograph	Bilateral opacities that are not fully explained by effusions, lobar/lung collapse, or nodules
Origin of edema	Respiratory failure is not fully explained by cardiac failure or fluid overload. An objective assessment (e.g., by echocardiography) is required to exclude hydrostatic edema if no risk factor is present
Oxygenation	Mild ARDS, 200 mmHg < PaO_2/FiO_2 ≤ 300 mmHg with PEEP ≥5 cm H_2O; moderate ARDS, 100 mmHg < PaO_2/FiO_2 ≤ 200 mmHg with PEEP ≥5 cm H_2O; severe ARDS, PaO_2/FiO_2 ≤ 100 mmHg with PEEP ≥5 cm H_2O

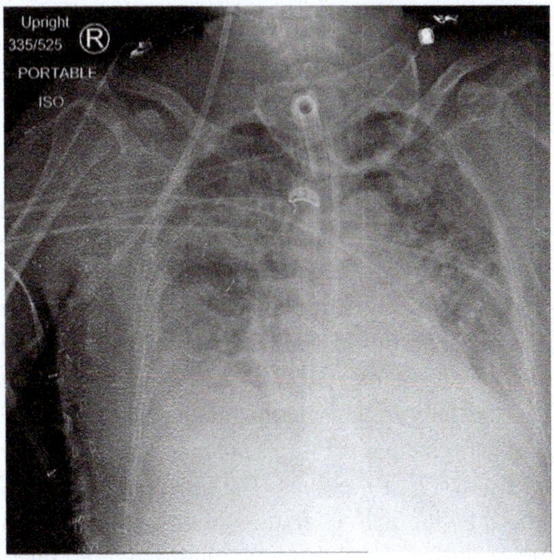

Fig. 1 Typical radiograph from an ARDS patient showing diffuse bilateral infiltrates

edema. Technically, these patients could be considered "volume overloaded." One study in burn patients [10] attempted to address this problem by using the clinical vignettes provided with the ARDS definition [15] and by making specific evaluations of clinical descriptions, use of diuretics, and echocardiography reports to rule out "volume overload" and hydrostatic pulmonary edema. That study found no difference in 24- and 48-h fluid resuscitation volumes between patients with no ARDS and those with ARDS [10]. Another study involving both combat casualty burns as well as civilian burns also was not able to identify any independent relationship between very high resuscitation volume (≥250 mL/kg/24 h) and the development of moderate or severe ARDS [11]. Thus, while it appears that resuscitation fluid volumes are not a cause of ARDS in burn patients, the clinician must be exceedingly careful to ensure that respiratory distress from suspected ARDS is not simply due to hydrostatic pulmonary edema from liberal fluid resuscitation.

4 Epidemiology

ARDS remains an epidemiologic challenge despite the various advances in developing a definition of ARDS [12]. There is no diagnostic test for ARDS such as a blood test or a biopsy. The PaO_2:FiO_2 ratio—essential to the diagnosis and determination of ARDS severity—can fluctuate substantially in the same patient on the same day just with changes in FiO_2 or positive end-expiratory pressure (PEEP) settings. The interpretation of the chest radiograph is fraught with difficulty and unreliability [12, 19]. Notwithstanding these important limitations, the reported incidence of ARDS in all patients over the past half century has ranged between 3.65 and 81.0 new cases per 100,000 person-years [12, 20, 21]. The recent Large Observational Study to Understand the Global Impact of Severe Acute Respiratory Failure (LUNG-SAFE) used the Berlin definition and found that the prevalence of ARDS was 10.4% of all ICU admissions and 23.4% of those that were mechanically ventilated [22]. This study showed that across all critically ill patients, ARDS is a global problem which is probably under-recognized. The most important risk factors appear to be pneumonia, non-pulmonary sepsis, aspiration, and trauma [12]. The mortality rate may be as high as 40% as reported in LUNG-SAFE22.

In the scenario of patients with burns that have been mechanically ventilated for at least 24–48 h, two studies found that the prevalence of ARDS using the Berlin definition ranges between 34% [11] and 43% [10]. The prevalence of moderate to severe ARDS was 29% in both studies [10, 11]. Older studies that used the AECC definitions found that the prevalence of ARDS in mechanically ventilated burn patients ranged between 40% 9 and 54% [8]. It is important to note that patients with ALI (PaO_2/FiO_2 200–300 Hg) were not included in those studies meaning that those prevalences represent what would be considered moderate to severe ARDS by the Berlin definition. This suggests that the prevalence of moderate to severe ARDS in burn patients has dropped over the past 15–20 years. One possible explanation, to be discussed under mechanical ventilation, may be the widespread adoption of strict lung-protective ventilation strategies, which were not in use during the earlier studies. The factors that have been identified as significant independent predictors for the development of moderate to severe ARDS in mechanically ventilated burn patients include the extent of full-thickness burn [10], as well as age, injury severity score, the presence of acute kidney injury, and pneumonia 11. Surprisingly, inhalation injury did not turn out to be a significant independent predictor of development of moderate or severe ARDS [10, 11]. The onset of ARDS usually takes place within the first week after the burn injury and occurred at a median of 4 days in the most recent studies on ARDS in burn patients [10, 11]. One study specifically examined the precipitating risk factor prior to onset of ARDS and found that the burn injury either alone or with inhalation injury preceded the onset of ARDS in 66% of cases, while ventilator-associated pneumonia (24%), sepsis (9%), and gastric aspiration (1%) were identified as the likely preceding primary event [10]. The mortality rates for burn patients that develop moderate or severe ARDS have been reported at 21–44% and 50–60%, respectively [10, 11]. Increasing severity of ARDS is associated with prolonged duration of mechanical ventilation as well as increased mortality [10, 11, 16].

5 Management Strategies for ARDS in the Burn Patient

The management of ARDS in any patient, including those with burns, is entirely supportive. At the present time there are no treatments that will halt or reverse the onset and progress of ARDS. Nevertheless, a variety of strategies to optimize the supportive care of patients with ARDS have been developed over the past two decades. Many of these approaches are guided by evidence from large high-quality randomized controlled trials (RCTs).

5.1 Conventional Mechanical Ventilation

The great paradox in mechanical ventilation of the patient with ARDS is that while mechanical ventilation is almost always needed, and is at times lifesaving, the process of mechanical ventilation inflicts further damage to the lungs affected by ARDS. This process is referred to as ventilator-induced lung injury (VILI). Thus, all current approaches to mechanical ventilation of patients with ARDS revolve around the goal of reducing VILI and in turn diminishing morbidity and mortality related to VILI while still providing life-sustaining oxygenation and gas exchange. One aspect of VILI occurs because large regions of the dependent portions of the lungs are unexpanded and not aerated, leaving only a small portion of remaining aerated lung (the "baby lung") [23] to receive the entire tidal volume of each mechanical breath. If large tidal volumes are used, alveoli in this region of the lung are subjected to repetitive and injurious cyclical stretch and over-distention, referred to as "volutrauma" [24]. Ventilation with high lung volumes can also produce gross barotrauma including pneumothoraces and pneumomediastinum. Another aspect of VILI occurs in other regions of the lung, especially at the interface between aerated and atelectatic lung, where alveoli are unstable and not held open through the tidal breath cycle. Here, low tidal volume ventilation exposes alveoli in these regions to repetitive cyclic opening and closing with each breath. This produces mechanical stress and strain forces that damage the alveoli, a process referred to as "atelectrauma" [24]. The injury produced by these various mechanical forces generates the release of pro-inflammatory mediators that inflict not only an additional traumatic insult to the alveolar-capillary units (referred to as "biotrauma") but also systemic translocation of these mediators as well as bacteria from the lung, leading to multiple organ damage [24].

Lung-protective ventilation strategies (LPVS) are used to limit VILI and have three key elements: small tidal volumes to limit volutrauma, the use of higher PEEP levels to reverse low lung volume atelectrauma, and the use of recruitment maneuvers (sustained application of high airway pressure) to open or "recruit" collapsed regions of the lung to make the lung more homogeneous. However, application of these principles is hampered by the heterogeneous nature of ARDS. The lung pathology not only may vary from patient to patient but also varies tremendously within the lungs of an individual patient. Some regions of the lung (typically the upper non-dependent portions) remain open, some areas may intermittently open and close, while other regions (typically the inferior-posterior dependent portions) remain closed and never receive any ventilation. Heterogeneity of the pathology leads to regional heterogeneity in the ventilation. For example, a lower tidal volume and lower PEEP strategy may reduce volutrauma to the open aerated regions of the lung but could contribute to atelectrauma in the unstable areas. Conversely, the use of a higher PEEP setting might reduce atelectrauma in one region while producing over-distention and tidal hyperinflation in another.

5.1.1 Low Tidal Volumes

This approach is designed to minimize over-distention of the open aerated parts of the lung affected by ARDS. The landmark ARMA trial by the ARDS Network Investigators found that the use of a 6 mL/kg predicted body weight (PBW) tidal volume (Vt) led to a significant 9% absolute reduction in mortality (40–31%) compared to the use of a 12 mL/kg PBW Vt in adults with ARDS [14]. Plasma levels of inflammatory biomarkers were reduced in the low Vt group, which suggested that less pulmonary biotrauma had occurred. Consequently it is recommended to maintain Vt as close to 6 mL/kg PBW as possible, during mechanical ventilation. Plateau pressures also should be kept <30 cm H_2O since this was a consistent intervention in the low Vt arm.

5.1.2 Higher PEEP

This approach is designed to keep unstable alveoli open and to avoid cyclic atelectrauma. Three large RCTs have been conducted to compare higher vs. lower PEEP settings while using a low tidal volume ventilation strategy [25–27]. These studies each used somewhat different approaches to determine higher vs. lower PEEP, and none individually showed any significant reduction in mortality with higher PEEP. However, a recent patient data level meta-analysis of these three trials found that in the subset of patients with moderate and severe ARDS ($PaO_2/FiO_2 \leq 200$ mmHg), higher PEEP settings (approximately 15 cm H_2O on day 1) were associated reduced time on the ventilator and improved survival [28]. The lowest acceptable limit of PEEP is probably 5 cm H_2O. Levels below this result in underinflation of the lung and are probably harmful. Several approaches have been described to determine the PEEP level. These include the use of a table that arbitrarily dictates PEEP based on the FiO_2, the use of the highest PEEP setting that optimizes oxygenation while still allowing an acceptable Vt and keeping the PPLAT within acceptable limits (generally ≤30 cm H_2O), and bedside manual titration of the PEEP based on assessment of compliance and "recruitability" of the lung.

5.1.3 Recruitment Maneuvers

During a recruitment maneuver, a higher than normal inflation pressure (usually ≥35 cm H_2O) is briefly applied to the lungs, typically for 20–40 s. This is done to "open the lung" and recruit atelectatic regions and lessen the overall heterogeneity of the ventilation. We do not know if the use of recruitment maneuvers leads to a better outcome from ARDS, and the intervention carries risks of causing hemodynamic compromise and barotrauma [24].

5.1.4 Special Considerations in the Burn Patient

Burn patients were not included in the major trials on ventilation during ARDS. Several unique characteristics of the major burns patient may affect the application of currently accepted lung-protective ventilation approaches. One is the reduced chest wall compliance that results from soft tissue edema from fluid resuscitation, restrictive eschar, or even tight skin grafts on the chest and abdomen. Another is inhalation injury which features narrowing or obstruction of the conducting airways and loss of surfactant in the alveoli. Yet another is the hypermetabolic response that is accompanied by a profound increase in minute ventilation. Notably, a small RCT involving burn patients with ARDS found that inadequate oxygenation and ventilation occurred in a large proportion of patients, especially those with an inhalation injury, when currently accepted low tidal volume ventilation strategies were employed [29].

The use of low tidal volumes in a burn patient with ARDS that has poor chest compliance and/or an inhalation injury with airway narrowing could contribute to the development of atelectasis from underinflation. One retrospective study spanning a 30 year period in pediatric burn patients with inhalation injury found that low tidal volume ventilation (mean 9 mL/kg) was associated with more atelectasis, longer periods of mechanical ventilation, and a higher incidence of ARDS than a higher tidal volume approach (mean 15 mL/kg) [30]. In our experience, in hypermetabolic burn patients with ARDS that already have abnormally high minute ventilation requirements, strict application of a 6 mL/kg PBW tidal volume sometimes leads to what appears to be "air hunger," dyssynchrony with the ventilator, and hypercapnia. While hypercapnia may be tolerated to an extent ("permissive hypercapnia"), adjustments to the ventilator mode and increases in inspiratory flow rate are often needed.

The altered chest wall mechanics in a burn patient with an edematous or eschar-restricted thorax or abdomen may affect the interpretation of plateau pressure and the setting of a PEEP level. The work of Talmor et al. [31] using trans-esophageal pressures to measure transpulmonary pressure is particularly important in this regard. The transpulmonary pressure (PTP) is the opening or distending pressure required to inflate the lung and is calculated as the difference between the alveolar pressure (PALV) and the surrounding pleural pressure (PPL), hence PTP = PALV—PPL.

PALV is easy enough to estimate during mechanical ventilation as the pressure in the proximal airway during an end-inspiratory pause in flow (i.e., the plateau pressure). Measurement of PPL on the other hand is problematic but can be approximated by measuring the pressure in the mid-esophagus using a specialized nasogastric tube with a pressure transducer.

It is conceivable that a burn patient on mechanical ventilation with a stiff chest wall from edema and eschar or intra-abdominal edema from large volume fluid resuscitation might have a PPL of approximately 25 cm H_2O. In this case, a plateau pressure of 30 cm H_2O, which otherwise would be considered at the upper limit of being acceptable, may not be that concerning because the PTP is only 30–25 = 5 cm H_2O. Recognition of this might allow more leeway with plateau pressure limits. Similarly, as was shown by Talmor et al. [31], the transpulmonary end-expiratory pressure in this case might be considerably lower than that set and recorded at the airway opening, meaning that a much higher PEEP setting is required.

5.2 Unconventional Mechanical Ventilation

Various unconventional modes of mechanical ventilation have been evaluated for patients with ARDS. The most widely known is high-frequency oscillatory ventilation (HFOV), in which very small, sub-dead space tidal volumes are delivered at high frequency (between 6 and 15 Hz) while maintaining a constant sustained mean airway pressure. HFOV can dramatically improve oxygenation and was found to significantly reduce mortality in a meta-analysis of eight RCTs, (total of 419 patients) [32], but two recent large RCTs both found that HFOV did not improve survival and may have contributed to worse outcomes among adult patients with ARDS [33, 34]. Consequently, HFOV is not recommended as part of the primary ventilation strategy in ARDS, but it is sometimes considered as a "rescue approach" for patients with refractory oxygenation failure. In the burn patient with ARDS, there are two unique considerations surrounding the use of HFOV. The first is that HFOV is generally unsuccessful in improving oxygenation when the patient has had a preceding inhalation injury [35]. This is probably because effective lung recruitment, which is the physiologic basis of HFOV, is impaired by narrowing or obstruction of the conducting airways. The second is that the recent large RCTs on HFOV did not include burn patients and enrolled large numbers of subjects with ARDS related to pneumonia [33, 34]. In many instances ARDS follows the burn injury itself rather than developing from pneumonia. Hypothetically, the lungs affected by burn-related ARDS may differ in terms of "recruitability" from the lungs where ARDS arises from pneumonia, based upon our understanding of ARDS heterogeneity and possible differences between "pulmonary" and "extrapulmonary" ARDS [36]. Thus we do not have a complete answer on whether HFOV may be suitable in some cases of burn-related ARDS.

High-frequency percussive ventilation (HFPV) using the volume diffusive respirator (VDR) delivers very small high-frequency tidal breaths with cyclic variations in mean airway pressure and regular passive exhalation to a predetermined baseline continuous positive airway pressure. This mode is a mainstay in the ventilatory care of patients with inhalation injury, but it has also been applied to burn patients with ARDS. A randomized controlled trial comparing HFPV to protective low tidal volume (LTV) conventional ventilation in burn patients with ARDS, found that a significantly higher proportion of patients in the LTV arm had inadequate oxygenation and ventilation and required "rescue" by crossover to HFPV [29]. This difference was even more pronounced in patients that had also sustained an inhalation injury.

Airway pressure release ventilation (APRV) is a mode in which patients breathe spontaneously at regularly fluctuating high and low levels of continuous positive airway pressure. The major benefit of this approach is that patients are less heavily sedated and breathe spontaneously, which appears to confer benefit to lung opening, maintenance of diaphragmatic activity, and hemodynamics. However, the use of spontaneous breathing modes such as APRV and pressure support ventilation during ARDS has not been extensively studied, and concerns surround the potential of generating very high transpulmonary pressures and tidal volumes with strong spontaneous breathing on these modes.

5.3 Prone Position

When a patient with ARDS is repositioned from supine to prone, the posterior and inferior lungs are freed from the weight of the heart and mediastinum, the lungs more naturally fill the thoracic cavity, the overall end-expiratory lung volume is increased, and there is an overall improvement in homogeneity of ventilation. This usually produces an increase in oxygenation by improving matching of ventilation and perfusion to the dorsal lung regions [24]. The most recent RCT found that >16 h/day of prone positioning in adults with severe ARDS (PaO_2:FiO_2 ratio <150 on a FiO_2 >0.6) led to significant reductions in 28- and 90-day mortality [37]. A 2015 Cochrane systematic review of RCTs on prone positioning in ARDS concluded that three groups of patients were most likely to derive a survival benefit from prone positioning (PP): those with severe hypoxemia, those where PP was instituted early, and those where PP was used >16 h/day [38]. PP is not without risk, and important potential complications include displacement, obstruction or loss of the airway, anterior pressure sores especially on the face, dislodgement of vascular access lines and chest tubes, and external pressure on the eyes with the risk of orbital compartment syndrome.

Special consideration must be given to prone positioning in a burn patient with ARDS. Loss of the airway in a patient with significant facial and/or neck edema with a difficult airway could be catastrophic. The same concern applies to loss of an indwelling vascular catheter in an edematous major burn patient with difficult vascular access. Anterior burns and recent skin grafts may be harmed during PP. The act of turning a massively burned and edematous patient prone is itself a difficult challenge. Undoubtedly PP in the burn patient with ARDS should only be considered in more extreme cases of oxygenation failure and only after due consideration of the above risks. Several experienced personnel under careful direction are needed to perform this intervention safely. One retrospective study has evaluated prone positioning in a cohort of burn patients and found that oxygenation was improved compared to baseline prior to being positioned prone. No airway dislodgements were reported though it should be noted that nearly 60% of the patients already had tracheostomies [39].

5.4 Neuromuscular Blocking Agents ("Paralytics")

Neuromuscular blocking agents (NMBAs) are sometimes used to paralyze the patient during severe ARDS to allow more precise delivery of low tidal volume ventilation and achieve better control over airway pressures and synchrony with the ventilator. There is no specific evidence to guide the use of NMBAs in burn patients with ARDS. In other critically ill patient populations with moderate to severe ARDS (i.e., a PaO_2:FiO_2 ratio <150), a meta-analysis of data from three RCTs found that initiation of a 48-h continuous infusion of cisatracurium within 36–48 h of ARDS diagnosis led to a significant reduction in 28-day mortality [40]. There does not appear to be any long-term risk of weakness from neuromyopathy from this intervention [41]. Thus, it is probably reasonable to consider a short course of pharmacological paralysis in burn patients early during severe ARDS, to facilitate strict adherence to protective low tidal volume and pressure-limited ventilation.

5.5 Inhaled Vasodilators

When a vasodilator is administered by inhalation, it selectively increases blood flow to the lung regions that are being ventilated, thus improving matching of ventilation and perfusion. The immediate effect is an improvement in oxygenation as measured by the PaO_2:FiO_2 ratio. The most widely studied agent is inhaled nitric oxide (iNO). A meta-analysis of 12 RCTs in adults with ARDS found that administration of iNO increased oxygenation but did not have any important effect on duration of ventilation or mortality [42]. Burn patients with ARDS similarly respond to iNO with an improvement in oxygenation [43], but there are no large-scale studies from which to determine any other effects on outcomes. Currently iNO is used as a "rescue agent" in patients with severe life-threatening oxygenation failure. It is usually started at 5 ppm and can be titrated up to 20 ppm. If no effect is seen after a short course, the agent is usually stopped. A newer but less well-studied agent that has similar effects on oxygenation is inhaled prostacyclin.

5.6 Other Pharmacologic Interventions

Numerous studies have attempted to alter the course and outcome of ARDS using a variety of anti-inflammatory drugs. A detailed review of this topic is beyond the scope of this chapter. However, a recent systematic review and meta-analysis of 23 RCTs conducted since 2003 in adults with ARDS found that the use of late low-dose methylprednisolone, neutrophil elastase inhibitors, *N*-acetylcysteine, granulocyte-macrophage colony-stimulating factor (GM-CSF), surfactant, or intravenous salbutamol had no effect on survival [40]. Consequently, none of these agents are recommended in the management of any patient with ARDS at this time.

5.7 Avoidance of Fluid Overload

While increased capillary permeability in the lung is a central component of ARDS, increased hydrostatic pressure can worsen extravascular lung water. Thus, there has been long-standing concern during the management of ARDS patients about avoiding fluid overload, in order to minimize deleterious hydrostatic forces. This concept was examined by the ARDS Network Investigators in a trial involving 1000 ARDS patients that were randomized to either a conservative fluid strategy (achieving approximately zero net daily fluid balance over 7 days) to a liberal fluid strategy (which achieved approximately 1 L/day positive fluid balance over 7 days) [44]. The conservative strategy led to better oxygenation and less time on the ventilator, although no significant survival benefit was identified. A subsequent meta-analysis of trials that compared fluid-conservative or "de-resuscitative" approaches to fluid liberal or "usual care" in ARDS found that fluid-conservative strategies led to significant increases in the number of ventilator-free days in hospital [45].

Translation of these findings to the burn patient is particularly difficult. We recognize that extremely large volumes of resuscitation fluid may need to be administered to a major burn patient by 48–72 h. Available studies show that ARDS onset occurs at a median of 4 days after burn injury [10, 11]. Hence, in many cases ARDS may overlap the resuscitation phase. Conservative fluid management and especially administration of diuretics have the potential to compromise burn resuscitation. Furthermore, most major burn patients have substantial insensible fluid losses from their wounds. Thus, determination of a daily fluid balance is inaccurate and often errs on the side of a falsely positive balance. Thus, application of a fluid-conservative strategy in a major burn patient with ARDS should be considered very carefully. This is not to say that there is a role for liberal fluid provision, but rather, strict attention should be given to providing the least amount of fluid that achieves adequate organ perfusion and function.

6 Managing the Burn Wound

It is axiomatic that deep partial-thickness and full-thickness burns should be excised and closed within 3–5 days of injury. The burn wound itself may be the inflammatory source that is stimulating the development of ARDS. In our experience, the median day of ARDS onset was postburn day 4, and in the majority of cases, the only identifiable risk factor for ARDS development was the burn wound [10]. Therefore, in a major burn patient, surgical debridement of the wounds should not be deferred because of respiratory deterioration related to ARDS. This approach requires an anesthesiologist that is experienced and familiar with the intraoperative and perioperative care of a critically ill patient with ARDS. We will sometimes use the patient's ICU ventilator in the OR during burn surgery, and we have gained considerable experience using HFOV as a temporary intraoperative ventilator approach in patients with moderate to severe ARDS [46]. Prone positioning in the OR to debride the large posterior surfaces is often necessary and does not need to be avoided. This often actually improves the oxygenation, which should not be surprising given our current understanding of the physiological changes induced by prone positioning in the ARDS patient.

Conclusions

Burn patients are at risk of developing ARDS. Approximately 30–40% of mechanically ventilated burn patients develop ARDS. Most of the approach to ARDS in the burn patient has been translated from an extensive body of research on ARDS in non-burn patients conducted over the last two decades. An important feature of ARDS in the burn population is that it appears to arise most often from the burn injury itself, in contrast to critically ill non-burn patients where ARDS predominantly arises from pneumonia and sepsis. Management of ARDS in the burn patient is largely supportive and includes the use of low tidal volume and pressure-limited mechanical ventilation, avoidance of fluid overload, and treatment of the primary source(s) that may be "driving" the lung process, including early excision of the burn wound and control of infective sources. Severe ARDS may require further intervention with ventilation in the prone position, short-term use of pharmacologic paralysis, and inhaled vasodilators. Burn patients that develop moderate to severe ARDS are at risk of more prolonged mechanical ventilation and higher mortality.

References

1. Ashbaugh DG, Bigelow DB, Petty TL, Levine BE (1967) Acute respiratory distress in adults. Lancet 2:319–323
2. Pruitt BA Jr, DiVincenti FC, Mason AD, Foley FD, Flemma RJ (1970) The occurrence and significance of pneumonia and other pulmonary complications in burned patients: comparison of conventional and topical treatments. J Trauma 10:519–531
3. Nash G, Foley FD, Langlinais PC (1974) Pulmonary interstitial edema and hyaline membranes in adult burn patients. Hum Pathol 5:149–160
4. Ware LB, Matthay MA (2000) The acute respiratory distress syndrome. N Engl J Med 342(18):1334–1349
5. Murray JF, Matthay MA, Luce JM, Flick MR (1988) An expanded definition of the adult respiratory distress syndrome. Am Rev Respir Dis 138(3):720
6. Bernard GR, Artigas A, Brigham KL, Carlet J, Falke K, Hudson L, Lamy M, Legall JR, Morris A, Spragg R (1994) The American-European Consensus Conference on ARDS: definitions, mechanisms, relevant outcomes, and clinical trial coordination. Am J Respir Crit Care Med 149:818–824
7. Hollingshead TC, Saffle JR, Barton RG, Craft BW, Morris SE (1993) Etiology and consequences of respiratory failure in thermally injured patients. Am J Surg 166:592–597
8. Dancey DR, Hayes J, Gomez M, Schouten D, Fish J, Peters W, Slutsky AS, Stewart TE (1999) ARDS in patients with thermal injury. Intensive Care Med 25:1231–1236
9. Liffner G, Bak Z, Reske A, Sjöberg F (2005) Inhalation injury assessed by score does not contribute to the development of acute respiratory distress syndrome in burn victims. Burns 31:263–268
10. Cartotto R, Li Z, Hanna S, Spano S, Wood D, Chung K, Camacho F (2016) The acute respiratory distress syndrome(ARDS) in mechanically ventilated burn patients: an analysis of risk factors, clinical features, and outcomes using the Berlin ARDS definition. Burns 42:1423–1432
11. Sine CR, Belenkiy SM, Buel AR, Waters JA, Lundy JB, Henderson JL, Stewart IJ, Aden JK, Liu NT,

Batchinsky A, Cannon JW, Cancio LC, Chung KK (2016) Acute respiratory distress syndrome in burn patients: a comparison of the Berlin and American-European definitions. J Burn Care Res 37:e461–e469
12. Pham T, Rubenfeld GD (2017) The epidemiology of acute respiratory distress syndrome: a 50th birthday review. Am J Resp Crit Care Med 195(7):860–870
13. Martin C, Papazian L, Payan MJ, Saux P, Gouin F (1995) Pulmonary fibrosis correlates with outcome in adult respiratory distress syndrome: a study in mechanically ventilated patients. Chest 107:196–200
14. Acute Respiratory Distress Syndrome Network, Brower RG, Matthay MA, Morris A, Schoenfeld D, Thompson BT, Wheeler A (2000) Ventilation with lower tidal volumes as compared with traditional tidal volumes for acute lung injury and the acute respiratory distress syndrome. N Engl J Med 342:1301–1308
15. Ranieri VM, Rubenfeld GD, Thompson BT, Ferguson ND, Caldwell E, Fan E, Camporota L, Slutsky AS (2012) Acute respiratory distress syndrome: the Berlin definition. J Am Med Assoc 307:2562–2533
16. Belenkiy SM, Buel AR, Cannon JW, Sine CR, Aden JK, Henderson JL et al (2014) Acute respiratory distress syndrome in wartime military burns: application of the Berlin criteria. J Trauma Acute Care Surg 76:821–827
17. Waters JA, Lundy JB, Aden JK, Sine CR, Buel AR, Henderson JL, Liu NT, Lundy JB, Renz EM, Batchinsky AI, Cancio LC, Chung KK (2015) A comparison of acute respiratory distress outcomes between military and civilian burn patients. Mil Med 180:56–59
18. Bordes J, la Croix G, Esnault P, Goutorhe P, Cotte J, Dantzer E, Meaudre E (2014) Comparison of the Berlin definition with the American-European Consensus definition for acute respiratory distress syndrome in burn patients. Burns 40:562–567
19. Meade MO, Cook RJ, Guyatt GH, Groll R, Kachura JR, Bedard M, Cook DJ, Slutsky AS, Stewart TE (2000) Interobserver variation in interpreting chest radiographs for the diagnosis of acute respiratory distress syndrome. Am J Resp Crit Care Med 161:85–90
20. Li G, Malinchoc M, Cartin-Ceba R, Venkata CV, Kor DJ, Peters SG, Hubmayr RD, Gajic O (2011) Eight year trend of acute respiratory distress syndrome : a population based study in Olmsted County, Minnesota. Am J Resp Crit Care Med. 183:59–66
21. Sigurdsson MI, Sigvaldason K, Gunnarsson TS, Moller A, Sigurdsson GH (2013) Acute respiratory distress syndrome; nationwide changes in incidence, treatment and mortality over 23 years. Acta Anaesthesiol Scand 57:37–45
22. Bellani G, Laffey JG, Pham T, Fan E, Brochard L, Esteban A, Gattinoni L, vanHaren F, Larsson A, McAuley DF et al (2016) Epidemiology, patterns of care, and mortality for patients with acute respiratory distress syndrome in intensive care units in 50 countries. J Am Med Assoc 315(8):788–800
23. Gattinoni L, Presenti A (2005) The concept of "baby lung". Intensive Care Med 31:776–784
24. Slutsky AS, Ranieri M (2013) Ventilator-induced lung injury. N Engl J Med 369:2126–2136
25. Brower RG, Lanken PN, MacIntyre N, Matthay MA, Morris A, Ancukiewicz M, Schoenfeld D, Thompson BT, National Heart, Lung, and Blood Institute ARDS Clinical Trials Network (2004) Higher vs lower positive end-expiratory pressures in patients with the acute respiratory distress syndrome. N Engl J Med 351:327–336
26. Meade MO, Cook DJ, Guyatt GH, Slutsky AS, Arabi YM, Copper DJ, Davies AR, Hand LE, Zhou Q, Thabane L, Austin P, Lapinsky S, Baxter A, Russell J et al (2008) Ventilation strategy using low tidal volumes, recruitment maneuvers, and high positive end-expiratory pressures for acute lung injury and acute respiratory distress syndrome; a randomized controlled study. J Am Med Assoc 299:637–645
27. Mercat A, Richard JC, Vielle B, Jaber S, Osman D, Diehl JH, Lefrant JY, Prat G, Richecoeur J, Nieszkowska A, Gervais C, Baudot J, Bouadma L, Brochard L, Expiratory Pressure (Express) Study Group (2008) Positive end-expiratory pressure setting in adults with acute lung injury and acute respiratory distress syndrome: a randomized controlled trial. J Am Med Assoc 299:646–655
28. Briel M, Meade M, Mercat A, Brower RG, Talmor D, Walter D, Slutsky AS, Pullenayegum E, Zhou Q, Cook D, Brochard L, Richard JC, Lamontagne F, Bhatnagar N, Stewart TE, Guyatt G (2010) Higher vs lower positive endexpiratory pressure in patients with acute lung injury and the acute respiratory distress syndrome: systematic review and meta-analysis. J Am Med Assoc 303:865–873
29. Chung KK, Wolf SE, Renz EM, Allan PF, Aden JK, Merrill GA, Shelhamer MC, King BT, White CE, Bell DG, Schwacha MG, Wanek SM, Wade CE, Holcomb JB, Blackbourne LH, Cancio LC (2010) High frequency percussive ventilation and low tidal volume ventilation in burns; a randomized controlled trial. Crit Care Med 38:1970–1977
30. Sousse LE, Herndon DN, Andersen CR, Ali A, Benjamin NC, Granchi T, Suman OE, Mlcak RP (2015) High tidal volume decreases adult respiratory distress syndrome, atelectasis, and ventilator days compared with low tidal volume in pediatric burned patients with inhalation injury. J Am Coll Surg 220:570–578
31. Talmor D, Sarge T, Malhotra A, O'Donnell CR, Ritz R, Lisbon A, Novack V, Loring SH (2008) Mechanical ventilation guided by esophageal pressure in acute lung injury. N Engl J Med 359:2095–2104
32. Sud S, Sud M, Friedrich JO, Meade MO, Ferguson ND, Wunsch H, Adhikari NK (2010) High frequency oscillation in patients with acute lung injury and acute respiratory distress syndrome (ARDS): systematic review and meta-analysis. BMJ 340:c2327
33. Ferguson ND, Cook DJ, Guyatt GH, Mehta S, Hand L, Austin P, Zhou Q, Matte A, Walter SD, Lamontagne F, Granton JT, Arabi YM, Arroliga AC, Stewart TE, Slutsky AS, Meade MO, OSCILLATE Trial Investigators; Canadian Critical Care Trials Group (2013) High frequency oscillation in early acute respiratory distress syndrome. N Engl J Med 368:795–805

34. Young D, Lamb SE, Shah S, MacKenzie I, Tunnicliffe W, Lall R, Rowan K, Cuthbertson BH, OSCAR Study Group (2013) High Frequency oscillation for acute respiratory distress syndrome. N Engl J Med 368:806–813
35. Cartotto R, Walia G, Ellis S, Fowler R (2009) Oscillation after inhalation: High frequency oscillatory ventilation in burn patients with the acute respiratory distress syndrome and co-existing smoke inhalation injury. J Burn Care Res 30:119–127
36. Gattinoni L, Pelosi P, Suter PM, Pedoto A, Vercesi P, Lissoni A (1998) Acute respiratory distress syndrome caused by pulmonary and extra-pulmonary disease: different syndromes? Am J Resp Crit Care Med 158:3–11
37. Guérin C, Reignier J, Richard JC, Beuret P, Gacouin A, Boulain T, Mercier E, Badet M, Mercat A, Baudin O, Clavel M, Chatellier D et al (2013) Prone positioning in severe acute respiratory distress syndrome. N Engl J Med 368:2159–2168
38. Bloomfield R, Noble DW, Sudlow A (2015) Prone position for acute respiratory failure in adults. Cochrane Database Syst Rev 11:CD008095
39. Hale DF, Cannon JW, Batchinsky AI, Cancio LC, Aden JK, White CE, Renz EM, Blackbourne LH, Chung KK (2012) Prone positioning improves oxygenation in adult burn patients with severe acute respiratory distress syndrome. J Trauma Acute Care Surg 72:1634–1639
40. Duggal A, Ganapathy A, Ratnapalan M, Adhikari NKJ (2015) Pharmacological treatments for acute respiratory distress syndrome: a systematic review. Minerva Anestesiol 81:567–588
41. Hraiech S, Forel JM, Papazian L (2012) The role of neuromuscular blockers in ARDS: benefits and risks. Curr Opin Crit Care 18:495–502
42. Adhikari NK, Burns KE, Friedrich JO, Granton JT, Cook DJ, Meade MO (2007) Effect of nitric oxide on oxygenation and mortality in acute lung injury. Systematic review and meta-analysis. BMJ 334:779
43. Musgrave MA, Fingland R, Gomez M, Fish J, Cartotto R (2000) The use of inhaled nitric oxide as adjuvant therapy in patients with burn injuries and respiratory failure. J Burn Care Rehabil 21(6):551–557
44. National Heart, Lung, and Blood Institute Acute Respiratory Distress Syndrome (ARDS) Clinical Trials Network, Wiedemann HP, Wheeler AP, Bernard GR, Thompson BT, Hayden D, deBoisblanc B, Connors AF Jr, Hite RD, Harabin AL (2006) Comparison of two fluid management strategies in acute lung injury. N Engl J Med 354:2564–2575
45. Silversides JA, Major E, Ferguson AJ, Mann EE, McAuley DF, Marshall JC, Blackwood B, Fan E (2017) Conservative fluid management or deresuscitation for patients with sepsis or acute respiratory distress syndrome following the resuscitation phase of critical illness: a systematic review and meta-analysis. Intensive Care Med 43:155–170
46. Walia G, Jada G, Cartotto R (2011) Anesthesia and intraoperative high-frequency oscillatory ventilation during burn surgery. J Burn Care Res 32(1):118–123

Chemical Burns to the Eye

Melvin A. Shiffman

1 Introduction

1.1 Chemical Burns

Chemical burns to the eye are divided into alkali burns, acid burns, and irritants. Substances with pH values less than 7 are acids, while numbers higher than 7 are alkaline; the higher or lower the number, the more acidic or basic a substance is and the more damage it can cause.

Alkali burns are more dangerous than acid burns. Alkalis have a high pH that can penetrate the surface of the eye and can cause severe injury to both the external structures like the cornea and the internal structures like the lens. Common alkaline substances contain the ammonium hydroxide, sodium hydroxide, lye (caustic potash), potassium hydroxide, magnesium, and lime. Some of the common alkaline substances include bleach, metal polish, oven cleaner, baking powder, and oven cleaner. Strong alkalis are corrosive and can break down the proteins that make up items such as grease and hair.

Acid burns from chemicals with a low pH and are usually less severe than alkali burns because they do not penetrate into the eye as readily as alkaline substances. The exception is a hydrofluoric acid burn, which is as dangerous as an alkali burn. Acids usually damage only the very front of the eye; however, they can cause serious damage to the cornea and also may result in blindness.

Irritants that have a neutral pH tend to cause more discomfort to the eye than actual damage.

Recovery from acid and alkali burns depends on the depth of the injury. The four grades of burns are:

Grade 1: Should recover fully.
Grade 2: There may be some scarring, but vision should recover.
Grade 3: Vision will usually be impaired to some degree.
Grade 4: Damage to vision will likely be severe.

2 Symptoms

Early signs and symptoms of a chemical eye burn are pain, redness, irritation, tearing, inability to keep the eye open, blurred vision, sensation of something in the eye, and swelling of the eyelids. There can be severe pain, epiphora, and blepharospasm [1]. Blurred vision is a true loss of vision that indicates a significant serious burn. Glaucoma and cataracts can occur but may be delayed by hours to days.

M.A. Shiffman, M.D., J.D.
Private Practice, Tustin, CA, USA
e-mail: shiffmanmdjd@gmail.com

Recent Clinical Techniques, Results, and Research in Wounds (2017)
DOI 10.1007/15695_2017_31,
Published Online: 24 October 2017

3 Medical Treatment in the Emergency Room

The physician should request the exact substance that splashed the eye in order to understand the severity. The immediate therapy is continued washing of the eye. No standard exists for the amount of washing required. Usually, least 1 L of fluid is used. Depending on the type of chemical involved, the pH of the eye should be determined, and the washing should continue until the pH returns to normal. Topical anesthetic eye drops are used to numb the eye to make washing less painful.

Any solid foreign material should be wiped or irrigated away in the eye. An eye examination using an eye chart should be used to determine how well the patient can see.

Eyelids are carefully assessed. Fluorescein may be used to help determine the extent of damage. The degree of limbal, corneal, and conjunctival involvement at the time of injury is critically associated with prognosis [2]. Until the surface of the eye heals, it is at a higher risk for an infection; therefore, topical antibiotics may be used in the form of eye drops or ointments. Any significant burn, especially an alkali or hydrofluoric acid burn, probably requires admission to the hospital. For more significant injuries, prolonged therapy with eye medication may be necessary in order heal the eye. Topical steroids are used to reduce inflammation and to facilitate healing early in the recovery period after a chemical injury. These medications should be used judiciously under the guidance of an ophthalmologist, because they can cause long-term complications, such as infection and glaucoma. Other medications used to support corneal repair include topical citrate and ascorbate drops, oral antibiotics, and vitamin C. If the eye pressure is too high, glaucoma medications may be used temporarily to control the pressure. Pain medications by the mouth may be necessary, and dilating eye drops are often also used to control pain and to aid recovery.

4 Surgery

If the eye has been seriously damaged, surgery may be needed. If the surface of the eye is severely damaged, limbal stem cells may be damaged and may require replacement to prevent surface scar. Surgery to the eyelids to restore good eyelid closure to protect the eye may be needed. If the cornea becomes opaque (or cloudy), a corneal transplant may be required. Cataracts can occur, and surgery may be needed depending on the degree of vision loss and whether it affects quality of life and ability to function. In children cataracts may need surgery because cataracts can interfere with the development of normal vision.

4.1 Amniotic Membrane Transplantation

Amniotic membrane transplantation (AMT) can be used both as a graft which can provide a basement membrane for epithelialization and/or as a patch where it acts as a biological bandage contact lens [3–6]. Arora et al. [6] concluded that "Amniotic membrane transplantation with fresh amniotic membrane increases patient comfort and reduces inflammation. In mild burns, AMT alone restores corneal and conjunctival surfaces. In moderate to severe burns, it probably reduces conjunctival scarring sequelae..." However, AMT does not prevent the limbal stem cell deficiency aftereffects that may require limbal stem cell transplantation. In the acute stage, amniotic membrane transplantation may have a protective role against progressive melting and perforation.

4.2 Hydrodelamination

Sugita and Kondo [7] used hydrodelamination by injecting saline solution into the cornea to enhance identification and removal of the deep stromal fibers. Because finding an actual cleavage plane over the Descemet's membrane (also called DM, posterior elastic lamina, posterior limiting lamina, lamina elastica posterior, and membrane of Demours [8]) is difficult, balance salt solution was injected into the four quadrants to make the trephined area opaque. A limbal paracentesis is performed to lower the intraocular pressure and to decrease the incidence of perforation during dissection. Then, lamellar dissection is performed down to the DM. A modification of this technique has been introduced by Ameyem and Anwar (2000) [9].

4.3 Layer-by-Layer Manual Dissection

The basic technique of layer-by-layer manual dissection is still useful in some cases such as preexisting corneal perforation, strong stroma to DM adhesion (e.g., deep stromal scarring), or inadequate visualization [10]. Partial, 2/3 total corneal thickness, trephination is performed and followed by stromal removal using a bevel-up crescent knife. "Layer-by-layer stromal dissection and resection is repeated as one approaches DM. In spite of being effective, this procedure is technically challenging, time consuming, leaves a relatively rough surface and has a high rate of perforation of DM" [10].

4.4 Viscoelastic Dissection Technique

The cornea is partially trephined to approximately two-thirds of its thickness, and then anterior stromal resection is performed. Air is injected into the anterior chamber, and the remaining stroma is dissected down to the DM. A small pocket is created, and ophthalmic viscoelastic device (OVD) is injected into the pocket to complete the detachment of DM from the posterior stroma. The procedure of recipient preparation is completed by excising the overlying stroma [11].

4.5 Corneal Transplantation

Corneal transplantation is performed for visual rehabilitation of patients with extensive stromal scarring and variability of corneal thickness and irregularity. Full-thickness transplants can be performed successfully, once the limbal stem cell deficiency has been addressed:

1. Tectonic keratoplasty is the surgical grafting of corneal material in an area where corneal tissue has been lost [12].
2. Penetrating keratoplasty is where a full thickness of the cornea is removed and replaced with donor tissue.
3. Tectonic penetrating keratoplasty is used as the last resort in burn patients in cases with severe thinning, large descemetoceles, and impending or frank corneal perforation.
4. Lamellar keratoplasty has evolved from partial removal of the corneal stroma to deep anterior lamellar keratoplasty (DALK), in which corneal stroma is removed down to DM [13].
5. Deep anterior lamellar keratoplasty (DALK) removes and replaces the pathologic corneal stroma while preserving host healthy endothelium, which eliminates the risk of endothelial graft rejection and has a reduced effect on the endothelial cell count [14–17].

4.6 Air-Assisted Manual Dissection (Archila's Technique)

Archila, in 1984 [18], used a technique that is considered to be the predecessor of other techniques of maximum depth dissection. "After partial thickness trephination, intrastromal air is injected until the cornea becomes opaque and then manual deep dissection is carried out down to the DM, which appears clear using either a sharp crescent or a blunt spatula. This step can be repeated as long as microbubbles are visible, making sure that there is still a layer of stroma that protects the DM against perforation" [18].

4.7 Anwar's Big-Bubble Technique

The big-bubble technique introduced by Anwar and Teichmann [19] provides a planned, safe, quick, and consistent exposure of DM by the injection of air deep into the stroma. The surface of the DM appears smooth after successful stromal resection. Approximately 80% of the corneal thickness is trephined, and a small-gauge needle attached to a 5 mL syringe is inserted into the deep stroma aiming toward the center of the cornea. Air is gently injected into the deep stroma until a round, well-demarcated big bubble is formed extending to the borders of trephination. After big-bubble formation, debulking of the anterior two-thirds of the corneal stroma is performed with a crescent blade. This is followed by a peripheral paracentesis and excision of the remaining stroma using blunt scissors [13].

4.8 Air-Guided Deep Stromal Dissection (Melles' Technique)

Melles et al. [20] introduced a technique of dissection in which the anterior chamber aqueous is completely replaced with an air bubble to generate a mirror reflection of the spatula inserted into the stromal pocket allowing determination of the depth of dissection and locating the DM. A half-depth scleral incision, 5.0 mm in width, is made 1–2 mm from the limbus at the 12-o'clock surgical position. A sclerocorneal tunnel is dissected extending 1.0 mm into the clear cornea. Through the scleral pocket, a beveled spatula is inserted and gradually advanced into the deep stroma until the mirror reflex of the tip of the spatula narrows to a fine line indicating a corneal depth of about 95%. The blunt spatula is advanced beyond the border of the ongoing trephination, and the air bubble is partially evacuated. The DM is kept away from the overlying stroma using an ophthalmic viscoelastic device (OVD) to displace the posterior corneal layers toward the iris to avoid damaging these layers during trephination. The preparation of the recipient bed is completed by trephination and excision of the anterior stroma [13].

Conclusions

Chemical burns of the eye and lids are treated as an emergency with adequate washing to completely remove the chemical. Examination should evaluate all aspects of the eye and lids and attempts be made to identify the chemical(s) that caused the burn to determine further treatment.

References

1. Fish IR, Davidson RS (2010) Management of ocular thermal and chemical injuries, including amniotic membrane therapy. Curr Opin Ophthalmol 21(4):317–321
2. Eslani M, Baradaran-Rafii A, Movahedan A, Djalilian AR (2014) The ocular surface chemical burns. J Ophthalmol 2014:Article ID 196827
3. Shimmura S, Shimazaki J, Ohashi Y, Tsubota K (2001) Antiinflammatory effects of amniotic membrane transplantation in ocular surface disorders. Cornea 20(4):408–413
4. Dua HS, Gomes JAP, King AJ, Maharajan VS (2004) The amniotic membrane in ophthalmology. Surv Ophthalmol 49(1):51–77
5. Bouchard CS, John T (2004) Amniotic membrane transplantation in the management of severe ocular surface disease: indications and outcomes. Ocul Surf 2(3):201–211
6. Arora R, Mehta D, Jain V (2005) Amniotic membrane transplantation in acute chemical burns. Eye (Lond) 19(3):273–278
7. Sugita J, Kondo J (1997) Deep lamellar keratoplasty with complete removal of pathological stroma for vision improvement. Br J Ophthalmol 81:184–188
8. Descemet's membrane - Wikipedia. https://en.wikipedia.org/wiki/Descemet%27s_membrane. Accessed 21 Jul 2017
9. Amayem AF, Anwar M (2000) Fluid lamellar keratoplasty in keratoconus. Ophthalmology 107:76–80
10. Tsubota K, Kaido M, Moden Y, Satake Y, Bissen-Miyajima H, Shimazaki J (1998) A new surgical

technique for deep lamellar keratoplasty with single running suture adjustment. Am J Ophthalmol 126:1–8
11. Melles GR, Lander F, Rietveld FJ, Remeijer L, Beekhuis WH, Binder PS (1999) A new surgical technique for deep stromal, anterior lamellar keratoplasty. Br J Ophthalmol 83:327–333
12. The American Heritage® ((2007) Medical dictionary. Houghton Mifflin Company, Boston
13. Karimian F, Feizi S (2010) Deep anterior lamellar keratoplasty: indications, surgical techniques and complications. Middle East Afr J Ophthalmol 17(1): 28–37
14. Panda A, Bageshwar LM, Ray M, Singh JP, Kumar A (1999) Deep lamellar keratoplasty versus penetrating keratoplasty for corneal lesions. Cornea 18: 172–175
15. Terry MA (2000) The evolution of lamellar grafting techniques over twenty-five years. Cornea 19:611–616
16. Watson SL, Ramsay A, Dart JK, Bunce C, Craig E (2004) Comparison of deep lamellar keratoplasty and penetrating keratoplasty in patients with keratoconus. Ophthalmology 111:1676–1682
17. Morris E, Kirwan JF, Sujatha S, Rostron CK (1998) Corneal endothelial specular microscopy following deep lamellar keratoplasty with lyophilised tissue. Eye 12:619–622
18. Archila EA (1984–1985) Deep lamellar keratoplasty dissection of host tissue with intrastromal air injection. Cornea 3:217–218
19. Anwar M, Teichmann KD (2002) Big-bubble technique to bare Descemet's membrane in anterior lamellar keratoplasty. J Cataract Refract Surg 28:398–403
20. Melles GR, Rietveld FJ, Beekhuis WH, Binder PS (1999) A technique to visualize corneal incision and lamellar dissection depth during surgery. Cornea 18:80–86

Severe Burns: Pathogenesis and Prevention of Infection

James C. Hurley

1 Introduction

Patients with severe burns are at high risk of developing infection. They often have prolonged length of stay in an intensive care unit-type environment during which they are at high risk of acquiring a serious infection. This chapter focuses on the infections and associated mortality risk occurring in patients with severe burns together with a critical review of the scant evidence base of management strategies for their detection and prevention [1, 2].

2 Pathogenesis

Intact skin is a major barrier to microbial invasion, and its disruption by a severe burn injury creates a major breech in host defenses (Fig. 1). Additional to being a physical barrier, the deeper layers of intact skin form the scaffolding for the host immune response to microbial invasion. These active and passive defensive properties of the skin are lost to a greater or lesser degree as part of a burn injury (Fig. 2).

Although the thermal injury itself often has the effect of sterilizing the burn wound surface, these surfaces eventually become colonized with a range of microorganisms. The colonized burn wound surface becomes a source for potential infection and sepsis. Sepsis relating to thermal injuries is believed to account for the majority of deaths among patients who survive the initial resuscitation phase.

The origins of the microorganisms which may contribute to subsequent infection are broadly classified as endogenous versus exogenous [3]. The endogenous microorganisms arise from the patient's own colonizing flora located within the bowel and also including that which remains within the skin following the thermal injury [4]. The exogenous flora arises from the patient's environment via cross transmission [5].

Additional to the skin damage of a thermal injury due to flame is the possibility of inhalation injury [6]. Inhalation injury may be a consequence of direct injury to the lower respiratory tract consequent to the inhalation of heat and steam. Compounding this direct lung injury is a chemical injury resulting in edema and bronchociliary damage which impairs clearance of bacteria. This together with endothelial damage leads to bacterial colonization with the potential for bronchopneumonia to develop. Inhalation injury typically becomes most apparent only in the days

J.C. Hurley, M.B.B.S., D.Med.Sc, M.Epi, Ph.D.
Department of Internal Medicine Service, Ballarat Health Services, Ballarat, Australia

Rural Health Academic Center, Melbourne Medical School, University of Melbourne,
Parkville, VIC, Australia
e-mail: jamesh@bhs.org.au; hurleyjc@unimelb.edu.au

Recent Clinical Techniques, Results, and Research in Wounds (2017)
DOI 10.1007/15695_2017_32, © Springer International Publishing AG
Published Online: 24 October 2017

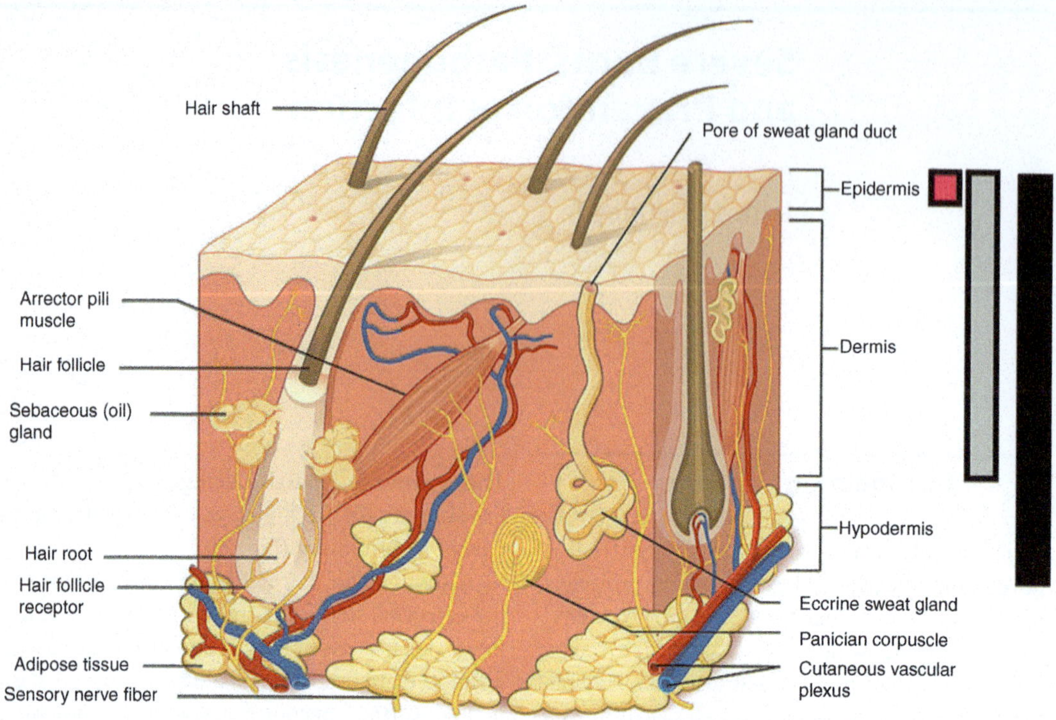

Fig. 1 A diagram of the structure of the skin and the corresponding extent of burn injury. The colored bars on the right indicate first-degree (*red*), second-degree (*gray*), and third-degree (*black*) burns. Diagram modified from https://commons.wikimedia.org/wiki/File:501_Structure_of_the_skin.jpg. Accessed 2/9/17

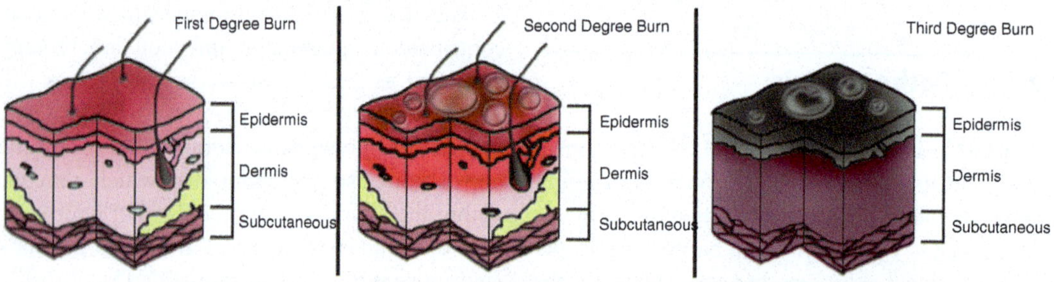

Fig. 2 Diagram of the extent of burn injury In: Burn. https://en.wikipedia.org/wiki/Burn. Accessed 2/9/17

after admission to hospital. The exact frequency of occurrence of inhalation injury is uncertain due to the lack of uniform defining criteria in many of the studies. However, it can be expected to be a common complication of burn injuries with a higher total body surface area injured and those requiring intensive care unit admission [6, 7]. The presence of inhalation injury is a risk factor for increased mortality [8, 9].

3 Prognosis

There are also a range of factors which increase the risk of fatal outcome in patients with severe burns. There are three principle risk factors identified for a fatal outcome being age over 60 years, total burn surface area (TBSA) over 40%, and the presence of inhalation injury [10]. The chart used to estimate the extent of burn injury is shown in Fig. 3.

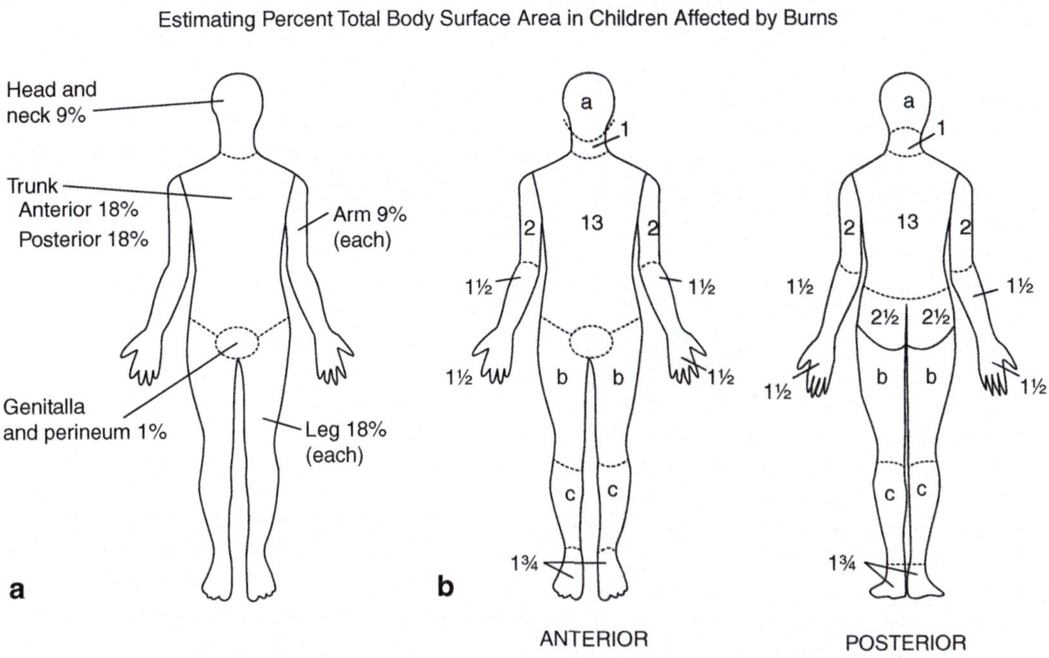

Relative percentage of body surface areas (% BSA) affected by growth

	0 yr	*1 yr*	*5 yr*	*10 yr*	*15 yr*
a–½ of head	9½	8½	6½	5½	4½
b–½ of 1 thigh	2¾	3¼	4	4¼	4½
c–½ of 1 lower leg	2½	2½	2¾	3	3¼

Fig. 3 Estimation of total body surface area (TBSA) of burn injury in children. *In: Burns (injury) Wikipedia.* https://simple.wikipedia.org/wiki/Burn_(injury). Accessed 2/9/17

The mortality risk of severe burn injuries is closely related to the total burn surface area (Fig. 4) [11–16]. Moreover, the length of hospital stay is similarly related. Each 1% increase in total burn surface area greater than 20% corresponds to an increase in hospital length of stay by approximately 1 extra day [12].

In a systematic review of over 180,000 burn injuries among 76 reports originating from European burn centers, a range of variables that might be associated with poor outcome were examined [7]. This mortality range noted in this review among these burn-injured patients, for which most but not all were hospitalized, was 1.4% and 18%. Of note, the most common cause of early mortality, being at less than 48 h after burn injury, was shock and inhalation injury. Late deaths after burn injury were commonly due to multi-organ failure in two thirds and respiratory complications in up to one third of deaths in these reports. However, the exact frequency of some of these complications is confounded by the uncertain prevalence of underlying premorbid conditions such as preexisting pulmonary disease due to smoking and age over 60 years.

Overall mortality appears to have fallen over the last four decades prior to 2016 [7, 14]. In some burn centers, the mortality has fallen by as much as a half [17, 18]. The exact reasons for the decline in mortality are not clear, but one possible factor is the decline in burn total body surface area injured among those requiring hospital admission. Another factor is the improvements in the care of patients with severe burns. A recent meta-analysis of six studies of early

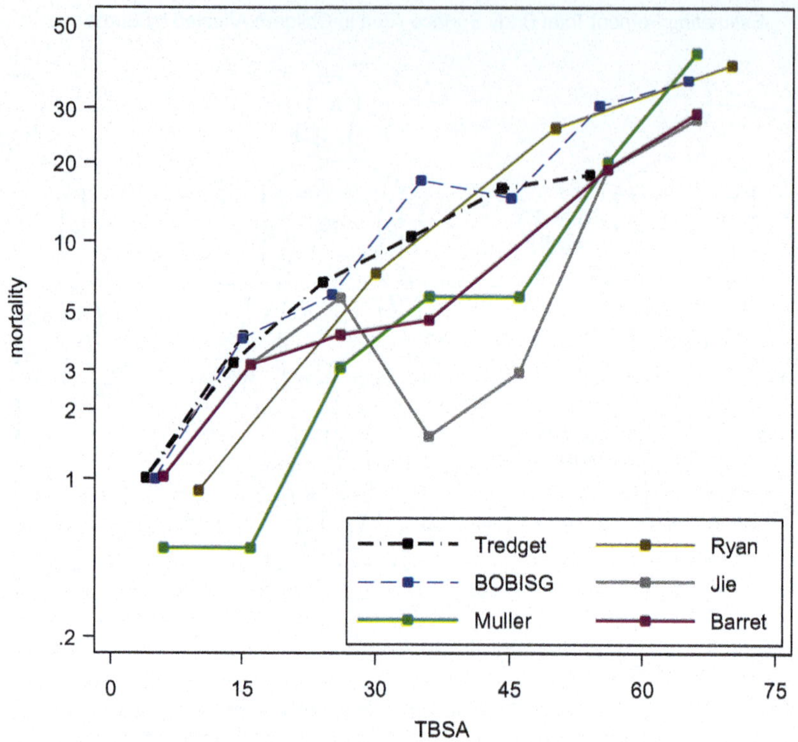

Fig. 4 Relationship between mortality proportion (note logit scale) and total burn surface area (TBSA) among adult patients (age >15 years) in six published studies; Tredget et al. 1990, Canada [11]; Ryan et al. 1998, USA [12]; Barret et al. 1998, Spain [13], Muller et al. 2001, Australia [14]; Jie et al. 2003, China [15] and Blot et al. 2008, Brussels [16]. The study populations ranged in size from 1705 to 5321 burns patients

excision of burns demonstrated that this practice is beneficial in reducing mortality and length of hospital stay [19]. The one possible detrimental consequence is the greater volume of blood loss and potential need for blood products. A recent multicenter study of blood transfusion use in patients with severe burns has demonstrated that the number of infections per patient increased with each unit of blood transfused (odds ratio, 1.13; $p < 0.001$; [20]).

4 Microbiology

The organisms responsible for infections in patients with severe burns have changed over the years [21–31]. In the pre-antibiotic era, *Streptococci* were a common cause of infection arising from burn wounds. In more recent times, infections due to *Pseudomonas* and *Staphylococci* are common. Most recently the USA300 strain of MRSA has emerged sporadically [26]. In particular, *Pseudomonas aeruginosa* has remained not only one of the commonest isolates among burns patients with bacteremia in the past 50 years but also has maintained a high associated mortality proportion [27]. Fungal infection occurs in patients with extended length of stay following severe burns and is associated with increased mortality [28–30]. The relationship between type of isolate and mortality risk is not simple and is discussed further below.

The diagnosis of infection complicating burn injury and the identification of the pathogenic microorganisms responsible for the infection are not simple [31]. The current "gold standard" for proving the presence and type of infection is a quantitative culture of a tissue biopsy together with a histological verification of the presence of microbial invasion [32–34]. This is of particular importance for difficult-to-treat infections such as fungal infections [35].

Unfortunately, quantitative tissue culture is not convenient enough to be routine, and surface swabs are frequently employed as type of surrogate marker. The reliability of surface swabs is uncertain, and comparative studies are difficult to interpret [33]. What studies are available indicates the potential for major discrepancies between surface swabs and tissue biopsy cultures with respect to both the type and the quantity of microorganisms. Also, the results of sequential swabs and biopsies may not agree over time. Moreover, a surface swab will not be able to indicate the presence or not of a concomitant inflammatory process to indicate the presence of an infection.

The exact rankings of microorganisms that occur vary in relation to the site of infection and the time since the burn injury [22]. Also, some bacteria acquired in the intensive care unit, such as *Acinetobacter* [36], are known to have regional variations in their incidence worldwide [37]. The exact prognostic significance of specific isolates may be difficult to determine given the vagaries in burn wound microbiology.

5 Epidemiology and Patient Risk Factors

The question arises as to the extent to which the presence of infection impacts on the mortality risk. This is most relevant in relation to bloodstream infections [38–44]. This is a question of great interest as it infers a preventable mortality fraction if only these infections could be prevented. A simplistic comparison of the mortality of those with bacteremia versus without, for example, would suggest that the mortality is higher versus those with bacteremia (Table 1) (Fig. 5). However, this simplistic comparison overlooks any factors which contributed both to the risk of bacteremia and also likely to the higher risk of mortality and hence confounds the analysis [40–46].

This question has importance beyond those with severe burn injuries, and the question has arisen in the context of the population of intensive care unit patients generally. It is an intriguing question given that only the minority of ICU patients with sepsis have a bloodstream infection detected, even among those with a fatal outcome. How much the detection of bacteremia influences the outcome of sepsis has been closely investigated in relation to Gram-negative bacteremias among the population of ICU patients in general, not limited to patients with severe burns. The answer is surprisingly elusive [46–52].

Outside of the context of burn-related infections, there is no doubt that severe bacteremic infections with pathogenic Gram-negative bacteria, for example, occurring in an outbreak setting in previously health people, as, for example, with

Table 1 Mortality of patients with severe burns injury and bacteremia

Author (year)	Ref.	Bacteremia[a]	TBSA	Patients	Mortality	
			(%)	(n)	(n)	(%)
Sittig et al. (1988)	[42]	Bacteremia	10	16	0	0
Sittig et al. (1988)	[42]	Bacteremia	30	19	3	16
Sittig et al. (1988)	[42]	Bacteremia	50	20	3	15
Sittig et al. (1988)	[42]	Bacteremia	70	25	6	36
Sittig et al. (1988)	[42]	Bacteremia	90	13	11	85
Brusselaers et al. (2010)	[39]	Bacteremia	41	76	9	12
Brusselaers et al. (2010)	[39]	No bacteremia	29	103	18	17
Appelgren et al. (2002)	[38]	Bacteremia	25	22	6	27
Appelgren et al. (2002)	[38]	No bacteremia	5	208	7	3
Mahar et al. (2010)	[41]	Pseudomonas	42	8	3	38
Mahar et al. (2010)	[41]	Gram negative	49	35	4	11
Ceniceros et al. (2015)	[40]	Bacteremia	40	73	18	25

[a]Bacteremia: In all studies except [41], the bacteremia included both Gram-negative and Gram-positive bacteremias. In [41] the outcome for patients with *Pseudomonas aeruginosa*, bacteremias were compared to those with non-*Pseudomonas* Gram-negative bacteremias

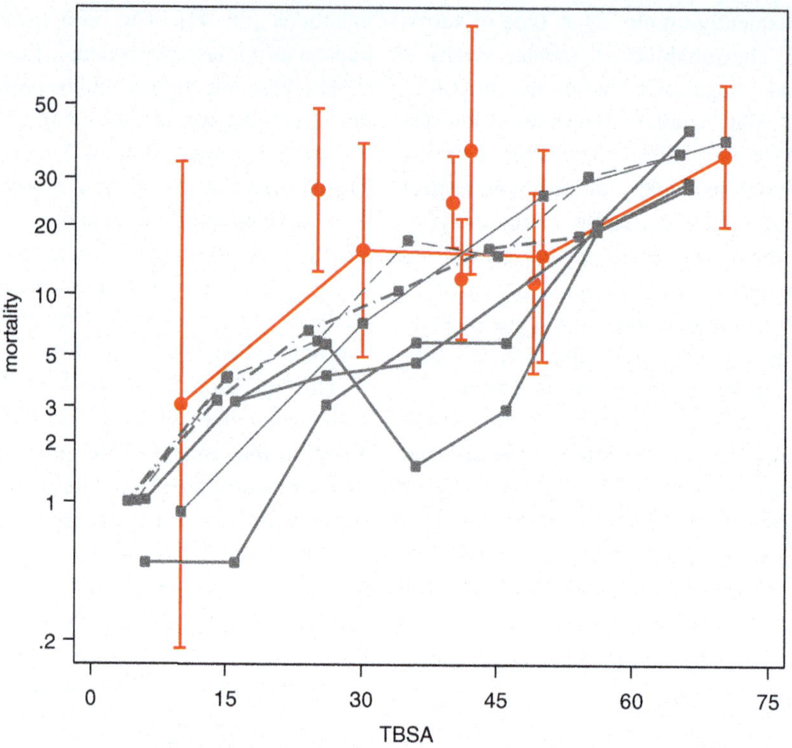

Fig. 5 Relationship between mortality proportion and 95% confidence intervals (note logit scale) and total burn surface area (TBSA) among adult patients (age >15 years) with bacteremia in published studies; Sittig et al. 1988 (continuous red line) [42]; Brusselaers et al. 2010 [39]; Mahar et al. 2010 [41]; Applegren et al. 2002 [38]; Ceniceros et al. 2015 (all red unconnected symbols) [40] and patients without bacteremia (*blue symbols*) [38, 39] as in Table 1. The relationship observed among six studies represented in Fig. 4 is presented for reference (*gray lines*)

Neisseria meningitidis, have high attributable mortality. Indeed even community-acquired GN bacteremias, of which 90% are Enterobacteriaceae, are associated with an adjusted RR of 1.5 (1.2–2.0) for mortality versus patients with negative blood cultures [53].

In contrast to previously healthy people, in the context of ICU-related infections including burn-related infections, the impact of acquisition of an opportunistic infection on mortality risk is dependent on underlying comorbidities. In attempting to estimate the attributable mortality associated with GN bacteremia among ICU patients in general, there are at least three interrelated factors to consider. These factors are the source of the GN bacteremia, the type of the Gram-negative bacteremia, and the method of statistical adjustment in matching for severity of underlying patient illness in deriving the estimate.

5.1 Source of the Gram-Negative Bacteremia

The site of origin of the GN bacteremia is an important prognostic determinant for the general population of ICU patients. A urinary tract site of origin is generally regarded as being of better prognosis than a non-urinary tract site of origin [54–56]. On the other hand, the prognosis is much worse for bacteremia for which the site of origin is pneumonia acquired in the intensive care unit. In a meta-analysis [57] of five studies of patients with ICU-acquired pneumonia and in particular ventilator-associated pneumonia, the presence of bacteremia (not necessarily Gram negative) is associated with an increased risk of mortality with an OR of 2.07 (95% CI 1.16–3.7) [58–60]. However, this question remains open as other large studies of pneumonia acquired in the intensive care unit (and not all included in the meta-analysis [57]) either have [61, 62] or have not [63, 64] been able to demonstrate a significant increased risk of mortality associated with the presence of bacteremia.

For the patient with severe burn injuries, the burn injury will serve as an additional potential source of infection, especially following burn injury manipulation [65]. This leads to considerations of early excision and skin grafting in the first week following the burn injury as a method for source control [66, 67]. This early intervention is regarded as the major advance in the treatment of patients with severe thermal injuries and the prevention of infection complications.

5.2 The Type of the Gram-Negative Bacteremia

Among critically ill patients with nosocomially acquired Gram-negative bacteremias including either *E. coli* [68], *Klebsiella* [69], *Acinetobacter baumannii* [70] and *Pseudomonas*, and other bacteremias [71–73], the difference in mortality between bacteremic case patients and matched controls (i.e., attributable mortality) is commonly less than 15% points. Polymicrobial bacteremias have a higher mortality risk. Other factors additional to the site of origin likely confound the mortality risk associated with different types of GN bacteremia.

The difficulty in attributing mortality risk to bacteremia can be illustrated by contrasting recent French [74] and Korean [75] studies of ICU patients. A multivariate analysis of risk factors for death among a cohort of 832 bacteremic patients with sepsis from a survey of 24 French hospitals revealed that five factors were found to be independently associated with an increased or decreased risk of death. The factors associated with increased risk of death include age, underlying patient illness severity, presence of severe sepsis or shock, whereas the factors associated with a decreased risk were a urinary tract source of infection and the type of bacteremia (Gram negative versus non- Gram negative) [75]. By contrast, a multivariate analysis of risk factors for death among 2286 bacteremic patients with sepsis from a survey of 18 Korean hospitals found that pathogens other than *E. coli* were associated with an increased risk of death after adjusting for illness severity and respiratory site of infection [75]. However, confounding the comparison of these cohorts, *Klebsiella* and *Pseudomonas* bacteremias were more common among the Korean cohort than the French cohort [74].

5.3 The Method of Statistical Adjustment

The execution and interpretation of studies that attempt to estimate attributable mortality associated with bacteremia or any other documented infection are not simple [47, 48, 76, 77]. There are two main methods to control for severity of underlying illness in attempting to define attributable mortality. The first is “control by design” such as a simple case-control-type study design [76]. This method is not commonly used however as controlling for disease severity is difficult to achieve given the large number of potential confounding factors for which matching is sought. The alternate approach to matching is “control by analysis” in which the severity of underlying illness is estimated and scored for each patient to produce a risk score. This score then serves as a basis to match case and control group patients for severity of illness [62, 77]. In the analysis of attributable risk, the method of risk factor adjustment is crucial to the estimates obtained, and there are at least five difficulties with this approach:

1. The most relevant severity score to choose may be conjectural.
2. The development of a risk score is not simple, and factors that determine its suitability may be unique to the population at hand. An important consideration is whether allowance was made for interaction effects in the development of any risk score.
3. The problematic choice of timing at which the severity score is made in relation to the presence of the documented infection of interest.
4. Of all the important factors that need to be controlled to obtain an unbiased estimate, not

all will be known for all patients. For example, the site of origin of the bacteremic infection may not be clear.
5. There may be additional factors that are presumably influential but remain as yet unknown. For example, the timing of administration and appropriateness of antibiotic therapy has emerged in more recent studies as additional significant factors but has infrequently been recorded in earlier studies [69–80].

In relation to the patient group with severe burn injuries, the mortality attributable risk associated with the detection of bacteremia remains somewhat unresolved. Mason et al. (1986) [25] investigated the mortality among 5877 patients admitted to a burn unit over a period of 25 years of whom 1481 had one or more positive blood cultures. They found the mortality was significantly increased by as much as 50% versus expected among those with a bacteremia due to either *Pseudomonas*, a yeast, or another Gram-negative but not in association with a Gram-positive bacteremia.

On the other hand, Brusselaers [39, 81] examined the impact of the detection of bloodstream infection on mortality using a logistic regression to assess the impact of various factors among patients matched on the Belgian Outcome in Burn Injury (BOBI) score with and without a bloodstream infection. The BOBI is a 10-point classification based on three major risk factors: age, TBSA, and inhalation injury. Age is divided into four risk categories (0–3 points) and TBSA into five risk categories (0–4 points), and the presence of inhalation injury is scored as three additional points. These investigators were careful in selecting a control group of patients without bloodstream infection blind to the patient outcome. Also, nonexposed patients were required to have a time to discharge at least equal to the time to event in the corresponding exposed patient. The findings from this study was that while age and TBSA remained significant predictors of mortality in the logistic regression model, surprisingly the detection of a bloodstream infection was not a significant predictor. This would imply that there was little to gain by preventing bacteremia in patients with severe burn injuries.In the context of burn-related infections and bacteremic ICU-acquired infections generally, there is, however, a different overall perspective from which to view the question of the mortality attributable to the bacteremia versus that due to the underlying illness in the context of burn-related infections and bacteremic ICU-acquired infections [82, 83]. Viewing this from an alternative perspective, among patients with systemic inflammatory response syndrome (SIRS), the morbidity and mortality are similar whether or not the SIRS is associated with documented infection, being a documented GN infection or another type of infection [49, 84]. This raises the presumption that for the patient group with SIRS without a documented infection, there is a missing mediator (or mediators) which accounts for the similar prognosis for those with, versus those without, a documented infection. Endotoxin and endotoxemia have long been suspected as having this role. However, the evidence for these "missing mediators" being endotoxemia is better established for pathogenic *Neisseria meningitides* than is the case for infection with opportunistic GN bacteria acquired in the ICU [85].In this regard, the role of endotoxemia in the patient with severe sepsis has long been the subject of speculation not only in the context of the patient with severe burns [85–88] but also in relation to severe sepsis generally [85, 87]. There is a theory that endotoxin originates from the intestinal tract of patients with severe burn injuries [88]. Endotoxin is measurable in plasma of patients with severe burn injury [89], and the levels are higher in those with larger [90] and more severe [91, 92] burns and reduced by burn excision [93]. This has led to a range of efforts to control endotoxin levels in blood of patients with severe burn injuries, but the results are mixed [94, 95].

6 Infection Diagnosis

The diagnosis of infection in a patient with severe burns relies on local and systemic features, and there are several local features that might be detected at the site of a burn to suggest the presence of an infection. These features include the appearance of pain, edema, and swelling occurring in all or part of the burn. There may also be malodor, discoloration, and pain to raise the suspicion of non-viability. Moreover, the adjacent non-injured skin may demonstrate the conventional signs of infection such as pain or tenderness, warmth, erythema, and swelling.

However, the diagnosis of infection in a patient with severe burns using the systemic features is difficult for several reasons [84]. Many of the indicators to the presence of an infection in patients without burns are less reliable in the patient with severe burns. For example, leukocytosis is commonly used in a range of settings as an indicator of infection, but in the patient with severe burns, the burn injury itself often will cause an elevation in the white cell count, and hence the detection of an elevated white cell count will have reduced specificity for an infection in this context.

Other markers have been used such as procalcitonin and other serum markers to assist in diagnosis [96–98], although not all have found this marker to be useful [99]. The challenge with these serum markers is to determine breakpoint values that are discriminatory between true sepsis and the nonspecific burn injury. A recent meta-analysis of nine studies of procalcitonin used as a diagnostic marker for burn wound-related sepsis [96] found that the pooled sensitivity and specificity were 0.74 and 0.88, respectively. However, the cutoff values used in the individual studies varied almost tenfold. Ideally these types of meta-analysis require multilevel techniques to derive summary estimates across disparate studies [100].

7 Infection Prevention

7.1 General

The prevention of infections in patients with severe burns is challenging. There are a range of strategies to prevent the development of infection in patients admitted to intensive care units in general. Many of these strategies also apply to patients with severe burns. Such methods include the care with placement and stewardship of invasive devices but with particular attention to central venous and other vascular access devices [101, 102].

As in ICU patients in general, the risk of bacteremia and other device-related infections is proportional to the number of lines and moreover to the number of device days. In one study, changing central venous lines every third rather than every fourth day leads to a reduction in frequency of bacteremia in patients with severe burn injury [102]. Another study examined the effect of substituting standard central venous catheters at day 3 with antibiotic-impregnated peripherally inserted central catheter (PICC) lines in patients admitted to a regional burn center. The comparison group was the 30 consecutive patients in a historical group that had received a standard PICC line. While the reduction in bacteremia between the study versus the control group appears to be impressive (0/19 vs. 15/30), the interpretation of this result is problematic for three reasons. Firstly, it is a somewhat small and non-randomized study, and the control group had a higher TBSA (31.1 vs. 18.3%, respectively). Moreover, there was no mortality in either group. Secondly, the study does not state how the blood cultures were obtained in this study and if they had been obtained through the PICC line that could have suppressed microbial growth in the blood culture sample. Finally, a standard practice in these types of studies is to adjust for time at risk by using the number of days of device use as the denominator, and this data was not available for this study [101].

Patients with severe burns are at high risk of acquiring colonizing bacteria from the environment including mattresses and hospital equipment such as hydrotherapy equipment [5, 103].

One of the largest studies of the patients' hospital environment and the incidence of bacteremia among patients with burns greater than 20% TBSA was undertaken at The US Army Institute of Surgical Research Burn Center [44]. The bacteremias and outcome of 1605 patients admitted to the burn center in the 10 years of an open ward (1974–1983) were compared to the subsequent

10 years (1984–1994) during which all 914 patients were admitted to a single-bed isolation environment. The mean age (31.1 years vs. 32.2 years, respectively), the mean TBSA (47.5 vs. 42.8%, respectively), and the management policies were similar in the two periods.

They observed a small reduction in the incidence of Gram-positive bacteremias (218/1605, 13.6 vs. 117/914, 12.8%, respectively) and also candidemia (107/1605, 6.7 vs. 49/914, 5.4%, respectively). However, there was a substantial reduction in not only Gram-negative bacteremias overall (500/1605, 31, vs. 110/914, 12%, respectively), and a reduction in problematic Gram-negative bacteremias such as *Pseudomonas* (268 vs. 31, respectively) and *Klebsiella pneumoniae* (193 vs. 37, respectively), but moreover, there was a reduction in the observed to predicted mortality ratio that was particularly apparent among those with a Gram-negative bacteremia (1.61 vs. 0.87, respectively). While the length of burn unit stay for these patients was not stated, the reductions for Gram-negative bacteremias are impressive and were attributed to more effective infection control implementation in the era of single-bed isolation [44].

However, the interpretation of these historically controlled studies is problematic. It is difficult to be certain the extent to which any improvement in infection prevention is related to changes in infection control practices or shorter length of stay in the ICU and how much may be due to burn wound management such as the widespread practice of early burn wound excision and possible grafting.

7.2 Antibiotic Prophylaxis

There have been a number of studies of various types of antibiotic prophylaxis to prevent infection in patients with severe burns either as perioperative administration given at the time of surgical debridement or administration given while the patient is at risk in the burn intensive care unit. The evidence for each strategy is limited, and the issue of antibiotic prophylaxis is controversial. In part this is due to the fact that the studies that have examined this question have used a range of patient inclusion criteria, antibiotic interventions, prophylaxis strategies, and end point definitions [104–115].

The two largest and most comprehensive systematic reviews of the evidence base for antibiotic prophylaxis in the burn patient group examined antibiotic prophylaxis in three broad context: as perioperative prophylaxis, as topical use on the wound, and as topical and systemic use given for the duration of time at risk in the burn unit. The two systematic reviews reached contrary findings [114, 115].

The first [114] reviewed 17 trials obtained after a systematic search of the literature for studies of antibiotic prophylaxis given to patients with severe burns. The second systematic review was a Cochrane review which was published in 2013 [115]. This systematic review used slightly wider literature search criteria and found 36 studies of interest published between 1968 and 2010.

With respect to perioperative prophylaxis, the first systematic review found that there was a reduction in wound infections, particularly those due to *Staphylococcus aureus* infection or colonization in association with the use of antistaphylococcal antibiotics. However, the Cochrane review found no evidence that perioperative prophylaxis influenced any of the primary or secondary outcomes of interest.

With respect to topical use on the wound, the two systematic reviews were largely in agreement. The first systematic review found no evidence of benefit in using topical antibiotic applied to the wound. The second systematic review concurred in that there was no evidence that the use of prophylactic, topical antibiotics versus other topical preparations, dressings, placebo, or no treatment reduced the risk of burn wound infection, invasive infections, or mortality.

The activity of topical silver-containing compounds in the prevention of burn injury infections has been of interest for many years as there is no doubt that the heavy metals have antibacterial effects that can be demonstrated in vitro [116]. However, these systemic reviews found that there may even be an increased risk of burn wound infection associated with the use of topical silver sulfadiazine (SSD) than those treated with more simple dressings (11 RCTs studied) [115]. The use of topical silver for preventing wound infection is the specific subject of further systematic reviews [117–119].

With respect to antibiotic prophylaxis given for the duration of time at risk in the burn unit, the two systematic reviews reached substantially contrary findings. The first systematic review found that when given for up to 14 days after admission (in five trials), there appeared to be a near halving in mortality (risk ratio 0.54, 95% confidence interval 0.34–0.87) (Fig. 3) [114]. The beneficial effect of systemic prophylaxis appeared to be due to a reduction in pneumonia (three studies).

On the other hand, the Cochrane review found that systemic antibiotic prophylaxis given for the duration of time at risk in the burn unit did not impact on mortality risk and was generally of no value (risk ratio 0.41:0.17–1.02) (2.8 of 117). There was the possibility that the incidence of pneumonia was reduced in one small study having only 40 patients who required mechanical ventilation in a burn unit [110].

The reason why these two systematic reviews appear to disagree on the overall summary findings is that the summary effect size derived was unstable in each review given the small number of studies. One of the five studies [107] contains over 100 of the 272 patients that constituted the evidence base for this end point and was particularly influential, as it constitutes as much as 41% of the weight in the summary effect. This single study achieved an apparent reduction in mortality of (risk ratio) 0.34:0.13–0.87 in association with the use of a combined intervention with topical antibiotics applied to the upper airway and, also parenterally, an intervention termed selective digestive decontamination (SDD). In both systematic reviews, this study is unique for several reasons. This study has a significant mortality reduction, it was one of the largest, it was conducted in a burn injury population for which the majority required mechanical ventilation, it was randomized, and it was placebo blinded through the use of a topical placebo.

The two reviews classified this large and influential study undertaken in burn-injured patients [107] differently due to the SDD intervention being a combined regimen of both systemic and parenteral antibiotics, and consequently the two reviews derived substantially different summary effect sizes in relation to the routine use of systemic antibiotic prophylaxis.

The two systematic reviews were in substantial agreement on two other findings. Both found studies for which there was evidence for increase in resistance to the antibiotics used for prophylaxis. In three trials, resistance to the antibiotic used for prophylaxis significantly increased (rate ratio 2.84:1.38–5.83).

Moreover, both systematic reviews found that the overall methodological quality of the trials was poor. Many of the studies had a high or uncertain risk of bias, and the amount of evidence overall was scant. Both systematic reviews appealed for further high-quality evidence before definitive treatment commendations regarding antibiotic prophylaxis can be made. They concurred that with this paucity of evidence, there was a need for large, well-designed, and robustly analyzed randomized controlled trials to address this issue.

In an attempt to progress the question of use of systemic antibiotic prophylaxis in the patient with severe burns, a Japanese group undertook an analysis of a nationwide database of 2893 patients admitted to 583 hospitals over the period July 2010 to March 2013 using 28-day all-cause mortality as the end point [104]. The antibiotic prophylaxis used was either a first-generation cephalosporin or ampicillin/sulbactam typically given for periods of up to 7 days. In this study, the subgroups that either did (692 patients) or did not (2201 patients) require mechanical ventilation were separately examined. This makes it by far the largest study of antibiotic prophylaxis in patients with severe burns. The likelihood that any individual patient received prophylactic antibiotics was scored. This propensity score was used as the basis for matching groups of patients that did versus did not receive antibiotic prophylaxis within each subgroup.

Tagami et al. [104] reported that prophylaxis with up to 7 days of parenteral antibiotic was associated with an impressive 10% point reduction in mortality but that this difference was apparent only for the patient group receiving mechanical ventilation. In this subgroup, the mortality proportions were 38.3% receiving prophylaxis versus 48.6% in those not treated. The substantially larger group of patients in the database not receiving mechanical ventilation showed no significant difference in mortality (5.8 vs. 7% for prophylaxis vs. control, respectively).

However, the mortality rate in the control group appears to be approximately 10% higher than comparable studies in the literature including two large studies of Japanese burn injury patients with inhalation injury [9, 17]. Each of these studies [9, 17] has over 1500 patients. The apparently impressive results of Tagami et al. [104] warrant closer scrutiny as the higher control group mortality rate is unexplained. The next four paragraphs here expand on a previously published critique [120] of this study [104].

The findings of Tagami et al. [104] resemble the promising findings from a range of methods for preventing ventilator-associated pneumonia (VAP) among the general population of mechanically ventilated ICU patients using a preventative strategy of topical antibiotics applied to the oropharynx of these patients. This strategy is selective antibiotic decontamination (SDD), which, in several studies and meta-analyses, appears to show a mortality benefit of 10% points [121] as is the case for the two studies that examined SDD in a population of burn-injured patients [106, 107].

However, a closer scrutiny of over 40 studies of SDD in the general population of high-risk ICU patients reveals that the median rates for candida in the respiratory tract [122], candidemia [123], VAP [124, 125], and even bacteremia [126] among the concurrent control groups from studies of SDD are surprisingly and inexplicably high. These rates among the control groups of the SDD studies are higher than that among nine other categories of control and intervention groups for studies of methods for VAP prevention not involving topical antibiotic use. The apparent effect of SDD on the event rates in these studies [122–126] requires a cautious interpretation as contextual mediations within these concurrent controlled studies cannot be excluded. Contextual effects cannot be observed in any single study examined in isolation and can only be seen in a comparison of observed rates within a study to an external benchmark.

In this regard, the broader evidence base for methods of preventing infection for patients with severe burn injuries receiving mechanical ventilation is summarized in Table 2 and Fig. 7 with attention not only to the summary effect but also to the mortality proportions in the component (control and intervention) groups of the studies. The data summary includes the two studies of antibiotic prophylaxis [107, 110] that were highly influential in the two systematic reviews above [114, 115] in addition to the study by Tagami et al. [104]. For external comparison are three studies of prevention methods other than antibiotics [127–129].Also provided are several nonconcurrent controlled and observational studies that provide comparative mortality data for the patient group with severe burn injury receiving mechanical ventilation [130–136] that provide a benchmark mortality incidence to serve as a reference (Table 2).

When the treatment effect is examined by a conventional meta-analysis technique (Fig. 6), there appears to be an approximately 50% reduction in mortality both for the summary effect derived from the studies of antibiotic methods and also for that derived from the studies of non-antibiotic methods of infection prevention. Of note in Fig. 6 is that the summary effect size on mortality prevention for these three studies of antibiotic methods is similar to that seen in each of the systematic reviews [114, 115]. The data shown in Fig. 7 provides the benchmark reference derived from the observational study groups to enable an external comparison of the mortality proportion derived from the component (i.e., control and intervention) groups of these studies

Table 2 Mortality for groups of patients with severe burn injury receiving mechanical ventilation

Author (year)	Ref.	Interventions[a]	Mechanical ventilation	Patients	Mortality	
			(%)	(n)	(n)	(%)
Groups of observational and nonconcurrent studies						
Brusselaers et al. (2012)	[6]	Nil	100	53	9	17
Cioffi et al. (1991)	[130]	Nil	100	54	10	19
Czaparan et al. (2015)	[131]	Nil	100	90	19	21
Fitzwater et al. (2003)	[82]	Nil	100	47	18	38
Lipovy et al. (2011)	[134]	Nil	100	127	18	14
Rue et al. (1993)	[135]	Nil	100	330	97	29
Tanizaki et al. (2012)	[136]	Nil	100	52	8	15
Hall et al. (2007)	[132]	HFPV	100	92	26	28
Hall et al. (2007)	[132]	CMV	100	130	56	43
Miller et al. (2009)	[133]	Heparin and NAC	100	16	1	6
Miller et al. (2009)	[133]	Nil	100	14	6	43
Nonantibiotic prevention methods *Control groups of concurrent controlled trials*						
Chung et al. (2010)	[129]	CMV	100	31	6	19
Garrel et al. 2003	[128]	Control feeds	100	19	8	42
Reper et al. (2002)	[129]	CMV	100	18	4	22
Nonantibiotic prevention methods *Intervention groups of concurrent controlled trials*						
Chung et al. (2010)	[129]	HFPV	100	31	6	19
Garrel et al. (2003)	[128]	Enteral glutamine	100	16	0	0
Reper et al. (2002)	[129]	HFPV	100	17	3	18
Antibiotic prevention methods *Control groups of concurrent controlled trials*						
De le Cal et al. (2005)	[107]	Placebo	80	54	15	28
Kimura et al. (1998)	[110]	Placebo	100	19	7	37
Tagami et al. (2016)	[104]	Nil	100	280	136	49
Antibiotic prevention methods *Intervention groups of concurrent controlled trials*						
De le Cal et al. (2005)	[107]	SDD	75	53	5	9
Kimura et al. (1998)	[110]	TMP-SMX	100	21	4	19
Tagami et al. (2016)	[104]	Iv Amp or Ceph	100	412	158	38

[a] *HFPV* high-frequency percussive ventilation; *CMV* conventional mechanical ventilation; *Heparin and NAC* intervention with nebulized heparin and N-acetyl-cysteine; *SDD* selective digestive decontamination; *TMP-SMX* trimethoprim-sulfamethoxazole; *Iv Amp or Ceph* intravenous ampicillin/sulbactam of a first-generation cephalosporin

versus from studies of comparable patients in the literature. In this comparison, two observations from the summary mortality proportion derived from the component groups emerge. The studies of antibiotic methods have control group mortality proportions that are approximately 10% higher versus both the control groups of the studies of nonantibiotic methods and benchmark reference derived from other studies (Fig. 7). By contrast, the mortality proportion for the control groups of the studies of nonantibiotic methods of infection prevention and, somewhat surprisingly, the corresponding intervention groups from the studies of antibiotic methods are all closer to the externally derived benchmark.

Hence, the summary effect size derived here for the three studies of antibiotic methods, being an apparent reduction (Fig. 6), is not so simple to

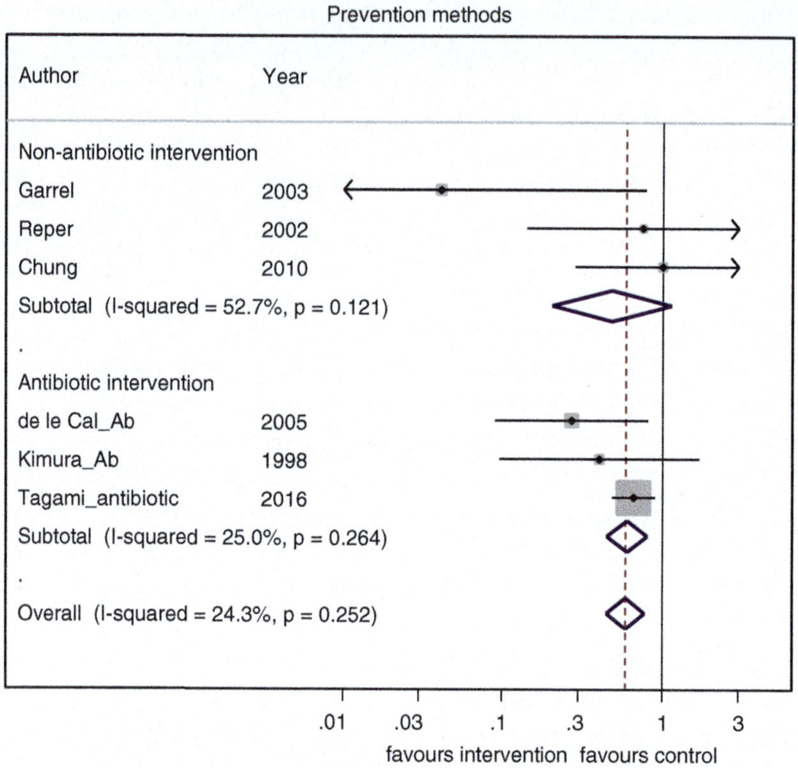

Fig. 6 Effect sizes for nonantibiotic- and antibiotic-based interventions for the prevention of mortality in six randomized controlled trials among patients with severe burn injuries for which the majority received mechanical ventilation. The size of the blocks is proportional to study size, the whiskers represent the summary specific 95% confidence intervals, and the diamonds represent the summary 95% confidence intervals. The overall effect for all six studies is represented by the vertical broken line

interpret (Fig. 7). An alternate interpretation is that the apparent reduction is attributable to a higher control group event rate rather than a lower intervention group rate. This interpretation is as with the overall evidence base of studies of the methods for VAP prevention such as SDD which involves topical antibiotic use [125]. The findings there also are consistent with a contextual effect leading to higher VAP, bacteremia, and candidemia rates within concurrent controlled studies of SDD. In those studies, the contextual effect is presumably a consequence of a change in the microbiome of the ICU resulting from the use of topical antibiotics in the intervention group patients. This presumably alters the risk of acquiring infection in the control group patients. This phenomenon where the patients not receiving antibiotics are placed at higher risk has been termed "herd peril" and is in contradistinction to "herd protection" where the minority of a population not receiving a vaccine is at placed at lower risk and is protected by the majority of the population receiving the vaccine [125].

The French Burn Society (Société Française d'Etude et de Traitement des Brûlures (SFETB)) formulated evidence-based guidelines for antibiotic use in patients with severe burns [137]. Their recommendation was for no antibiotics without proven infection. More specifically in relation to prophylaxis, they recommended that antibiotic prophylaxis be used in patients needing invasive surgery (excisions, flaps, etc.) but not in dressing changes. These guidelines also note that the patient with severe burns will often have profoundly altered physiological parameters that affect the pharmacokinetics of most

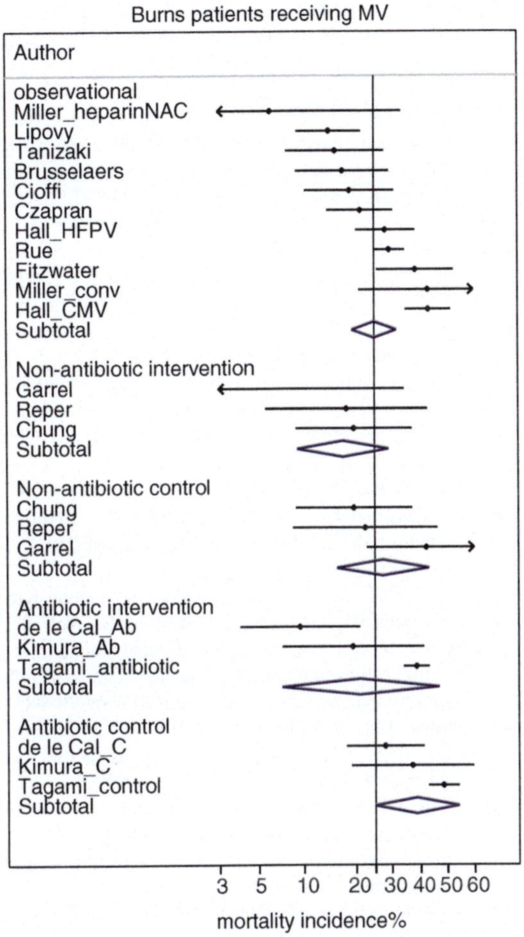

Fig. 7 Caterpillar plot of group-specific (*small diamonds*) and summary (*large open diamonds*) mortality proportions and 95% confidence intervals for groups from studies of patients with burn injury of patients receiving mechanical ventilation (MV) from studies as in Fig. 6. The center line represents the summary mortality incidence derived from 11 additional groups from observational and nonconcurrent control studies as in Table 2

drugs. This makes dosing of antibiotic (as well as other drugs) to achieve adequate antibiotic levels in serum challenging [138, 139]. For example, patients with severe burn injury have a higher clearance of vancomycin compared to patients without severe burn injury [138]. There can be major variations in dosing requirements both between patients with and without burn injuries but also for patients with burn injuries over time [140].

Conclusions

This chapter has examined the risks of acquiring severe infection in patients with severe burn injuries in the intensive care unit environment. The evidence base for using antibiotics to prevent this acquisition is open to alternate interpretations, and two recent systematic reviews of the very limited evidence base disagree with respect to any value. Crucially, it remains to be established whether prophylactic antibiotic use among patients with severe burns is safe. This review has not examined the role of specific antibiotics in the treatment of infections related to severe burn injuries. That is the subject of a proposed systematic review [141].

Financial Support This research has been supported by the Australian Government Department of Health and Ageing through the Rural Clinical Training and Support (RCTS) program.

References

1. Murray CK (2015) Burns. In: Bennett JE, Dolin R, Blaser MJ (eds) Mandell, Douglas, and Bennett's principles and practice of infectious diseases, 8th edn. Saunders Elsevier, St. Louis, pp 3505–3509
2. Church D, Elsayed S, Reid O, Winston B, Lindsay R (2006) Burn wound infections. Clin Microbiol Rev 19(2):403–434
3. Sharma BR (2007) Infection in patients with severe burns: causes and prevention thereof. Infect Dis Clin North Am 21(3):745–759
4. Erol S, Altoparlak U, Akcay MN, Celebi F, Parlak M (2004) Changes of microbial flora and wound colonization in burned patients. Burns 30(4):357–361
5. Shirani KZ, McManus AT, Vaughan GM, McManus WF, Pruitt BA, Mason AD (1986) Effects of environment on infection in burn patients. Arch Surg 121(1):31–36
6. Brusselaers N, Logie D, Vogelaers D, Monstrey S, Blot S (2012) Burns, inhalation injury and ventilator-associated pneumonia: value of routine surveillance cultures. Burns 38(3):364–370
7. Brusselaers N, Monstrey S, Vogelaers D, Hoste E, Blot S (2010) Severe burn injury in Europe: a systematic review of the incidence, etiology, morbidity, and mortality. Crit Care 14(5):R188
8. Smith DL, Cairns BA, Ramadan F, Dalston JS, Fakhry SM, Rutledge R, Meyer AA, Peterson HD (1994) Effect of inhalation injury, burn size, and

age on mortality: a study of 1447 consecutive burn patients. J Trauma Acute Care Surg 37(4):655–659
9. Suzuki M, Aikawa N, Kobayashi K, Higuchi R (2005) Prognostic implications of inhalation injury in burn patients in Tokyo. Burns 31(3):331–336
10. Clark CJ, Reid WH, Gilmour WH, Campbell D (1986) Mortality probability in victims of fire trauma: revised equation to include inhalation injury. Br Med J 292:1303–1305
11. Tredget EE, Shankowsky HA, Taerum TV, Moysa GL, Alton JD (1990) The role of inhalation injury in burn trauma. A Canadian experience. Ann Surg 212(6):720–727
12. Ryan CM, Schoenfeld DA, Thorpe WP, Sheridan RL, Cassem EH, Tompkins RG (1998) Objective estimates of the probability of death from burn injuries. N Engl J Med 338(6):362–366
13. Barret JP, Gomez P, Solano I, Gonzalez-Dorrego M, Crisol FJ (1999) Epidemiology and mortality of adult burns in Catalonia. Burns 25(4):325–329
14. Muller MJ, Pegg SP, Rule MR (2001) Determinants of death following burn injury. Br J Surg 88(4):583–587
15. Jie X, Baoren C (2003) Mortality rates among 5321 patients with burns admitted to a burn unit in China: 1980–1998. Burns 29(3):239–245
16. Blot S (2008) Development and validation of a model for prediction of mortality in patients with acute burn injury: the Belgian Outcome in Burn Injury Study Group. Br J Surg 96(1):111–117
17. Kobayashi K, Ikeda H, Higuchi R, Nozaki M, Yamamoto Y, Urabe M, Shimazaki S, Sugamata A, Aikawa N, Ninomiya N, Sakurai H (2005) Epidemiological and outcome characteristics of major burns in Tokyo. Burns 31(1):S3–S11
18. Dokter J, Vloemans AF, Beerthuizen GI, Van der Vlies CH, Boxma H, Breederveld R, Tuinebreijer WE, Middelkoop E, van Baar ME (2014) Epidemiology and trends in severe burns in the Netherlands. Burns 40(7):1406–1414
19. Ong YS, Samuel M, Song C (2006) Meta-analysis of early excision of burns. Burns 32(2):145–150
20. Palmieri TL, Caruso DM, Foster KN, Cairns BA, Peck MD, Gamelli RL, Mozingo DW, Kagan RJ, Wahl W, Kemalyan NA, Fish JS (2006) Effect of blood transfusion on outcome after major burn injury: a multicenter study. Crit Care Med 34(6):1602–1607
21. Altoparlak U, Erol S, Akcay MN, Celebi F, Kadanali A (2004) The time-related changes of antimicrobial resistance patterns and predominant bacterial profiles of burn wounds and body flora of burned patients. Burns 30(7):660–664
22. Bahemia IA, Muganza A, Moore R, Sahid F, Menezes CN (2015) Microbiology and antibiotic resistance in severe burns patients: a 5 year review in an adult burns unit. Burns 41(7):1536–1542
23. Öncül O, Öksüz S, Acar A, Ülkür E, Turhan V, Uygur F, Ulçay A, Erdem H, Özyurt M, Görenek L (2014) Nosocomial infection characteristics in a burn intensive care unit: analysis of an eleven-year active surveillance. Burns 40(5):835–841
24. Pruitt BA, McManus AT (1992) The changing epidemiology of infection in burn patients. World J Surg 16(1):57–67
25. Wibbenmeyer L, Danks R, Faucher L, Amelon M, Latenser B, Kealey GP, Herwaldt LA (2006) Prospective analysis of nosocomial infection rates, antibiotic use, and patterns of resistance in a burn population. J Burn Care Res 27(2):152–160
26. Wibbenmeyer LA, Kealey GP, Latenser BA, Diekema DJ, Williams IM, Coffman SL, Winokur PL, Kroeger JS, Lewis RW, Herwaldt LA (2008) Emergence of the USA300 strain of methicillin-resistant Staphylococcus aureus in a burn-trauma unit. J Burn Care Res 29(5):790–797
27. McManus AT, Mason AD, McManus WF, Pruitt BA (1985) Twenty-five year review of Pseudomonas aeruginosabacteremia in a burn center. Eur J Clin Microbiol Infect Dis 4(2):219–223
28. Miranda BH, Ali SN, Jeffery SL, Thomas SS (2008) Two stage study of wound microorganisms affecting burns and plastic surgery inpatients. J Burn Care Res 29(6):927–932
29. Horvath EE, Murray CK, Vaughan GM, Chung KK, Hospenthal DR, Wade CE, Holcomb JB, Wolf SE, Mason AD Jr, Cancio LC (2007) Fungal wound infection (not colonization) is independently associated with mortality in burn patients. Ann Surg 245(6):978–985
30. Moore EC, Padiglione AA, Wasiak J, Paul E, Cleland H (2010) Candida in burns: risk factors and outcomes. J Burn Care Res 31(2):257–263
31. Pruitt BA Jr (1984) The diagnosis and treatment of infection in the burn patient. Burns 11(2):79–91
32. Kallstrom G (2014) Are quantitative bacterial wound cultures useful? J Clin Microbiol 52(8):2753–2756
33. Steer JA, Papini RP, Wilson AP, McGrouther DA, Parkhouse N (1996) Quantitative microbiology in the management of burn patients. I. Correlation between quantitative and qualitative burn wound biopsy culture and surface alginate swab culture. Burns 22(3):173–176
34. McManus AT, Kim SH, McManus WF, Mason AD, Pruitt BA (1987) Comparison of quantitative microbiology and histopathology in divided burn-wound biopsy specimens. Arch Surg 122(1):74–76
35. Spebar MJ, Walters MJ, Pruitt BA Jr (1982) Improved survival with aggressive surgical management of noncandidal fungal infections of the burn wound. J Trauma 22(10):867–868
36. Atilla A, Tomak L, Katrancı AO, Ceylan A, Kılıç SS (2015) Mortality risk factors in burn care units considering the clinical significance of Acinetobacter infections. Ulus Travma Acil Cerrahi Derg 21(1):34–38
37. Hurley JC (2016) World-wide variation in incidence of Acinetobacter associated ventilator associated pneumonia: a meta-regression. BMC Infect Dis 16(1):577
38. Appelgren P, Björnhagen V, Bragderyd K, Jonsson CE, Ransjö U (2002) A prospective study of infections in burn patients. Burns 28(1):39–46
39. Brusselaers N, Monstrey S, Snoeij T, Vandijck D, Lizy C, Hoste E, Lauwaert S, Colpaert K, Vandekerckhove L, Vogelaers D, Blot S (2010) Morbidity and mortal-

ity of bloodstream infections in patients with severe burn injury. Am J Crit Care 19(6):e81–e87
40. Ceniceros A, Pértega S, Galeiras R, Mourelo M, López E, Broullón J, Sousa D, Freire D (2016) Predicting mortality in burn patients with bacteraemia. Infection 44(2):215–222
41. Mahar P, Padiglione AA, Cleland H, Paul E, Hinrichs M, Wasiak J (2010) Pseudomonas aeruginosa bacteraemia in burns patients: risk factors and outcomes. Burns 36(8):1228–1233
42. Sittig K, Deitch EA (1988) Effect of bacteremia on mortality after thermal injury. Arch Surg 123(11):1367–1370
43. Mason AD, McManus AT, Pruitt BA (1986) Association of burn mortality and bacteremia: a 25-year review. Arch Surg 121(9):1027–1031
44. McManus AT, Mason AD, McManus WF, Pruitt BA (1994) A decade of reduced gram-negative infections and mortality associated with improved isolation of burned patients. Arch Surg 129(12):1306–1309
45. Bryan CS (1989) Clinical implications of positive blood cultures. Clin Microbiol Rev 2(4):329–335
46. Prowle JR, Echeverri JE, Ligabo EV, Sherry N, Taori GC, Crozier TM, Hart GK, Korman TM, Mayall BC, Johnson PD, Bellomo R (2011) Acquired bloodstream infection in the intensive care unit: incidence and attributable mortality. Crit Care 15(2):R100
47. Cosgrove SE, Carmeli Y (2003) Studies of bloodstream infection outcomes: reading between the lines. Infect Control Hosp Epidemiol 24(12):884–886
48. Blot S, De Bacquer D, Hoste E, Depuydt P, Vandewoude K, De Waele J, Benoit D, De Schuijmer J, Colardyn F, Vogelaers D (2005) Influence of matching for exposure time on estimates of attributable mortality caused by nosocomial bacteremia in critically ill patients. Infect Control Hosp Epidemiol 26(4):352–356
49. Zahar JR, Timsit JF, Garrouste-Orgeas M, Francais A, Vesin A, Descorps-Declere A, Dubois Y, Souweine B, Haouache H, Goldgran-Toledano D, Allaouchiche B, Azoulay E, Adrie C (2011) Outcomes in severe sepsis and patients with septic shock: pathogen species and infection sites are not associated with mortality. Crit Care Med 39(8):1886–1895
50. Garrouste-Orgeas M, Timsit JF, Tafflet M, Misset B, Zahar JR, Soufir L, Lazard T, Jamali S, Mourvillier B, Cohen Y, De Lassence A, Azoulay E, Cheval C, Descorps-Declere A, Adrie C, Costa de Beauregard MA, Carlet J, OUTCOMEREA Study Group (2006) Excess risk of death from intensive care unit-acquired nosocomial bloodstream infections: a reappraisal. Clin Infect Dis 42(8):1118–1126
51. Januel JM, Harbarth S, Allard R, Voirin N, Lepape A, Allaouchiche B, Guerin C, Lehot JJ, Robert MO, Fournier G, Jacques D, Chassard D, Gueugniaud PY, Artru F, Petit P, Robert D, Mohammedi I, Girard R, Cêtre JC, Nicolle MC, Grando J, Fabry J, Vanhems P (2010) Estimating attributable mortality due to nosocomial infections acquired in intensive care units. Infect Control Hosp Epidemiol 31(4):388–394
52. Thompson DS (2008) Estimates of the rate of acquisition of bacteraemia and associated excess mortality in a general intensive care unit: a 10 year study. J Hosp Infect 69(1):56–61
53. Sogaard M, Norgaard M, Pedersen L, Sorensen HT, Schonheyder HC (2011) Blood culture status and mortality among patients with suspected community-acquired bacteremia: a population-based cohort study. BMC Infect Dis 11:139
54. Laupland KB, Gregson DB, Church DL, Ross T, Pitout JD (2008) Incidence, risk factors and outcomes of Escherichia coli bloodstream infections in a large Canadian region. Clin Microbiol Infect 14(11):1041–1047
55. Lefort A, Panhard X, Clermont O, Woerther PL, Branger C, Mentre F, Fantin B, Wolff M, Denamur E (2011) Host factors and portal of entry outweigh bacterial determinants to predict the severity of Escherichia coli bacteremia. J Clin Microbiol 49(3):777–783
56. Johnson JR, Kuskowski MA, O'Bryan TT, Maslow JN (2002) Epidemiological correlates of virulence genotype and phylogenetic background among Escherichia coli blood isolates from adults with diverse-source bacteremia. J Infect Dis 185(10):1439–1447
57. Siempos II, Vardakas KZ, Kyriakopoulos CE, Ntaidou TK, Falagas ME (2010) Predictors of mortality in adult patients with ventilator-associated pneumonia: a meta-analysis. Shock 33(6):590–601
58. Agbaht K, Diaz E, Munoz E, Lisboa T, Gomez F, Depuydt PO, Blot SI, Rello J (2007) Bacteremia in patients with ventilator-associated pneumonia is associated with increased mortality: a study comparing bacteremic vs. nonbacteremic ventilator-associated pneumonia. Crit Care Med 35(9):2064–2270
59. Garnacho-Montero J, Ortiz-Leyba C, Fernández-Hinojosa E, Aldabó-Pallás T, Cayuela A, Marquez-Vácaro JA, Garcia-Curiel A, Jiménez-Jiménez FJ (2005) Acinetobacter baumannii ventilator-associated pneumonia: epidemiological and clinical findings. Intensive Care Med 31:649–655
60. Iregui M, Ward S, Sherman G, Fraser VJ, Kollef MH (2002) Clinical importance of delays in the initiation of appropriate antibiotic treatment for ventilator-associated pneumonia. Chest 122:262–268
61. Kollef KE, Schramm GE, Wills AR, Reichley RM, Micek ST, Kollef MH (2008) Predictors of 30-day mortality and hospital costs in patients with ventilator-associated pneumonia attributed to potentially antibiotic-resistant gram-negative bacteria. Chest 134:281–287
62. Magret M, Lisboa T, Martin-Loeches I, Manez R, Nauwynck M, Wrigge H, Cardellino S, Diaz E, Koulenti D, Rello J (2011) Bacteremia is an independent risk factor for mortality in nosocomial pneumonia: a prospective and observational multicenter study. Crit Care 15(1):R62
63. Luna CM, Videla A, Mattera J, Vay C, Famiglietti A, Vujacich P, Niederman MS (1999) Blood cultures have limited value in predicting severity of illness

and as a diagnostic tool in ventilator-associated pneumonia. Chest 116(4):1075–1084
64. Muscedere JG, McColl C, Shorr A, Jiang X, Marshall J, Heyland DK (2008) Determinants of outcome in patients with a clinical suspicion of ventilator-associated pneumonia. J Crit Care 23(1):41–49
65. Sasaki TM, Welch GW, Herndon DN, Kaplan JZ, Lindberg RB, Pruitt BA Jr (1979) Burn wound manipulation-induced bacteremia. J Trauma Acute Care Surg 19(1):46–48
66. Herndon DN, Barrow RE, Rutan RL, Rutan TC, Desai MH, Abston S (1989) A comparison of conservative versus early excision therapies in severely burned patients. Ann Surg 209(5):547–552
67. Sørensen B, Fisker NP, Steensen JP, Kalaja E (1984) Acute excision or exposure treatment? Final results of a three-year randomized controlled clinical trial. Scand J Plast Reconstr Surg 18(1):87–93
68. Blot S, Vandewoude K, Hoste E, De Waele J, Kint K, Rosiers F, Vogelaers D, Colard yn F (2003) Absence of excess mortality in critically ill patients with nosocomial Escherichia coli bacteremia. Infect Control Hosp Epidemiol 24(12):912–915
69. Blot SI, Vandewoude KH, Colardyn FA (2002) Clinical impact of nosocomial Klebsiella bacteremia in critically ill patients. Eur J Clin Microbiol Infect Dis 21(6):471–473
70. Blot S, Vandewoude K, Colardyn F (2003) Nosocomial bacteremia involving Acinetobacter baumannii in critically ill patients: a matched cohort study. Intensive Care Med 29(3):471–475
71. Blot S, Vandewoude K, De Bacquer D, Colardyn F (2002) Nosocomial bacteremia caused by antibiotic-resistant gram-negative bacteria in critically ill patients: clinical outcome and length of hospitalization. Clin Infect Dis 34(12):1600–1606
72. Blot S, Vandewoude K, Hoste E, Colardyn F (2003) Reappraisal of attributable mortality in critically ill patients with nosocomial bacteraemia involving Pseudomonas aeruginosa. J Hosp Infect 53(1):18–24
73. Blot SI, Vandewoude KH, Colardyn FA (2003) Evaluation of outcome in critically ill patients with nosocomial Enterobacter bacteremia: results of a matched cohort study. Chest 123(4):1208–1213
74. Brun-Buisson C, Doyon F, Carlet J (1996) Bacteremia and severe sepsis in adults: a multicenter prospective survey in ICUs and wards of 24 hospitals. French Bacteremia-Sepsis Study Group. Am J Respir Crit Care Med 154(3 Pt 1):617–624
75. Kang CI, Song JH, Chung DR, Peck KR, Ko KS, Yeom JS, Ki HK, Son JS, Lee SS, Kim YS, Jung SI, Kim SW, Chang HH, Ryu SY, Kwon KT, Lee H, Moon C, Korean Network for Study of Infectious Diseases (KONSID) (2011) Risk factors and pathogenic significance of severe sepsis and septic shock in 2286 patients with gram-negative bacteremia. J Infect 62(1):26–33
76. Wunsch H, Linde-Zwirble WT, Angus DC (2006) Methods to adjust for bias and confounding in critical care health services research involving observational data. J Crit Care 21(1):1–7
77. Timsit JF, Fosse JP, Troche G, De Lassence A, Alberti C, Garrouste-Orgeas M, Bornstain C, Adrie C, Cheval C, Chevret S (2002) Calibration and discrimination by daily logistic organ dysfunction scoring comparatively with daily sequential organ failure assessment scoring for predicting hospital mortality in critically ill patients. Crit Care Med 30(9):2003–2013
78. MacArthur RD, Miller M, Albertson T, Panacek E, Johnson D, Teoh L, Barchuk W (2004) Adequacy of early empiric antibiotic treatment and survival in severe sepsis: experience from the MONARCS trial. Clin Infect Dis 38(2):284–288
79. McGregor JC, Rich SE, Harris AD, Perencevich EN, Osih R, Lodise TP Jr, Miller RR, Furuno JP (2007) A systematic review of the methods used to assess the association between appropriate antibiotic therapy and mortality in bacteremic patients. Clin Infect Dis 45(3):329–337
80. Paul M, Shani V, Muchtar E, Kariv G, Robenshtok E, Leibovici L (2010) Systematic review and meta-analysis of the efficacy of appropriate empiric antibiotic therapy for sepsis. Antimicrob Agents Chemother 54(11):4851–4863
81. Brusselaers N, Hoste EA, Monstrey S, Colpaert KE, De Waele JJ, Vandewoude KH, Blot SI (2005) Outcome and changes over time in survival following severe burns from 1985 to 2004. Intensive Care Med 31(12):1648–1653
82. Fitzwater J, Purdue GF, Hunt JL, O'keefe GE (2003) The risk factors and time course of sepsis and organ dysfunction after burn trauma. J Trauma Acute Care Surg 54(5):959–966
83. Vogelaers D, Lambert ML, Blot S (2011) Impact estimates of nosocomial bloodstream infection: looking from a different angle. Crit Care 15(3):169
84. Greenhalgh DG, Saffle JR, Holmes JH IV, Gamelli RL, Palmieri TL, Horton JW, Tompkins RG, Traber DL, Mozingo DW, Deitch EA, Goodwin CW (2007) American Burn Association consensus conference to define sepsis and infection in burns. J Burn Care Res 28(6):776–790
85. Hurley JC (2013) Endotoxemia: correlation with gram negative bacteremia and association with outcome. D Med Sc thesis, University of Melbourne. http://repository.unimelb.edu.au/10187/17991. Accessed 14 Feb 2017
86. Munster AM, Meek M, Winchurch RA, Dickerson C (1993) A new sepsis scale for burns: correlation with endotoxin and host response. In: Faist E, Meakins JL, Schildberg FW (eds) Host defense dysfunction in Trauma, shock and sepsis. Springer, Berlin, pp 843–849
87. Hurley JC (1995) Endotoxin: methods of detection and clinical correlates. Clin Microbiol Rev 8:268–292
88. Munster AM (1999) Is endotoxin an important factor in burn patients? Curr Opin Crit Care 5(4):290–292

89. Konigova R, Konickova Z, Bouska I (1979) Clinical forms of endotoxemia in burns. Scand J Plast Reconstr Surg 13(1):61–62
90. Winchurch RA, Thupari JN, Munster AM (1987) Endotoxemia in burn patients: levels of circulating endotoxins are related to burn size. Surgery 102(5):808–812
91. Endo S, Inada K, Kikuchi M, Yamada Y, Kasoi T, Kondo M, Hoshi S, Yamashita H, Suzuki M, Yoshida M (1992) Are plasma endotoxin levels related to burn size and prognosis? Burns 18(6):486–489
92. Heggers JP, Goodheart R, Carino E, McCoy L, Ramirez RJ, Maness C (1998) Is the limulus amebocyte lysate the sole predictor of septic episodes in major thermal injuries? J Burn Care Rehabil 19(6):512–515
93. Dobke MK, Simoni J, Ninnemann JL, Garrett J, Harnar TJ (1989) Endotoxemia after burn injury: effect of early excision on circulating endotoxin levels. J Burn Care Rehabil 10(2):107–111
94. Munster AM, Moran KT, Thupari J, Allo M, Winchurch RA (1987) Prophylactic intravenous immunoglobulin replacement in high-risk burn patients. J Burn Care Rehabil 8(5):376–380
95. Munster AM, Xiao GX, Guo Y, Wong LA, Winchurch RA (1989) Control of endotoxemia in burn patients by use of polymyxin B. J Burn Care Res 10(4):327–330
96. Ren H, Li Y, Han C, Hu H (2015) Serum procalcitonin as a diagnostic biomarker for sepsis in burned patients: a meta-analysis. Burns 41(3):502–509
97. Lavrentieva A, Kontakiotis T, Lazaridis L, Tsotsolis N, Koumis J, Kyriazis G, Bitzani M (2007) Inflammatory markers in patients with severe burn injury: what is the best indicator of sepsis? Burns 33(2):189–194
98. Lavrentieva A, Papadopoulou S, Kioumis J, Kaimakamis E, Bitzani M (2012) PCT as a diagnostic and prognostic tool in burn patients. Whether time course has a role in monitoring sepsis treatment. Burns 38(3):356–363
99. Paratz JD, Lipman J, Boots RJ, Muller MJ, Paterson DL (2014) A new marker of sepsis post burn injury? Crit Care Med 42(9):2029–2036
100. Hurley JC (2011) Meta-analysis of studies of diagnostic tests: developments in how the ROC 'works'. Arch Pathol Lab Med 135:1585–1590
101. Armstrong SD, Thomas W, Neaman KC, Ford RD, Paulson J (2013) The impact of antibiotic impregnated PICC lines on the incidence of bacteremia in a regional burn center. Burns 39(4):632–635
102. King B, Schulman CI, Pepe A, Pappas P, Varas R, Namias N (2007) Timing of central venous catheter exchange and frequency of bacteremia in burn patients. J Burn Care Res 28(6):859–860
103. Özkurt Z, Altoparlak Ü, Yilmaz SI, Erol S, Özden K, Akçay MN (2012) Reducing hospital infection rates in the burn unit by adherence to infection control measures: a six-year experience. Turkish J Med Sci 42(1):17–24
104. Tagami T, Matsui H, Fushimi K, Yasunaga H (2016) Prophylactic antibiotics may improve outcome in patients with severe burns requiring mechanical ventilation: propensity score analysis of a Japanese nationwide database. Clin Infect Dis 62(1):60–66
105. Durtschi MB, Orgain C, Counts GW, Heimbach DM (1982) A prospective study of prophylactic penicillin in acutely burned hospitalized patients. J Trauma Acute Care Surg 22(1):11–14
106. Barret JP, Jeschke MG, Herndon DN (2001) Selective decontamination of the digestive tract in severely burned pediatric patients. Burns 27(5):439–445
107. de La Cal MA, Cerdá E, García-Hierro P, Van Saene HK, Gómez-Santos D, Negro E, Lorente JA (2005) Survival benefit in critically ill burned patients receiving selective decontamination of the digestive tract: a randomized, placebo-controlled, double-blind trial. Ann Surg 241(3):424–430
108. Deutsch DH, Miller SF, Finley RK Jr (1990) The use of intestinal antibiotics to delay or prevent infections in patients with burns. J Burn Care Res 11(5):436–442
109. Ergün O, Celik A, Ergün G, Özok G (2004) Prophylactic antibiotic use in pediatric burn units. Eur J Pediatr Surg 14(06):422–426
110. Kimura A, Mochizuki T, Nishizawa K, Mashiko K, Yamamoto Y, Otsuka T (1998) Trimethoprim-sulfamethoxazole for the prevention of methicillin-resistant Staphylococcus aureus pneumonia in severely burned patients. J Trauma Acute Care Surg 45(2):383–387
111. Levine BA, Petroff PA, Slade CL, Pruitt BA (1978) Prospective trials of dexamethasone and aerosolized gentamicin in the treatment of inhalation injury in the burned patient. J Trauma Acute Care Surg 18(3):188–193
112. Steer JA, Papini RP, Wilson AP, McGrouther DA, Nakhla LS, Parkhouse N (1997) Randomized placebo-controlled trial of teicoplanin in the antibiotic prophylaxis of infection following manipulation of burn wounds. Br J Surg 84(6):848–853
113. Ugburo AO, Atoyebi OA, Oyeneyin JO, Sowemimo GO (2004) An evaluation of the role of systemic antibiotic prophylaxis in the control of burn wound infection at the Lagos University Teaching Hospital. Burns 30(1):43–48
114. Avni T, Levcovich A, Ad-El DD, Leibovici L, Paul M (2010) Prophylactic antibiotics for burns patients: systematic review and meta-analysis. Br Med J 340:c241
115. Barajas-Nava LA, López-Alcalde J, RoquéiFiguls M, Solà I, BonfillCosp X (2013) Antibiotic prophylaxis for preventing burn wound infection. Cochrane Database Syst Rev 6(6):CD008738
116. Said J, Dodoo CC, Walker M, Parsons D, Stapleton P, Beezer AE, Gaisford S (2014) An in vitro test of the efficacy of silver-containing wound dressings against Staphylococcus aureus and Pseudomonas aeruginosa in simulated wound fluid. Int J Pharm 462(1):123–128
117. Aziz ZS, Abu SF, Chong NJ (2012) A systematic review of silver-containing dressings and topical sil-

ver agents (used with dressings) for burn wounds. Burns 38(3):307–318
118. Storm-Versloot MN, Vos CG, Ubbink DT, Vermeulen H (2010) Topical silver for preventing wound infection. Cochrane Database Syst Rev 17(3):CD006478
119. Vermeulen H, van Hattem JM, Storm-Versloot MN, Westerbos SJ (2007) Topical silver for treating infected wounds (Review). Cochrane Database Syst Rev 24(1):CD005486
120. Hurley JC (2016) Prophylactic antibiotics for severe burns: are they safe? Clin Infect Dis 62(9):1191–1193
121. Hurley JC (1995) Prophylaxis with enteral antibiotics in ventilated patients: selective decontamination or selective cross infection? Antimicrob Agents Chemother 39:941–947
122. Hurley JC (2016) Impact of selective digestive decontamination on respiratory tract Candida. Eur J Clin Microbiol Infect Dis 35(7):1121–1135
123. Hurley JC (2015) ICU-acquired candidemia within selective digestive decontamination studies: a meta-analysis. Intensive Care Med 41(11):1877–1885
124. Hurley JC (2011) Paradoxical ventilator associated pneumonia incidences among selective digestive decontamination studies versus other studies of mechanically ventilated patients: benchmarking systematic review data. Crit Care 15:R7
125. Hurley JC (2014) Ventilator Associated Pneumonia prevention methods using topical antibiotics: herd protection or herd peril? Chest 146(4):890–898
126. Hurley JC (2014) Topical antibiotics as a major contextual hazard toward bacteremia within selective digestive decontamination studies: a meta-analysis. BMC Infect Dis 14(1):714
127. Chung KK, Wolf SE, Renz EM, Allan PF, Aden JK, Merrill GA, Shelhamer MC, King BT, White CE, Bell DG, Schwacha MG (2010) High-frequency percussive ventilation and low tidal volume ventilation in burns: a randomized controlled trial. Crit Care Med 38(10):1970–1977
128. Garrel D, Patenaude J, Nedelec B, Samson L, Dorais J, Champoux J, D'elia M, Bernier J (2003) Decreased mortality and infectious morbidity in adult burn patients given enteral glutamine supplements: a prospective, controlled, randomized clinical trial. Crit Care Med 31(10):2444–2449
129. Reper P, Wibaux O, Van Laeke P, Vandeenen D, Duinslaeger L, Vanderkelen A (2002) High frequency percussive ventilation and conventional ventilation after smoke inhalation: a randomised study. Burns 28(5):503–508
130. Cioffi WG Jr, Rue LW 3rd, Graves TA, McManus WF, Mason AD Jr, Pruitt BA Jr (1991) Prophylactic use of high-frequency percussive ventilation in patients with inhalation injury. Ann Surg 213(6):575–582
131. Czapran A, Headdon W, Deane AM, Lange K, Chapman MJ, Heyland DK (2015) International observational study of nutritional support in mechanically ventilated patients following burn injury. Burns 41(3):510–518
132. Hall JJ, Hunt JL, Arnoldo BD, Purdue GF (2007) Use of high-frequency percussive ventilation in inhalation injuries. J Burn Care Res 28(3):396–400
133. Miller AC, Rivero A, Ziad S, Smith DJ, Elamin EM (2009) Influence of nebulized unfractionated heparin and N-acetylcysteine in acute lung injury after smoke inhalation injury. J Burn Care Res 30(2):249–256
134. Lipovy B, Rihova H, Gregorova N, Hanslianova M, Zaloudikova Z, Kaloudova Y, Brychta P (2011) Epidemiology of ventilator-associated tracheobronchitis and vantilator-associated pneumonia in patients with inhalation injury at the Burn Centre in Brno (Czech Republic). Ann Burns Fire Disasters 24(3):120–125
135. Rue LW, Cioffi MW, Mason AD, McManus CW, Pruitt CB (1993) Improved survival of burned patients with inhalation injury. Arch Surg 128(7):772–780
136. Tanizaki S, Suzuki K (2012) No influence of burn size on ventilator-associated pneumonia in burn patients with inhalation injury. Burns 38(8):1109–1113
137. Ravat F, Le-Floch R, Vinsonneau C, Ainaud P, Bertin-Maghit M, Carsin H, Perro G (2011) Antibiotics and the burn patient. Burns 37(1):16–26
138. Dolton M, Xu H, Cheong E, Maitz P, Kennedy P, Gottlieb T, Buono E, McLachlan AJ (2010) Vancomycin pharmacokinetics in patients with severe burn injuries. Burns 36(4):469–476
139. Blanchet B, Jullien V, Vinsonneau C, Tod M (2008) Influence of burns on pharmacokinetics and pharmacodynamics of drugs used in the care of burn patients. Clin Pharmacokinet 47(10):635–654
140. Weinbren MJ (1999) Pharmacokinetics of antibiotics in burn patients. J Antimicrob Chemother 44(3):319–327
141. Lu J, Yang M, Zhan M, Xu X, Yue J, Xu T (2016) Antibiotics for treating infected burn wounds. Cochrane Libr 2:CD012084

Comparison of Antemortem Clinical Diagnosis and Postmortem Findings in Burn-Related Deaths

Hüseyın Balandız and Burak Gümüs

1 Introduction

Skin is the largest organ of our body, and the exposure of high temperatures to a body will cause severe damage to the skin and the other tissues/organs. Because of this, severe or not, burn injuries that can result in mortality are still very important health problems in the world. It is estimated that approximately six million patients seek medical treatment for burns annually in the world [1]. Also burns are the most expensive traumatic injuries because of long hospitalization and expensive wound treatment [2, 3]. It was reported that the incidence of major burns is 0.2–2.9 per 100,000 individuals with flash burns, scalds, and contact burns being the most common types of burns [1]. Although the mortality rates of burns have decreased in the world due to the development and increased numbers of specialist burn centers and the medical advances in this area, burns are still quite mortal if the clinicians do not make the right diagnoses and do not give the right treatments to the patients.

H. Balandız (✉) · B. Gümüs
GATA Adli Tıp Anabilim Dalı Başkanlığı, Etlik, Ankara, Turkey
e-mail: huseyinbalandiz@gmail.com

2 Burns Can Be Divided into Categories [4]

2.1 Flame Burns

There is a contact between the flame and the body. Also, flash burns may be assessed under this topic, which is caused by the initial ignition from the flash fires of the explosion of gases, petrochemicals, or fine particulate material.

2.2 Contact Burns

There is a physical contact between the body and hot objects like a stove, etc.

2.3 Radiant Heat Burns

These burns are caused by heat waves and there is not any contact between body and flame/hot objects.

2.4 Scalding Burns

These burns are caused by contact with hot liquids, especially with hot water and hot oil.

Recent Clinical Techniques, Results, and Research in Wounds (2018)
https://doi.org/10.1007/15695_2018_111, © Springer International Publishing AG
Published Online: 05 July 2018

2.5 Chemical Burns

These burns are caused by contact with chemicals (acidic and basic materials).

2.6 Microwave and Electricity (Low-/High-Voltage) Burns

These burns are less well known.

3 Burn Injuries

Burn injuries are the fourth most common type of trauma all over the world, following traffic accidents, falls, and interpersonal violence [5], and the accidental burn injury is the commonest manner of burns [6]. Flame burn is the most common cause of burns [7–9], and inhalation burns are often accompanied by the flame burns [10, 11]. Higher mortality in burn injuries is associated with older age, the extent of the burn surface area, the presence of inhalation injury, pulmonary injury, sepsis, prolonged intubation, and the presence of concurrent diseases [1, 7, 9, 12].

A clinician must not forget that all burn-related deaths are forensic cases and these deaths must absolutely be autopsied. Besides a medicolegal autopsy is mandatory to these deaths, postmortem examinations will help the clinician to verify their treatments and clinical approach.

4 Discrepancies Between Premortem Diagnoses and Postmortem Examination

There are only a few studies on the comparison of antemortem clinical diagnoses and postmortem findings in burn-related deaths in the literature [9, 10, 12, 13].

In Krishnan et al.'s study [10], the mortality of burns was 1.9% (92 deaths out of 4745 admissions for acute burns), and flame burns (84%) and scalding (8%) were the common burn types. In the assessment of 55 patients who underwent a medicolegal autopsy, multi-organ failure (MOF) was clinically thought to be the leading cause of death, and septic shock (53.8%) was determined to be the primary trigger for MOF. Among the deaths, 51.2% had an inhalational injury. The other clinical causes of deaths were respiratory failure (9%, $n = 2$ ARDS, $n = 1$ pneumonia, $n = 1$ hemopneumothorax and ARDS, $n = 1$ wean due to their pre-burn chronic obstructive lung disease), primary gastrointestinal failure (9%, $n = 2$ ischemic bowel, $n = 1$ toxic megacolon, $n = 2$ liver failure), cardiac deaths (9%, $n = 1$ myocardial infarction, $n = 4$ cardiac arrest due to poor cardiac indices), and one death from brain death. Clinically, 61.8% of 55 patients had a sepsis diagnosis and only 9 of the septic patients had positive blood cultures. *Pseudomonas aeruginosa* was the predominant causative organism from wounds. Following organisms were fungal infections (*Candida* and *Aspergillus*) and sensitive staphylococcal (*Staphylococcus aureus*) infections.

Of the 55 patients, 85% had a postmortem examination, and "burns," "burns and smoke inhalation," or "burns and associated symptoms" were the most primary cause of death issued in death certificates. The authors think that the causes of death in death certificates are not compatible with the clinical notes. For example, in two instances, patients clearly died of a clinical diagnosis of ischemic bowel, while in death certificate the cause of death was "burns" and "burns and associated symptoms" [10].

In Kallinen et al.'s study [9], the mortality rate was 5.4% (74 deaths out of 1370 admissions with burns). There were 71 patients who underwent medicolegal autopsies. There was a complete agreement between premortem clinical diagnoses and autopsy findings in 86% of patients. Only ten (14.1%) autopsies revealed diagnostic differences: respiratory, gastrointestinal, and cardiovascular. Six of the diagnostic discrepancies were major (pneumonia [the most], hepatic cirrhosis, myocardial infarction, liver and spleen failure, pulmonary embolism, acute respiratory distress syndrome) and would have altered the clinical approach if known at the time.

In Tuğcu et al.'s study [12], there were a total of 450 deaths and 31 (6.9%) of them were burn-related. Twelve of the burn-related deaths underwent a medicolegal autopsy, and half of them had a diagnosis of pneumonia at autopsy that remained clinically unrecognized.

Fish et al. [13] mentioned that 18% (16 of 88) of patients had diagnostic discrepancies between premortem diagnoses and postmortem examination, and 4 (4.5%) patients had major missed diagnoses.

There are significant diagnostic discrepancies between the premortem clinical diagnoses and autopsy findings. A judicial autopsy is mandatory for burn-related deaths, but it is also very necessary and helpful for a clinician to review his/her clinical approach for burn patients. In judicial autopsies, the brain, chest, and abdomen are opened and all of the organs are examined externally. Besides, histopathological examinations of the organs, toxicological analysis of the body fluids (blood, urine, eye fluid, gall fluid, etc.) and tissues, microbiological examinations of tissues, and any other essential medical examinations that are necessary are done in an autopsy. In consequence of all these postmortem examinations, the accurate "cause of death" and the other situations that aid to death is revealed. So, the judicial autopsy is both useful for clinician and jurisdiction.

5 Difficulties in Medico-legal Approach of Burn-related Deaths

Although a judicial autopsy is mandatory for a burn-related death, there are still some problems with the outcomes. In most countries, there is not any or enough collaboration of feedback and communication with the clinicians who treated the patient antemortem and the forensic experts who examined the body postmortem. The postmortem examination of a burn-related death should give a useful feedback to the clinician for reconsidering his/her antemortem clinical approach and treatment of the burned patients. Obtaining autopsy reports of burn-related deaths is very hard for a clinician. The clinician works at a hospital that is bound to the Ministry of Health, and the medical examiners work for the jurisdiction that is bound to the Ministry of Justice. These two different institutions are independent of each other. But, there must be an online system which the clinicians could see the autopsy reports and postmortem examinations of their patients. Or there must be an obligatory feedback system to the clinicians about the postmortem examinations. Our suggestion to the clinicians is run after the autopsy report and postmortem examinations even if it did not come in front of you spontaneously.

If we look from the viewpoint of forensic medicine, another problem is the death certificates and the "cause of death" parts that are issued by the medical examiner. The coroners, medical examiners, or forensic experts must issue the death certificates correctly and meticulously. It is not enough and suitable to give a cause of death just only "burns" or "burns and associated symptoms." If a death certificate includes a correct "cause of death," with the full histopathologic, toxicological, and microbiological examinations, it will help the clinician to review his/her treatment and diagnoses. The purpose of an autopsy is not only to give a "cause of death." An autopsy should also provide a useful clinical data, reveal diagnostic discrepancies, and provide a useful educational recourse to clinical services [10].

Conclusions

Burn injuries are important cause of mortality, and all of the burn-related deaths should undergo medicolegal autopsy. The findings revealed by the autopsy could make significant contributions to the treatment of burn cases with the interdisciplinary data sharing between clinicians and forensic experts.

References

1. Brusselaers N, Monstrey S, Vogelaers D, Hoste E, Blot S (2010) Severe burn injury in Europe: a systematic review of the incidence, etiology, morbidity, and mortality. Crit Care 14(5):R188

2. Sanchez JL, Pereperez SB, Bastida JL, Martinez MM (2007) Cost-utility analysis applied to the treatment of burn patients in a specialized center. Arch Surg 142(1):50–57
3. de Roche R, Lüscher NJ, Debrunner HU, Fischer R (1994) Epidemiological data and costs of burn injuries in workers in Switzerland: an argument for immediate treatment in burn centres. Burns 20(1):58–60
4. DiMaio VJ, DiMaio D (2001) Forensic pathology, 2nd edn. CRC Press LLC, Boca Raton
5. Pekka S, Knight B (2004) The pathology of burns. In: Pekka S, Knight B (eds) Bernard knight's forensic pathology, 3rd edn. Oxford University Press Inc., New York, p 322
6. van Rijn OJ, Bouter LM, Meertens RM (1989) The aetiology of burns in developed countries: review of the literature. Burns 15(4):217–221
7. Kumar V, Mohanty MK, Kanth S (2007) Fatal burns in Manipal area: a 10 year study. J Forensic Legal Med 14(1):3–6
8. Kallinen O, Maisniemi K, Böhling T, Tukiainen E, Koljonen V (2012) Multiple organ failure as a cause of death in patients with severe burns. J Burn Care Res 33(2):206–211
9. Kallinen O, Partanen TA, Maisniemi K, Böhling T, Tukiainen E, Koljonen V (2008) Comparison of premortem clinical diagnosis and autopsy findings in patients with burns. Burns 34(5):595–602
10. Krishnan P, Frew Q, Green A, Martin R, Dziewulski P (2013) Cause of death and correlation with autopsy findings in burns patients. Burns 39(4):583–588
11. Gomez R, Murray CK, Hospenthal DR, Cancio LC, Renz EM, Holcomb JB, Wade CE, Wolf SE (2009) Causes of mortality by autopsy findings of combat casualties and civilian patients admitted to a burn unit. J Am Coll Surg 208(3):348–354
12. Tuğcu H, Zor F, Toygar M, Balandız H (2015) Comparison of antemortem clinical diagnosis and postmortem findings in burn-related deaths. Ulus Travma Acil Cerrahi Derg 21(6):491–495
13. Fish J, Hartshorne N, Reay D, Heimbach D (2000) The role of autopsy on patients with burns. J Burn Care Rehabil 21(4):339–344

The Effect of Natural Extracts on Laser Burn Wound Healing

Zouhir Sahnoun, Sana Bardaa, and Tarek Rebaï

1 Introduction

Remarkable advances have been made in the use of the laser in medicine and surgery since the 1990s especially in the field of dermatology. Laser efficacy is now recognized in the treatment of several diseases such as angiomas, nevus spilus, and telangiectasia as well as against superficial pigmented lesions. The laser has also been recognized as an effective treatment for common skin diseases. Laser treatment is used too in the field of esthetic dermatology to reduce facial wrinkles and skin irregularities, such as blemishes or acne scars, and to treat alopecia. The different indications of the lasers depend on the laser wavelength [1]. Although there are various types of lasers, the most common used lasers in dermatology are erbium and carbon dioxide (CO_2). Both lasers could vaporize the damaged surface skin cells. In the field of esthetic dermatology, laser resurfacing is one of the most widely used lasers.

Despite the development of CO_2 laser technology and the introduction of fractionated CO_2 laser for a better balance effectiveness – tolerance – some side effects still occur even with the best technology and physician care and sometimes may be severe, like scarring and dyschromia which are cosmetically disturbing to patients [2]. Overall, patients undergoing cosmetic surgery have less tolerance to side effects than patients treated by medically indicated procedures. Appropriate treatment of the skin following a laser application especially with a cosmetic aim is vital to ensure a speedy recovery while minimizing the risk of adverse effects, in particular infections.

In this chapter, we present a definition of the principle of laser treatment, a short list of indications and side effects of laser treatment, and a succinct review of different therapeutics used in the treatment of the resurfacing laser side effect by focusing on studies that evaluate the effects of natural derivatives of medicinal plants on post-laser wounds.

2 Definition of Laser

Laser stands for light amplification by stimulated emission of radiation. It is a solid, liquid, or gaseous environment in which we excite electrons of atoms with an external source. These electrons return in orbit to a stable state to emit a beam of monochrome coherent light, it's a laser beams with very high photon intensity and focused into very small spots [3]. In the medical field, laser types use high peak powers and short pulse widths to remove selectively any kind of pigments without damage to the surrounding tissue [4].

Z. Sahnoun (✉) · S. Bardaa · T. Rebaï
Laboratory of Pharmacology, Faculty of Medicine of Sfax, University of Sfax, Sfax, Tunisia

Recent Clinical Techniques, Results, and Research in Wounds (2018)
https://doi.org/10.1007/15695_2018_113, © Springer International Publishing AG
Published Online: 22 August 2018

2.1 How a Laser Acts on the Skin

Laser acts on the skin according two effects:

1. A non-specific thermal effect corresponding to a non-specific burn by carbonization of the targets without respecting the surrounding tissues.
2. A specific photochemical effect that corresponds to the specific destruction of a single target without destroying the other surrounding elements: For instance, the red dye laser will destroy the red blood cells and the vessels without damaging the underlying epidermis. It is used to treat angioma planes [3].

2.2 Types of Lasers

The multiplication of lasers, changes in wavelengths, and the variability of operating make the classification and choice of applications harder.

The biological targets of lasers are blood, melanin, and water that absorb light energy differently depending on the wavelength of the incident photon energy. According to the environment target in the beginning, we obtain a chromophore that absorbs a specific laser wavelength. For example, both CO_2 laser at 10.600 nm and an erbium-YAG laser have water as a chromophore [5].

Three types of lasers are highly used in dermatology:

1. Abrasion lasers (CO_2 and erbium -YAG) (yttrium aluminum garnet)
2. Lasers for vascular lesions (YAG-KTP and pulsed dye laser (PDL))
3. Lasers for pigmentation (ND YAG QS,QS Alexandrite, Ruby QS) [3]

CO_2 laser has water as a chromophore target that exists uniformly in soft tissues. But, it could be considered as tissue-selective since it is used only as tissue ablative with minimal involvement of the surrounding normal tissue [5].

Currently, laser classes include mainly nonablative and ablative lasers in both fractionated and nonfractionated varieties. Nonablative lasers conserve the epidermis and target the dermal tissues to enhance collagen formation. They are considered as soft treatment as they reduce the adverse event profile and recovery time. However, ablative lasers are more aggressive and are similar to a skin peel with higher adverse event profile and prolonged recovery time. These lasers target water molecules in the epidermis, causing vaporization of skin cells and retraction of the dermis with collagen formation. Fractionated lasers are designed to target microscopic treatment zones to create columns of thermal injury with adjacent normal skin. This procedure improves skin texture and promotes wound healing compared with nonfractionated lasers without the high side effect profile of ablative lasers [6].

Although there are various types of lasers, in this chapter we will describe laser resurfacing which is the one of the most widely used lasers in the field of esthetic dermatology. The two most commonly used lasers in dermatology are erbium and carbon dioxide (CO_2). Both lasers could vaporize the damaged surface skin cells.

2.2.1 Carbon Dioxide (CO_2) Laser

The CO_2 laser is a gaseous laser. The excitement of the gas produces a radiation that acts on the tissular structures of the skin. Carbon dioxide (CO_2) laser is an ablative laser device producing energy at a wavelength of 10,600 nm. It was one of the earliest laser systems developed in 1964 to treat scars and aging skin. This device was quickly known as an excellent surgical laser noticed in many indications due to its high capacity to absorb water [7].

The full ablative resurfacing aimed to remove the epidermis and leave a partially coagulated tissue in the dermis that could initiate the wound healing process. This zone is known as residual thermal damage and considered as the main driver of laser rejuvenation through resurfacing [8]. In fact, full ablative laser resurfacing is still the efficient standard for facial rejuvenation [9]. However, the high incidence of side effects such as pigmentation variability and permanent scarring has limited its use in dermatology practice [10–12]. This kind of CO_2 laser treatment induces severe oozing and crusting followed by prolonged erythema, infection, and herpes simplex lesions [13].

In 2000, the side effect issues following ablative laser resurfacing ceased, thanks to a number of nonablative skin rejuvenation lasers. They were based on the theory of delivering controlled dermal damage under a cooled and intact epidermis to speed up the skin regeneration. Despite the improvement of dermal histology, the epidermis did not show any recovery progress [14]. To overcome this issue, it was mandatory to develop and mix both approaches frankly ablative and completely nonablative using a scanner in order to set the new technology of fractional laser rejuvenation [15]. The latter optimized device was established by using a nonablative approach with 1540 nm laser pulses generating micronecrotic zones of dermis coagulation under a certain intact epidermis. In the process, some skin microdamage occurred before epidermal renewal, which could not be avoided.

Ablative fractional laser resurfacing (AFR) is an extremely promising tool to accommodate a multidisciplinary functional and skin restoration of patients [16, 17]. AFR ensures the control of tissue vaporization by inducing dermal coagulation that goes in greater depths than that of traditional laser devices. Accordingly, AFR produces higher tissue contraction rates and collagen production amounts than those recorded with nonablative devices. AFR has several advantages over traditional CO_2 laser resurfacing including the fact of a very low risk of scarring and/or hypopigmentation. Few studies have reported that AFR treatment limitations are likely related to inappropriate treatment techniques or setting issues [18, 19].

Indications for the Carbon Dioxide Laser

The CO_2 laser has many indications as it could be used for almost anything surgical [20]. Some of the main indications will be listed in this subsection.

Skin Lesions

The clinical indications of the CO_2 laser include a number of techniques which are incision, vaporization, and coagulation that achieve hemostasis and ensure a dry field. The CO_2 laser can be prescribed for the treatment of nevus cells, seborrheic keratosis. Xanthelasmas and syringomas could also be treated with the CO_2 laser. Furthermore, the CO_2 laser has been used in the treatment of some malignant tumors, such as basal cell epithelioma that has an increased tendency of metastasize [21].

Warts

Verruca vulgaris is the common known wart that has a predilection to show up on the fingers and toes especially in children. The CO_2 laser allows to ablate and vaporize the wart medullar portion till normal tissue morphology [22].

Toenail Disease

Recently, the use of CO_2 laser has been advocated in the treatment of nails, in particular toenails. According to Lim et al. [23], toenail diseases, onychodystrophy, for example, lend themselves well to CO_2 laser treatment.

Anti-aging

Fractional laser treatment represents the most commonly known indication for facial wrinkles [24]. Lines and wrinkles could be treated by both fractional ablative and nonablative lasers [24, 25]. Lapidoth et al. [26] reported the efficacy of ablative fractionated Er:YAG laser in the treatment of photoaging.

2.2.2 Erbium Laser Resurfacing

Erbium laser resurfacing is used to eliminate surface levels and to treat deep lines and wrinkles. It could be more efficient for darker skin than CO_2 laser. One of the advantages of erbium laser resurfacing is minimum burning of surrounding tissue. The common side effects of this type of laser are redness, swelling, and bruising that regress faster than with CO_2 laser resurfacing [27].

3 Side Effects of Lasers

The therapeutic use of laser has become frequent both in the cosmetic and dermatological fields. It becomes the basic treatment in some skin pathologies. The development of CO_2 lasers is aimed to achieve excellent results with a favorable side effect profile. The potential complications associated with CO_2 laser treatments are well-described in the literature [10]. They are usually benign, but in some cases they may be serious requiring strict monitoring and sometimes preventive measures to avoid their occurrence [28].

3.1 Pain

During the laser procedure of the skin, topical anesthetics are usually applied before starting a laser treatment to minimize the pain as much as possible. But, the patient feels discomfort after the treatment [29].

3.2 Erythema

Erythema is a very common side effect of laser skin treatments. For nonablative lasers, it usually stays for 2–3 days but can persist up to 1 week. However, it is more intensive and prolonged for traditional ablative lasers which would physically vaporize the top layer of the skin, leaving it raw for 3–4 weeks until it heals on its own [29–31]. It may be due to inappropriate laser settings, infection, aggressive debridement between laser passes, and contact dermatitis. This adverse effect can regress faster if using a pulsed dye laser or intense pulsed light device [28].

3.3 Post-treatment Edema

Post-treatment edema is patient-dependent. It lasts on average 1–3 days; it may exceed a week in some patients. The use of ice at 10-min intervals for the first 24-h postoperative laser or topical systemic corticosteroids following treatment is advocated to avoid the risk of edema [32].

3.4 Bruising

The use of higher fluencies may lead to occasional bruising often occurring 3 days following laser treatment [33]. To reduce the risk of such a side effect, it is recommended in the immediate postoperative time to avoid nonsteroidal anti-inflammatory drugs and blood thinners.

3.5 Dyschromia

Not every patient's skin is suitable for laser treatment. Usually, lasers work better on people with lighter skin tones than on people with darker skin tones, but both kinds of skin tones have a risk of hypopigmentation or hyperpigmentation. The incidence of hyperpigmentation is considerably less with fractional resurfacing assuming reasonable treatment parameters than that with ablative lasers [34]. Nevertheless, fractional lasers are certainly capable of causing disruption of melanogenesis which leads to hypopigmentation [10, 28].

3.6 Infections

An intact skin is an effective barrier against infection. But laser treatment in particular the ablative one affects the microbiotic balance of the skin causing a high risk of surinfection. The microorganisms involved in the cutaneous infection can be bacteria, fungi, and viruses. The germs often implicated are *Staphylococcus*, *Pseudomonas*, *Klebsiella*, and *Enterobacter* [28]. Thus, most patients are treated with antibiotics and the antiviral drug is usually selected for herpes simplex [35].

3.7 Blistering, Scabbing, and/or Crusting

These are moderate to severe side effects of cosmetic lasers and light-based facial treatments. Most of the time, it is as if the patient had a sunburn post-laser, but sometimes blistering, scabbing, and even crusting can occur on his face. These symptoms must be left alone to heal on their own [36].

3.8 Scarring

Scarring is the most dreaded side effect [18]. Several factors may be involved in the appearance of cutaneous scarring lesions. Manuskiatti et al. [37] documented in their study a 3.8% incidence of scarring caused only by infection. Choi et al. [38] showed also that the more aggressive treatments with higher energies and an increased number of passes can provide dramatic clinical results such as scarring. The neck and chest are more susceptible to scarring than the face [39].

3.9 Other Complications

Other potential complications related to laser treatments are well-described in the literature and include pruritus, milia, acneiform eruption, and contact dermatitis [10]. The latter may be either irritant or allergic in nature [28].

4 Post-laser Care

The laser treatments are known as efficient tools to cure common skin diseases. However, they lead to several postoperative side effects mainly redness and swelling. These effects prolong the wound healing period which requires both pre- and post-laser care. The laser care management reduces the local systems, speeds up re-epithelialization, and enhances wound healing with minimal irritation [40]. In fact, the number of studies reports a high recorded infection rate that ranges from 6 to 8% for ablative resurfacing-treated patients [41]. Since the last few years, interest in the post-laser care has increased rapidly, and nowadays it is considered as an important step to keep the skin moist, clean, and healthy. So, synthetic drugs such as antibiotics and moisturizing products have been the subject of several studies. However, few publications exist in the literature which describe the effect of natural extracts on laser burn wound healing.

4.1 Synthetic and Probiotic Post-care

The first attempts of the treatment of laser skin complications amid patient-tested synthetic drugs which have been the subject of several studies. For instance, West et al. [42] study of post-laser resurfacing highlighted the beneficial topical effect of hydroquinone, tretinoin, and/or glycolic acid preparations on hyperpigmentation. The latter is considered as the most noted complication following carbon dioxide (CO_2) laser resurfacing. A previous study carried out by Lowe et al. [43] has also shown a good effect on hyperpigmentation of oral anti-herpes simplex medications, antibiotics, and skin lightening agents for pretreated laser resurfacing combined with topical retinoids and acetic acid for post-treated laser. However, the study of Zimber et al. [44] proved that the diluted acetic acid is not effective and petrolatum remains the standard treatment for laser wound care.

Petrolatum as the trolamine provide a moist environment that promotes fibroblastic proliferation and prevents the infectious contamination of the wound site. In a study of 20 patients undergoing CO_2 fractional laser resurfacing of the perioral area, Sarnoff [40] compared the wound healing efficacy of petrolatum contained in Aquaphor Healing Ointment (AHO) formulation and Biafine Topical Emulsion (BTE) (trolamine) treatment. All patients received antiviral and antibiotic medication before and after laser treatment. The AHO formulation seems to be more efficient on the parameters of laser irritation than BTE. However, in the study of Rendon et al. [45], statistically significant improvements have been observed with BTE in erythema and edema and in physicians' assessment of global re-epithelialization compared to white petrolatum. According to Sarnoff [40], the AHO formulation has an advantage to associate petrolatum, lipid barriers, and humectants. The latter ingredient holds moisture, and the wound exudates are drawn into the ointment and away from skin which could explain the reduction of the crust.

Another clinical study was conducted by Ehsani et al. [46] to evaluate the healing potential of Cicactive (CICA) gel on 15 patients with photoaged facial skin who were treated with erbium resurfacing laser. CICA gel which is composed mainly of sodium alginate, hydroxyprolisilane, and D-panthenol showed better healing effect than silver sulfadiazine reference cream. The tested gel seems also able to alleviate the discomfort of patient and to improve post-laser treatment complications such as erythema. Aldraibi et al. [47] have reported a significant reduction of postoperative erythema and swelling amid skin type IV–VI patients treated with a topical corticosteroid (TCS) cream (betamethasone dipropionate) 10 min before the alexandrite prelaser and twice a day for 5 days post-laser. We think that this type of anti-inflammatory treatment administered not associated with the antibiotics for an extended period can expose the patient to infectious risks. In fact, the use of steroidal anti-inflammatory drugs after ablative laser resurfacing could have locoregional immunosuppressive consequences that affect the balance of skin microbiota and promote the multiplication of pathogens increasing thus the risk of surinfection.

Moreover, the role of the human microbiota (the whole of the microorganisms (bacteria, viruses, fungi, yeasts) living in a specific environment) in maintaining good body health is a topical issue. Most recent studies have focused on the human intestinal microbiota, but far less research have been carried out on skin microbiota. The cutaneous microflora is fundamental for the homeostasis of the skin. It controls innate immunity as well as the barrier function [48, 49]. The imbalance of commensal ecosystem could lead to skin diseases such as acne [50] and atopic dermatitis [51]. Thus, understanding the involvement of the skin microbiota in several skin pathologies is vital. The prebiotic and probiotics seem to improve the balance of the microbiota and can be a second therapeutic alternative to the treatment of many skin disorders. A recent study conducted by Zoccali et al. [52] has assessed the wound healing potential of a topical probiotic cream on 42 patients receiving fractional CO_2 laser. The cream containing DermaACB (based on probiotic-derived active principles) has been administered twice a day for a couple of week in a postoperative laser care. Compared to antibiotic and hyaluronic acid reference creams, DermaACB cream significantly reduced postoperative erythema and swelling.

4.2 Natural Post Laser Care in Rat

The third attempt in the treatment of cutaneous laser side effects focused on the use of medicinal plants. For decades, plants have been used as a main *source* of medicines to treat a wide variety of ailments. With the considerable progress in the pharmaceutical industry, synthetic drugs replaced plants making as such phytotherapy an outdated practice with doubtful effects. However, given the limited availability of medications in wound healing, only 1–3% of the drugs in the Western pharmacopeia are dedicated to the treatment of skin diseases [53], and the use of traditional medicines reappeared as an alternative form of health care. A study carried out by Payyappallimana in 2010 [54] estimated that traditional medicine covers the primary health-care needs of 80% of the world's population.

In the literature, various studies have demonstrated the efficiency of phytochemical constituents, herbal formulations, and natural extracts in wound care treatment. Yet, only few studies have been recently carried out to assess the healing effect of medicinal plants on post-laser wound treatment.

A comparative study conducted on rats by Aliasl et al. [55] has shown that *Arnebia euchroma* has a better wound healing than petrolatum and silver sulfadiazine used as references to treat fractional CO_2 laser wounds. It significantly decreases erythema and crusting on the 9th day and enhances epithelial confluence and general wound appearance scores on the 7th and the 9th days. This wound healing effect is attributed to the anti-inflammatory and antimicrobial properties of *Arnebia euchroma* ointment. This cream seems to improve re-epithelization, fibroblast proliferation, and vascularization of the injured tissues.

Our research team is also interested in medicinal plants given their attested anti-inflammatory, antioxidant, and antibacterial properties. According to Bardaa et al. [56] and Khedir et al. [57], "CYTOL BASIC" (a reference cream emulsion based on *Vitis vinifera* (grape) seed oil) could promote wound healing effect of CO_2 fractional laser burns. Conducting research on rats having partial-thickness fractional CO_2 laser burns, these authors [56, 57] have shown, for the first time, the wound healing potential of the oils extracted from the prickly pear, pumpkin, linseed, and *Pistacia lentiscus*. During the trial, the rats treated with these oils have a better general wound appearance and crusting compared to the control and the reference groups. In fact, the wound healing effect of these oils on laser burns lasted only 7–8 days [56, 57]. Treated with pumpkin oil, the mechanical wounds took 11 days to recover [56, 58], while the thermal wounds took 33 days [59]. Indeed, several factors such as the type of trauma, the extent of the damage, and the depth of the lesion can affect the duration of wound healing [60]. Locoregional zones at the level of thermal wounds can be deeply affected. The inflammation, the ionic imbalance, the congestion, and the capillary thrombosis are more severe in thermal wounds than in laser or mechanical wounds. In addition, thermal wounds provoke an important blood aggregation which could be a nutriment for bacteria that colonize the burn. The excessive multiplication of pathogens could cause the absorption of oxygen, the decrease of the wound pH, and the formation of microthromboses. This induces a state of local tissue hypoxia which inhibits phagocytosis and increases the wound infection delaying as such wound healing [61, 62]. So, the short healing time observed following laser burn could be at least partly explained by the presence of partially preserved healthy skin with epithelial annex areas that allow a rapid regeneration of the dermis and epidermis [63].

The wound healing effect of the prickly pear, the linseed, the pumpkin, and the lentiscus oils is attributed to their compounds mainly polyunsaturated fatty acids (oleic, linoleic, and linolenic acids), tocopherols, and sterols. The antibacterial and antioxidant activities of these oils in synergy might also contribute to their wound healing effects. Moreover, the rapid reduction of laser burn size observed in both studies could be attributed to the barrier lipid formed by the tested oils. They seem to provide a moist environment that enhances cell migration and wound healing. All the tested oils don't provoke neither irritation nor infections for the treated groups [56, 57].

So, we think that these oils could be considered as an effective treatment for immediate post-operative laser skin resurfacing. Human clinical studies are in progress to confirm experimental findings on rats.

4.3 Natural Post-laser Care in Patient

In the literature there are only four works focused on natural products use on human subjects. Alonso et al. [64] tested the effect of topical Arnica Gel on the bruising of 19 patients divided into pretreatment and posttreatment groups. They all have facial telangiectases treated with pulsed dye laser. No significant difference was observed in the prevention or treatment of bruising between the vehicle and the topical Arnica. The small number of subjects is the major limitation of this study.

Conducting a study on two human subjects, Huber et al. [65] showed the good effect of Arnica ethanolic extract, known as Combudoron, on second-degree burns induced by erbium-YAG laser. This study is also limited since it was carried out on two patients only which doesn't prove neither the efficacy of Combudoron nor the reliability of the study.

Aliasl et al. study [66] compared the effect of *Arnebia euchroma* ointment (AEO) made up from *A. euchroma* roots and sesame (*Sesamum indicum*) oil with petrolatum on post-laser resurfacing wound. AEO and petrolatum were applied for 1 week to 47 subjects having Fitzpatrick skin phototype and facial atrophic acne scars treated with MIXEL-CO_2 fractional laser. Although the

AEO is known to be an effective burn drug, it seems to be not as efficient as the petrolatum for acne laser treatment. In fact, post-laser wounds are drier than other burn wounds because CO_2 laser vaporizes intracellular and extracellular water [67]. Thus, AEO might be combined with moisturizing materials to improve the wound healing conditions of post-laser wounds. The authors also attribute this result to the small size of the study sample among other reasons.

Conducting a study on 50 patients having photoaging skin damage treated with fractional laser resurfacing, a recent study of Grippaudo [68] proved that the ionic hydrogel (Procutase®) based on plant-derived peptides, natural hydrophilic polymers, and ionized trace metals was an efficient treatment of minor and superficial burns. According to the author, the ionic hydrogel creates a moist environment that promotes fibroblastic proliferation and prevents the infection of the wound site. We think that ionic hydrogel is a mixture of natural active ingredients so it cannot be assimilated to a plant extract.

Conclusions

The studies initiated to evaluate the effect of natural extracts on laser burn wound healing are rare and also inconclusive mainly for methodological reasons. Moreover, according to several published works, the use of antibiotic prophylaxis for post-laser resurfacing care is still controversial [69–71], and the pretreatment protocols using antibiotic and antiviral prophylaxis are non-univocal [72]. Since traditional medicines is currently more and more recognized, we believe that medicinal plants can be an alternative therapy for the treatment of laser's adverse effects on the skin. Unlike synthetic medicines which hold one active ingredient, medicinal plants have several properties at a time that in synergy could be efficient for wound healing especially in treatment of laser cutaneous complications.

References

1. Omi T, Numano K (2014) The role of the CO_2 laser and fractional CO2 laser in dermatology. Laser Ther 23(1):49–60
2. Hunzeker CM, Weiss ET, Geronemus RG (2009) Fractionated CO2 laser resurfacing: our experience with more than 2000 treatments. Aesthet Surg J 29:317–322
3. Michaud D (2006) Les lasers en dermatologie, 2nd edn. DOIN Publishing, Paris
4. Anderson RR, Parrish JA (1983) Selective photothermolysis, precise microsurgery by selective absorption of pulsed radiation. Science 220:524–527
5. Itzkan I, Drake EH (1997) History of lasers in medicine. In: Arndt KA, Dover JS, Olbricht SM (eds) Lasers in cutaneous and aesthetic surgery. Lippincott-Raven, Inc., Philadelphia, pp 3–10
6. Richter AL, Barrera J, Markus RF, Brissett A (2014) Laser skin treatment in non-Caucasian patients. Facial Plast Surg Clin North Am 22(3):439–446
7. Kaplan I (2010) The CO2 surgical laser. Photomed Laser Surg 28(6):847–848
8. Ross EV, Barnette DJ, Glatter RD, Grevelink JM (1999) Effects of overlap and pass number in CO2 laser skin resurfacing: a study of residual thermal damage, cell death, and wound healing. Lasers Surg Med 24(2):103–112
9. Chwalek J, Goldberg DJ (2011) Ablative skin resurfacing. Curr Probl Dermatol 42:40–47
10. Bernstein LJ, Kauvar AN, Grossman MC, Geronemus RG (1997) The short- and long-term side effects of carbon dioxide laser resurfacing. Dermatol Surg 23(7):519–525
11. Nanni CA, Alster TS (1998) Complications of carbon dioxide laser resurfacing. An evaluation of 500 patients. Dermatol Surg 24(3):315–320
12. Alster T, Hirsch R (2003) Single-pass CO2 laser skin resurfacing of light and dark skin: extended experience with 52 patients. J Cosmet Laser Ther 5(1):39–42
13. Ragland HP, McBurney E (1996) Complications of resurfacing. Semin Cutan Med Surg 15(3):200–207
14. Goldberg DJ (2002) Nonablative dermal remodeling: does it really work? Arch Dermatol 138(10):1366–1368
15. Geronemus RG (2006) Fractional photothermolysis: current and future applications. Lasers Surg Med 38(3):169–176
16. Perry A, Elston J, Reynolds H, Hawley L, Kroonen L, Uebelhoer NS, Shumaker PR (2014) Ablative fractional photothermolysis in the treatment of scar contractures of the wrists and forearms: a retrospective data analysis. J Am Acad Dermatol 71(4):841–842
17. Issler-Fisher AC, Fisher OM, Smialkowski AO, Li F, van Schalkwyk CP, Haertsch P, Maitz PK (2017) Ablative fractional CO2 laser for burn scar reconstruction: an extensive subjective and objective short-term outcome analysis of a prospective treatment cohort. Burns 43(3):573–582
18. Ross RB, Spencer J (2008) Scarring and persistent erythema after fractionated ablative CO2 laser resurfacing. J Drugs Dermatol 7(11):1072–1073
19. Fife DJ, Fitzpatrick RE, Zachary CB (2009) Complications of fractional CO2 laser resurfacing: four cases. Lasers Surg Med 41(3):179–184
20. Kaplan I (2007) The CO_2 laser as a versatile surgical modality. Laser Ther 16:25–38

21. Mirza FN, Khatri KA (2017) The use of lasers in the treatment of skin cancer: a review. J Cosmet Laser Ther 10:1–8
22. Oni G, Mahaffey PJ (2011) Treatment of recalcitrant warts with the carbon dioxide laser using an excision technique. J Cosmet Laser Ther 13(5):231–236
23. Lim EH, Seo YJ, Lee JH, Im M (2013) Onychodystrophy treated using fractional carbon dioxide laser therapy and topical steroids: new treatment options for nail dystrophy. Dermatol Surg 39(12):1931–1933
24. Rahman Z, Alam M, Dover JS (2006) Fractional laser treatment for pigmentation and texture improvement. Skin Therapy Lett 11(9):7–11
25. Bass LS (2005) Rejuvenation of the aging face using Fraxel laser treatment. Aesthet Surg J 25(3):307–309
26. Lapidoth M, Yagima Odo ME, Odo LM (2008) Novel use of erbium:YAG (2,940-nm) laser for fractional ablative photothermolysis in the treatment of photodamaged facial skin: a pilot study. Dermatol Surg 34(8):1048–1053
27. Preissig J, Hamilton K, Markus R (2012) Current laser resurfacing technologies: a review that delves beneath the surface. Semin Plast Surg 26(3):109–116
28. Ramsdell WM (2012) Fractional CO_2 laser resurfacing complications. Semin Plast Surg 26(3):137–140
29. Roynesdal AK, Björnland T, Barkvoll P, Haanaes HR (1993) The effect of soft-laser application on postoperative pain and swelling. A double-blind, crossover study. Int J Oral Maxillofac Surg 22(4):242–245
30. Rokhsar CK, Fitzpatrick RE (2005) The treatment of melasma with fractional photothermolysis: a pilot study. Dermatol Surg 31(12):1645–1650
31. Metelitsa AI, Alster TS (2010) Fractionated laser skin resurfacing treatment complications: a review. Dermatol Surg 36(3):299–306
32. Cervelli V, Gentile P, Spallone D, Nicoli F, Verardi S, Petrocelli M, Balzani A (2010) Ultrapulsed fractional CO2 laser for the treatment of post-traumatic and pathological scars. J Drugs Dermatol 9(11):1328–1331
33. Fife DJ, Zachary CB (2009) Delayed pinpoint purpura after fractionated carbon dioxide treatment in a patient taking ibuprofen in the postoperative period. Dermatol Surg 35(3):553
34. Tan KL, Kurniawati C, Gold MH (2008) Low risk of postinflammatory hyperpigmentation in skin types 4 and 5 after treatment with fractional CO2 laser device. J Drugs Dermatol 7(8):774–777
35. Fisher AA (1996) Lasers and allergic contact dermatitis to topical antibiotics, with particular reference to bacitracin. Cutis 58(4):252–254
36. Royston SL, Wright PA, Widdowson DC, Wareham WJ, Strike PW (2008) Adverse effects reported in epilatory ruby laser treatment. Lasers Med Sci 23(1):35–39
37. Manuskiatti W, Fitzpatrick RE, Goldman MP (1999) Long-term effectiveness and side effects of carbon dioxide laser resurfacing for photoaged facial skin. J Am Acad Dermatol 40(3):401–411
38. Choi B, Barton J, Chan E, Thomsen SL, Welch AJ (1998) Infrared imaging of CO_2 laser ablation: implications for laser skin resurfacing. Proc SPIE 3245:344–351
39. Avram MM, Tope WD, Yu T, Szachowicz E, Nelson JS (2009) Hypertrophic scarring of the neck following ablative fractional carbon dioxide laser resurfacing. Lasers Surg Med 41(3):185–188
40. Sarnoff DS (2011) A comparison of wound healing between a skin protectant ointment and a medical device topical emulsion after laser resurfacing of the perioral area. J Am Acad Dermatol 64(3 Suppl):36–43
41. Hantash BM, Mahmood MB (2007) Fractional photothermolysis: a novel aesthetic laser surgery modality. Dermatol Surg 33(5):525–534
42. West TB, Alster TS (1999) Effect of pretreatment on the incidence of hyperpigmentation following cutaneous CO2 laser resurfacing. Dermatol Surg 25(1):15–17
43. Lowe NJ, Lask G, Griffin ME (1995) Laser skin resurfacing. Pre- and posttreatment guidelines. Dermatol Surg 21(12):1017–1019
44. Zimber MP, Mansbridge JN, Taylor M, Stockton T, Hubka M, Baumgartner M, Rheins L, Hubka K, Brandt EN, Kellar R, Naughton GK (2012) Human cell-conditioned media produced under embryonic-like conditions result in improved healing time after laser resurfacing. Aesthet Plast Surg 36(2):431–437
45. Rendon M, Cardona L, Benitez A (2008) The safety and efficacy of trolamine/sodium alginate topical emulsion in postlaser resurfacing wounds. J Drugs Dermatol 7(Suppl):S23–S28
46. Ehsani AH, Miresmaeli M, Montaser KL, Ahmadi H, Hoseini M (2011) Efficacy of cicactive® versus silver sulfadiazine 0.1% cream on facial wound healing in patients treated with erbium-yag resurfacing laser: a single-blind randomized clinical trial (letter to editor). Iran. J Dermatol 14:119–120
47. Aldraibi MS, Touma DJ, Khachemoune A (2007) Hair removal with the 3-msec alexandrite laser in patients with skin types IV-VI: efficacy, safety, and the role of topical corticosteroids in preventing side effects. J Drugs Dermatol 6(1):60–66
48. Grice EA, Kong HH, Renaud G, Young AC, NISC Comparative Sequencing Program, Bouffard GG, Blakesley RW, Wolfsberg TG, Turner ML, Segre JA (2008) A diversity profile of the human skin microbiota. Genome Res 18(7):1043–1050
49. Martín R, Miquel S, Langella P, Bermúdez-Humarán LG (2014) The role of metagenomics in understanding the human microbiome in health and disease. Virulence 5(3):413–423
50. Bek-Thomsen M, Lomholt HB, Scavenius C, Enghild JJ, Brüggemann H (2014) Proteome analysis of human sebaceous follicle infundibula extracted from healthy and acne-affected skin. PLoS One 9(9):e107908
51. Blanchet-Réthoré S, Bourdès V, Mercenier A, Haddar CH, Verhoeven PO, Andres P (2017) Effect of a lotion containing the heat-treated probiotic strain lactobacillus johnsonii NCC 533 on Staphylococcus aureus colonization in atopic dermatitis. Clin Cosmet Investig Dermatol 10:249–257
52. Zoccali G, Cinque B, La Torre C, Lombardi F, Palumbo P, Romano L, Mattei A, Orsini G, Cifone

MG, Giuliani M (2016) Improving the outcome of fractional CO2 laser resurfacing using a probiotic skin cream: preliminary clinical evaluation. Lasers Med Sci 31(8):1607–1611
53. Kumar B, Vijayakumar M, Govindarajan R, Pushpangadan P (2007) Ethnopharmacological approaches to wound healing—exploring medicinal plants of India. J Ethnopharmacol 114(2):103–113
54. Payyappallimana U (2010) Role of traditional medicine in primary health care: an overview of perspectives and challenging. https://www.researchgate.net/publication/284697212_Role_of_Traditional_Medicine_in_Primary_health_care. Accessed 9 Jan 2017
55. Aliasl J, Barikbin B, Khoshzaban F, Naseri M, Sedaghat R, Kamalinejad M, Talei D, Emadi F, Akbari Z, Aliasl F, Jalaly NY, Mohseni-Moghaddam P (2015) Effect of Arnebia euchroma ointment on post-laser wound healing in rats. J Cosmet Laser Ther 17(1):41–45
56. Bardaa S, Chabchoub N, Jridi M, Moalla D, Mseddi M, Rebai T, Sahnoun Z (2016) The effect of natural extracts on laser burn wound healing. J Surg Res 201(2):464–472
57. Khedir SB, Bardaa S, Chabchoub N, Moalla D, Sahnoun Z, Rebai T (2017) The healing effect of Pistacia lentiscus fruit oil on laser burn. Pharm Biol 55(1):1407–1414
58. Bardaa S, Ben Halima N, Aloui F, Ben Mansour R, Jabeur H, Bouaziz M, Sahnoun Z (2016) Oil from pumpkin (Cucurbita pepo L.) seeds: evaluation of its functional properties on wound healing in rats. Lipids Health Dis 15:73
59. Bardaa S, Moalla D, Ben Khedir S, Rebai T, Sahnoun Z (2016) The evaluation of the healing proprieties of pumpkin and linseed oils on deep second-degree burns in rats. Pharm Biol 54(4):581–587
60. Hess CT (2011) Checklist for factors affecting wound healing. Adv Skin Wound Care 24(4):192
61. Lakhel A, Pradier JP, Brachet M, Duhoux A, Duhamel P, Fossat S (2008) Chirurgie des brûlures graves au stade aigu. In: EMC Techniques Chirurgicales – Chirurgie Plastique Reconstructrice et Esthétique. Elsevier SAS, Paris, pp 45–157
62. Guo S, DiPietro L (2010) Factors affecting wound healing. J Dental Res 89(3):219–229
63. Beylot C (2009) Lasers ablatifs et lasers fractionnels. Ann de Derm et de Vénér 135(1):189–194
64. Alonso D, Lazarus MC, Baumann L (2002) Effects of topical arnica gel on post-laser treatment bruises. Dermatol Surg 28(8):686–688
65. Huber R, Bross F, Schempp C, Gründemann C (2011) Arnica and stinging nettle for treating burns - a self-experiment. Complement Ther Med 19(5):276–280
66. Aliasl J, Khoshzaban F, Barikbin B, Naseri M, Kamalinejad M, Emadi F, Razzaghi Z, Talei D, Yousefi M, Aliasl F, Barati M, Mohseni-Moghaddam P, Hasheminejad SA, Esmailzad NH (2014) Comparing the healing effects of Arnebia euchroma ointment with petrolatum on the ulcers caused by fractional CO2 laser: a single-blinded clinical trial. Iran Red Crescent Med J 16(10):e16239
67. Chapas AM, Brightman L, Sukal S, Hale E, Daniel D, Bernstein LJ, Geronemus RG (2008) Successful treatment of acneiform scarring with CO2 ablative fractional resurfacing. Lasers Surg Med 40(6):381–386
68. Grippaudo FR (2016) Ionic hydrogel monotherapy and in combination with antiviral-antibiotic prophylaxis, in the post-procedure Management of Fractional Laser-Treated Patients. J Clin Aesthet Dermatol 9(11):23–28
69. Friedman PM, Geronemus RG (2000) Antibiotic prophylaxes in laser resurfacing patients. Dermatol Surg 26:695–697
70. Alster TS (2000) Against antibiotic prophylaxis for cutaneous laser resurfacing. Dermatol Surg 26:697–698
71. Graber EM, Tanzi EL, Alster TS (2008) Side effects and complications of fractional laser photothermolysis: experience with 961 treatments. Dermatol Surg 34:301–307
72. Jalian HR, Jalian CA, Avram MM (2013) Common cause of injury and legal action in laser surgery. JAMA Dermatol 149:188–193

Part II

Infections

Malnutrition Predicts Infectious and Wound Complications Following Posterior Lumbar Spinal Fusion

Ankur S. Narain, Fady Y. Hijji, Krishna T. Kudaravalli, Kelly H. Yom, and Kern Singh

1 Introduction

The current aging of the population will require more patients to be treated for degenerative spinal disorders both now and in the future [1]. Posterior lumbar spinal fusion is one of the most popular operative techniques for this purpose, and it will be increasingly utilized as the incidence of spinal pathology increases. As such, it is of utmost importance to characterize the outcomes and morbidity associated with this type of procedure.

Postoperative surgical site infection (SSI), along with other infectious complications, is of significant concern after posterior lumbar fusion procedures. Previous investigations have determined the incidence of postoperative SSI after spinal procedures to be between 4 and 17% [2–12]. Postoperative SSI is associated with significant morbidity and prolonged length of inpatient stay [2, 4, 5, 7, 13–19]. Furthermore, infectious complications are also associated with significant costs to physicians and the overall healthcare system [2, 5, 7]. Previous studies have estimated the monetary cost per encounter for postoperative SSI to range from $26,977 to $961,722 [20].

Due to the clinical and financial burden associated with postoperative SSI, the identification of modifiable risk factors has been an important topic of investigation. One particular risk factor that has received significant attention is nutritional status. Previous studies have demonstrated that up to 40% of the hospitalized population and up to 42.4% of orthopedic patients are malnourished [21–28]. Within the general surgery literature, malnutrition has been extensively studied and has been demonstrated to have a clear association with postoperative SSI [29, 30]. Multiple investigations have also been performed in the literature pertaining to spine surgery, with the purpose of this chapter being to review those studies along with their clinical implications.

2 Definition and Evaluation of Malnutrition

Malnutrition can be defined by a variety of different measurement techniques and screening tools (Table 1). One method to define malnutrition involves utilization of anthropometric measurements [24, 31, 32]. These measurements include such indices as body mass index (BMI), body fat characteristics, and thigh, calf, or mid-upper arm circumference [33–37]. In regard to BMI, malnutrition is defined as either a BMI < 18.5 kg/m^2 or a reduced age-specific BMI associated with recent weight loss [38]. For muscle circumference,

A.S. Narain • F.Y. Hijji • K.T. Kudaravalli
K.H. Yom • K. Singh, M.D. (✉)
Department of Orthopaedic Surgery, Rush University Medical Center, Chicago, IL, USA
e-mail: kern.singh@rushortho.com

Recent Clinical Techniques, Results, and Research in Wounds (2017)
DOI 10.1007/15695_2017_35, © Springer International Publishing AG
Published Online: 24 October 2017

>40% reductions in arm circumference in relation to sex-specific standards is considered to be associated with malnutrition [39].

Table 1 Commonly utilized criteria for determination of malnutrition [15, 24, 26, 27, 31–37, 39, 40, 42, 44, 45]

Measurement	Criteria for malnutrition
Anthropometric measurements	
Body mass index	<18.5 kg/m^2
Mid-upper arm circumference	>40% reduction from sex-specific standard
Screening questionnaires	
NRS-2002	Score ≥ 3
MNA-Short Form	Score = 8–11—at risk Score ≤ 7—malnourished
Laboratory values	
Albumin	<3.5 g/dL
Prealbumin	<20 mg/dL
Transferrin	<200 mg/dL
Total lymphocyte count	<1500 cells/mm^3

NRS-2002 Nutritional risk screening 2002, *MNA* Mini Nutritional Assessment

Screening questionnaires have also been developed with the purpose of identifying patients who are at risk for malnutrition. One such screening tool used for inpatients is the Nutritional Risk Screening 2002 (NRS-2002), developed by the European Society for Clinical Nutrition and Metabolism (Table 2) [40]. This scale utilizes a two-stage scoring system taking into account a patient's BMI, recent weight loss, percentage of normal food intake, and severity of disease. Scores ≥3 are associated with being nutritionally at risk, with recommendations for nutritional intervention. Wang et al. [41], in a study of 432 spinal surgery patients screened via NRS-2002, demonstrated that 11.6% of inpatients were nutritionally at risk, while 12.7% were malnourished.

Another screening questionnaire is the Mini Nutritional Assessment-Short Form (MNA-SF), which was specifically designed for use in the elderly patient population (Fig. 1) [42]. This scale produces a score out of 14 from a 6-question survey assessing a patient's food intake, recent

Table 2 (A) NRS-2002 initial screening [40]; (B) NRS-2002 final screening [40]

A. NRS-2002 initial screening [40]			
	Yes?		No?
BMI < 20.5?			
Weight loss in the last 3 months?			
Reduced dietary intake in the last week?			
Severely ill? (i.e., requires intensive therapy)			
If "yes" to any question → proceed to part B If "no" to all questions → rescreen weekly BMI = body mass index			

B. NRS-2002 final screening [40]			
Nutritional status		Severity of disease	
Absent (Score = 0)	Normal	Absent (Score = 0)	Normal dietary requirements
Mild (Score = 1)	Weight loss >5% over 3 months OR 50–75% normal food intake over the last week	Mild (Score = 1)	Hip fracture, acute exacerbation of chronic disorders (cirrhosis, COPD)
Moderate (Score = 2)	Weight loss > 5% over 2 months OR BMI 18.5 – 20.5 + general condition impairment OR 25–60% normal food intake over the last week	Moderate (Score = 2)	Abdominal surgery, stroke
Severe (Score = 3)	Weight loss >5% over the last month OR BMI < 18.5 + general condition impairment OR 0–25% normal food intake over the last week	Severe (Score = 3)	Head trauma, bone marrow transplantation, ICU patients
If >70 years old: add 1 to total score Score ≥ 3: nutritionally at risk Score < 3: weekly rescreening recommended			

BMI body mass index, *COPD* chronic obstructive pulmonary disease, *ICU* intensive care unit

Mini Nutritional Assessment

MNA®

Nestlé NutritionInstitute

Last name: First name:

Sex: Age: Weight, kg: Height, cm: Date:

Complete the screen by filling in the boxes with the appropriate numbers. Total the numbers for the final screening score.

Screening

A Has food intake declined over the past 3 months due to loss of appetite, digestive problems, chewing or swallowing difficulties?
0 = severe decrease in food intake
1 = moderate decrease in food intake
2 = no decrease in food intake ☐

B Weight loss during the last 3 months
0 = weight loss greater than 3 kg (6.6 lbs)
1 = does not know
2 = weight loss between 1 and 3 kg (2.2 and 6.6 lbs)
3 = no weight loss ☐

C Mobility
0 = bed or chair bound
1 = able to get out of bed / chair but does not go out
2 = goes out ☐

D Has suffered psychological stress or acute disease in the past 3 months?
0 = yes 2 = no ☐

E Neuropsychological problems
0 = severe dementia or depression
1 = mild dementia
2 = no psychological problems ☐

F1 Body Mass Index (BMI) (weight in kg) / (height in m)² ☐
0 = BMI less than 19
1 = BMI 19 to less than 21
2 = BMI 21 to less than 23
3 = BMI 23 or greater ☐

IF BMI IS NOT AVAILABLE, REPLACE QUESTION F1 WITH QUESTION F2.
DO NOT ANSWER QUESTION F2 IF QUESTION F1 IS ALREADY COMPLETED.

F2 Calf circumference (CC) in cm
0 = CC less than 31
3 = CC 31 or greater ☐

Screening score ☐☐
(max. 14 points)

12-14 points: ☐ Normal nutritional status
8-11 points: ☐ At risk of malnutrition
0-7 points: ☐ Malnourished

Save
Print
Reset

Fig. 1 The Mini Nutritional Assessment-Short Form questionnaire used to screen for malnutrition in elderly patients [42, 59–62]

weight loss, mobility, psychological or acute stress, neuropsychological problems, and anthropometric measurements such as BMI or calf circumference. Scores between 8 and 11 indicate a risk for malnutrition, while scores ≤7 indicate malnourishment. Murphy et al. [43], in a survey of 49 female patients on an orthopedic ward, found that 73% of patients were characterized as either "at risk" or "malnourished" based on Mini Nutritional Assessment score.

Despite the prevalence of anthropometric and questionnaire-based screening tools, serologic laboratory tests still represent the gold standard for assessment of malnutrition. Laboratory values commonly used to detect malnutrition include prealbumin, albumin, transferrin, total serum protein, total lymphocyte count, and hematocrit [15, 26, 27, 44, 45]. Of those, the preferred laboratory test remains serum albumin level, with a value <3.5 g/dL indicating inadequate nutritional status in the majority of published studies [26, 29, 31, 44]. Prealbumin level has also been gaining in popularity as a possible test for malnutrition, as it has been postulated to be a more accurate depiction of nutritional status due to its shorter half-life compared to albumin [27].

3 Pathophysiology of Malnutrition and Infectious Complications

While many previous studies in the general surgical literature have demonstrated an association between malnutrition and postoperative SSI, no definitive pathophysiologic link has been determined. Two mechanisms are likely at play, with the first involving an association between malnutrition and impaired wound healing [46–48]. Previous studies have indicated that malnutrition is associated with decreased fibroblast proliferation and reduced collagen synthesis capacity [49]. Specifically, collagen synthesis is impaired because states of malnutrition are postulated to reduce the hydroxylation of proline and lysine that is necessary for those amino acids to be incorporated into connective tissue. The second mechanism likely involves an association between malnutrition and an impaired immune response [24, 29, 31]. Malnutrition has been demonstrated to be associated with reductions in innate immune cell activation and increases in apoptosis [50, 51]. This impairment in macrophage-mediated immunity can hinder both the innate and adaptive immune responses against potential pathogens which patients are exposed to postoperatively. Furthermore, reduced serum albumin levels seen in malnourished states may lead to increased tissue edema due to reduced colloid osmotic pressure, creating an ideal environment for bacterial propagation [29].

4 Malnutrition and Postoperative Wound Infections: Supporting Evidence

Many studies have been published on the topic of malnutrition and postoperative SSIs after posterior spinal fusion procedures, with the earliest literature being compromised of small case series and case-control studies [52, 53]. Stambough et al. [52] performed one of the earliest studies, in an examination of 19 patients treated for deep wound infections after spinal arthrodesis procedures. The authors determined that 16/19 (84.2%) patients were malnourished as defined by total lymphocyte count (<2000 cells/mL). After treatment with antibiotics and surgical debridement, 84.2% of patients did not require hardware removal, and 94.4% has successful fusions. Jevsevar and Karlin also undertook an early investigation of malnutrition in a study of 44 patients with cerebral palsy undergoing spinal fusion for scoliosis [53]. Patients were stratified by nutritional status, with malnutrition defined by both serum albumin levels (<3.5 g/dL) and total lymphocyte count (<1500 cells/mL). Those patients classified as malnourished not only exhibited higher rates of postoperative infection but also experienced longer endotracheal intubation times and longer overall lengths of hospital stay.

More recent investigations have focused on larger patient populations in retrospective cohort or case-control studies [24, 26, 27, 44]. Klein et al. [26], in a study of 114 patients undergoing elective lumbar decompression and fusion, described 13 cases of infectious complications with 10 deep wound infections. Of these infectious complications, 84.6% occurred in patients classified as malnourished. Furthermore, malnourishment was identified as a significant predictor of infectious complications on multivariate, stepwise regression analysis. Similar findings were demonstrated by Adogwa et al. [44], who determined that malnutrition was associated with superficial SSI in a study of 136 patients undergoing either posterior or anterior spinal fusion. Upon subgroup analysis, the authors also demonstrated that preoperative albumin levels were a significant predictor of postoperative complications in elective surgery but not in nonelective cases. In regard to the use of prealbumin as a test for malnutrition, Salvetti et al. [27] performed a case-control study of 106 patients undergoing posterior spinal procedures. The authors found that prealbumin level < 20 mg/dL was a significant predictor for postoperative infection (hazard ratio = 2.12).

While the majority of previous studies were derived from single-center retrospective case series, the advent of administrative databases has allowed the most recent investigations to be conducted with sample sizes of adequate statistical power [31, 54]. Schoenfeld et al. [54] conducted a study of 5857 patients undergoing spinal fusions from the National Surgical Quality Improvement Program (NSQIP) database. In this population, the rate of postoperative wound infection was approximately 2%. Malnutrition as defined by serum albumin level was found to be associated with an increased risk of both postoperative wound infection (odds ratio [OR] = 2.4) and mortality (OR = 13.8). Bohl et al. [31] performed a similar study utilizing the NSQIP database, with a sample of 4310 patients undergoing posterior lumbar fusion. In this sample, the prevalence of malnutrition as defined by serum albumin levels was 4.8%. Furthermore, malnutrition was associated with significantly increased risks of postoperative wound dehiscence and SSI. Additionally, malnourished patients had an increased rate of unplanned hospital readmission within the first 30 postoperative days compared to patients with normal nutritional status.

While most of the literature supports an association between malnutrition and SSI after posterior spinal fusion, contradictory studies do exist [55, 56]. In a case-control study of 60 patients undergoing spinal laminectomy or fusion, Apisarnthanarak et al. determined that malnutrition was not a significant predictor of postoperative infection [55]. A similar finding was also described by Klekamp et al. [56], in an investigation of 70 spinal surgery patients with 19 cases of deep wound infection. While these studies may call into question the association between malnutrition and postoperative infection, they do represent only a small minority of the available evidence. Furthermore, these studies represent small case series that may be statistically underpowered compared to the larger case series and administrative database studies that support an association.

5 Treatment and Prevention of Postoperative Wound Infections

In the case of a postoperative wound infection, treatment modalities remain the same irrespective of the nutritional status of the patient. Specifically, first-line therapy entails the combination of wound care, antibiotics, and early wound irrigation and debridement. Controversy does exist, however, regarding the necessity for hardware removal in patients who have undergone posterior spinal fusion. The literature supports the preservation of posterior instrumentation, with Mok et al. [19] and Stambough et al. [52] demonstrating fusion and maintenance of neurologic status in most patients treated with early debridement and antibiotics alone.

In regard to the prevention of SSI and wound complications, there has been significant interest in evaluating the effect of nutritional modification preoperatively. It has been proposed in multiple studies that a comprehensive nutritional plan should be utilized more frequently before spinal fusion procedures [24, 44]. Components of this plan would include preoperative screening for malnutrition, dietary counseling to alter food habits, and oral or intravenous supplementation as deemed clinically necessary. While relatively few studies have been published, those that do exist in the general surgical and orthopedic literature support the efficacy of preoperative supplementation [30, 57]. Eneroth et al. [57] performed a prospective, randomized controlled trial of 80 patients hospitalized with hip fractures. Patients were randomized to receive either a normal hospital diet or a hospital diet along with a 1400 kcal oral and intravenous supplement. The supplementation group not only had near-optimal energy and fluid intake during their inpatient stay but also had decreased rates of complications and mortality up to 4-month post-discharge. In a study of 120 abdominal surgery patients who were severely malnourished (NRS-2002 score $\geq$ 5), Jie et al. [30] demonstrated that those who received 7 days of preoperative enteral or parenteral dietary supplementation had both lower complication rates and shorter length of inpatient stay postoperatively. Interestingly, this trend was not present when a sub-analysis of patients with NRS scores of 3–4 was performed. While the results of these studies are promising, more investigation is required in spine-specific populations before supplementation can be widely utilized in patients undergoing posterior lumbar fusion.

Postoperative nutritional supplementation via total parenteral nutrition (TPN) has also been proposed as a preventative measure against SSI, particularly in cases of multi-segment fusions or staged anterior-posterior fusions [45, 58]. The rationale of this approach entails utilizing protein and energy-rich supplementation to return postoperative nutritional parameters to approximately baseline levels more rapidly. However, the efficacy of this approach has not been supported by the literature. Lapp et al. [45] conducted a study of 48 patients undergoing multi-segment spinal fusions randomized to receive or not receive TPN postoperatively. The authors determined that there were no significant differences between groups in terms of total postoperative complications. Furthermore, the same result was observed when only those patients who received posterior fusions were analyzed. Similarly, Hu et al. [58] conducted a randomized trial of 40 patients undergoing staged anterior-posterior fusion procedures. While patients that were randomized to not receive TPN had greater decreases in albumin and prealbumin postoperatively, there were no significant differences observed in the incidence of wound complications. While these studies provide evidence against the use of TPN after spinal procedures, more specific investigations must be performed in populations comprised of patients undergoing more common short-segment posterior lumbar fusions.

Conclusions

Surgical site infections and other wound complications represent a significant clinical and financial burden after posterior lumbar fusion procedures. Preoperative malnutrition has been identified in the majority of the literature as a prominent risk factor for the development of SSI. As malnutrition is modifiable, practitioners should consider more carefully screening for and assessing the nutritional status of their patients preoperatively. While multiple screening modalities exist, serum albumin level remains the gold standard for characterizing nutritional status. In cases of confirmed preoperative malnutrition, practitioners and patients should consider interventions including dietary counseling and oral dietary supplementation. Further research, including high-level prospective studies, is necessary to fully elucidate the effects of pre- and postoperative nutritional supplementation on the modification of postoperative risk for infectious wound complications.

References

1. Fehlings MG, Tetreault L, Nater A, Choma T, Harrop J, Mroz T, Santaguida C, Smith JS (2015) The aging of the global population: the changing epidemiology of disease and spinal disorders. Neurosurgery 77(Suppl 4):S1–S5
2. Bible JE, Biswas D, Devin CJ (2011) Postoperative infections of the spine. Am J Orthop (Belle Mead NJ) 40(12):E264–E271
3. Faciszewski T, Winter RB, Lonstein JE, Denis F, Johnson L (1995) The surgical and medical perioperative complications of anterior spinal fusion surgery in the

thoracic and lumbar spine in adults. A review of 1223 procedures. Spine (Phila Pa 1976) 20(14):1592–1599
4. Fang A, Hu SS, Endres N, Bradford DS (2005) Risk factors for infection after spinal surgery. Spine (Phila Pa 1976) 30(12):1460–1465
5. Gerometta A, Rodriguez Olaverri JC, Bitan F (2012) Infections in spinal instrumentation. Int Orthop 36(2):457–464
6. Glassman SD, Dimar JR, Puno RM, Johnson JR (1996) Salvage of instrumental lumbar fusions complicated by surgical wound infection. Spine (Phila Pa 1976) 21(18):2163–2169
7. Kurtz SM, Lau E, Ong KL, Carreon L, Watson H, Albert T, Glassman S (2012) Infection risk for primary and revision instrumented lumbar spine fusion in the Medicare population. J Neurosurg Spine 17(4):342–347
8. Linam WM, Margolis PA, Staat MA, Britto MT, Hornung R, Cassedy A, Connelly BL (2009) Risk factors associated with surgical site infection after pediatric posterior spinal fusion procedure. Infect Control Hosp Epidemiol 30(2):109–116
9. Olsen MA, Mayfield J, Lauryssen C, Polish LB, Jones M, Vest J, Fraser VJ (2003) Risk factors for surgical site infection in spinal surgery. J Neurosurg 98(2 Suppl):149–155
10. Olsen MA, Nepple JJ, Riew KD, Lenke LG, Bridwell KH, Mayfield J, Fraser VJ (2008) Risk factors for surgical site infection following orthopaedic spinal operations. J Bone Joint Surg Am 90(1):62–69
11. Pull ter Gunne AF, Cohen DB (2009) Incidence, prevalence, and analysis of risk factors for surgical site infection following adult spinal surgery. Spine (Phila Pa 1976) 34(13):1422–1428
12. Weinstein MA, McCabe JP, Cammisa FP Jr (2000) Postoperative spinal wound infection: a review of 2,391 consecutive index procedures. J Spinal Disord 13(5):422–426
13. Calderone RR, Garland DE, Capen DA, Oster H (1996) Cost of medical care for postoperative spinal infections. Orthop Clin North Am 27(1):171–182
14. de Lissovoy G, Fraeman K, Hutchins V, Murphy D, Song D, Vaughn BB (2009) Surgical site infection: incidence and impact on hospital utilization and treatment costs. Am J Infect Control 37(5):387–397
15. Glotzbecker MP, Riedel MD, Vitale MG, Matsumoto H, Roye DP, Erickson M, Flynn JM, Saiman L (2013) What's the evidence? Systematic literature review of risk factors and preventive strategies for surgical site infection following pediatric spine surgery. J Pediatr Orthop 33(5):479–487
16. Ho C, Skaggs DL, Weiss JM, Tolo VT (2007) Management of infection after instrumented posterior spine fusion in pediatric scoliosis. Spine (Phila Pa 1976) 32(24):2739–2744
17. Kowalski TJ, Berbari EF, Huddleston PM, Steckelberg JM, Mandrekar JN, Osmon DR (2007) The management and outcome of spinal implant infections: contemporary retrospective cohort study. Clin Infect Dis 44(7):913–920
18. Labbe AC, Demers AM, Rodrigues R, Arlet V, Tanguay K, Moore DL (2003) Surgical-site infection following spinal fusion: a case-control study in a children's hospital. Infect Control Hosp Epidemiol 24(8):591–595
19. Mok JM, Guillaume TJ, Talu U, Berven SH, Deviren V, Kroeber M, Bradford DS, Hu SS (2009) Clinical outcome of deep wound infection after instrumented posterior spinal fusion: a matched cohort analysis. Spine (Phila Pa 1976) 34(6):578–583
20. Hedequist D, Haugen A, Hresko T, Emans J (2009) Failure of attempted implant retention in spinal deformity delayed surgical site infections. Spine (Phila Pa 1976) 34(1):60–64
21. Bruun LI, Bosaeus I, Bergstad I, Nygaard K (1999) Prevalence of malnutrition in surgical patients: evaluation of nutritional support and documentation. Clin Nutr 18(3):141–147
22. Cuervo M, Garcia A, Ansorena D, Sanchez-Villegas A, Martinez-Gonzalez M, Astiasaran I, Martinez J (2009) Nutritional assessment interpretation on 22,007 Spanish community-dwelling elders through the Mini Nutritional Assessment test. Public Health Nutr 12(1):82–90
23. Inoue Y, Miki C, Kusunoki M (2004) Nutritional status and cytokine-related protein breakdown in elderly patients with gastrointestinal malignancies. J Surg Oncol 86(2):91–98
24. Jensen JE, Jensen TG, Smith TK, Johnston DA, Dudrick SJ (1982) Nutrition in orthopaedic surgery. J Bone Joint Surg Am 64(9):1263–1272
25. Kaiser MJ, Bauer JM, Ramsch C, Uter W, Guigoz Y, Cederholm T, Thomas DR, Anthony PS, Charlton KE, Maggio M, Tsai AC, Vellas B, Sieber CC (2010) Frequency of malnutrition in older adults: a multinational perspective using the mini nutritional assessment. J Am Geriatr Soc 58(9):1734–1738
26. Klein JD, Hey LA, CS Y, Klein BB, Coufal FJ, Young EP, Marshall LF, Garfin SR (1996) Perioperative nutrition and postoperative complications in patients undergoing spinal surgery. Spine (Phila Pa 1976) 21(22):2676–2682
27. Salvetti DJ, Tempel ZJ, Gandhoke GS, Parry PV, Grandhi RM, Kanter AS, Okonkwo DO (2015) Preoperative prealbumin level as a risk factor for surgical site infection following elective spine surgery. Surg Neurol Int 6(Suppl 19):S500–S503
28. Sungurtekin H, Sungurtekin U, Balci C, Zencir M, Erdem E (2004) The influence of nutritional status on complications after major intraabdominal surgery. J Am Coll Nutr 23(3):227–232
29. Hennessey DB, Burke JP, Ni-Dhonochu T, Shields C, Winter DC, Mealy K (2010) Preoperative hypoalbuminemia is an independent risk factor for the development of surgical site infection following gastrointestinal surgery: a multi-institutional study. Ann Surg 252(2):325–329
30. Jie B, Jiang ZM, Nolan MT, Zhu SN, Yu K, Kondrup J (2012) Impact of preoperative nutritional support on clinical outcome in abdominal surgical patients at nutritional risk. Nutrition 28(10):1022–1027
31. Bohl DD, Shen MR, Mayo BC, Massel DH, Long WW, Modi KD, Basques BA, Singh K (2016)

Malnutrition predicts infectious and wound complications following posterior lumbar spinal fusion. Spine (Phila Pa 1976) 41(21):1693–1699
32. Cross MB, Yi PH, Thomas CF, Garcia J, Della Valle CJ (2014) Evaluation of malnutrition in orthopaedic surgery. J Am Acad Orthop Surg 22(3):193–199
33. Bistrian BR, Blackburn GL, Sherman M, Scrimshaw NS (1975) Therapeutic index of nutritional depletion in hospitalized patients. Surg Gynecol Obstet 141(4):512–516
34. Frisancho AR (1974) Triceps skin fold and upper arm muscle size norms for assessment of nutrition status. Am J Clin Nutr 27(10):1052–1058
35. Gurney JM, Jelliffe DB (1973) Arm anthropometry in nutritional assessment: nomogram for rapid calculation of muscle circumference and cross-sectional muscle and fat areas. Am J Clin Nutr 26(9):912–915
36. Ruiz L, Colley JR, Hamilton PJ (1971) Measurement of triceps skinfold thickness. An investigation of sources of variation. Br J Prev Soc Med 25(3):165–167
37. Schutte K, Tippelt B, Schulz C, Rohl FW, Feneberg A, Seidensticker R, Arend J, Malfertheiner P (2015) Malnutrition is a prognostic factor in patients with hepatocellular carcinoma (HCC). Clin Nutr 34(6):1122–1127
38. Cederholm T, Bosaeus I, Barazzoni R, Bauer J, Van Gossum A, Klek S, Muscaritoli M, Nyulasi I, Ockenga J, Schneider SM, de van der Schueren MA, Singer P (2015) Diagnostic criteria for malnutrition—An ESPEN Consensus Statement. Clin Nutr 34(3):335–340
39. Pratt WB, Veitch JM, McRoberts RL (1981) Nutritional status of orthopedic patients with surgical complications. Clin Orthop Relat Res 155:81–84
40. Kondrup J, Rasmussen HH, Hamberg O, Stanga Z, Ad Hoc EWG (2003) Nutritional risk screening (NRS 2002): a new method based on an analysis of controlled clinical trials. Clin Nutr 22(3):321–336
41. Wang N, Dong Y, Huo T, Shao Y, Xing W, Li S (2016) Nutritional risk, malnutrition and nutritional support among hospitalized patients in orthopedics/spinal surgery of a Hohhot teaching hospital. Asia Pac J Clin Nutr 25(2):273–282
42. Rubenstein LZ, Harker JO, Salva A, Guigoz Y, Vellas B (2001) Screening for undernutrition in geriatric practice: developing the short-form mini-nutritional assessment (MNA-SF). J Gerontol A Biol Sci Med Sci 56(6):M366–M372
43. Murphy MC, Brooks CN, New SA, Lumbers ML (2000) The use of the Mini-Nutritional Assessment (MNA) tool in elderly orthopaedic patients. Eur J Clin Nutr 54(7):555–562
44. Adogwa O, Martin JR, Huang K, Verla T, Fatemi P, Thompson P, Cheng J, Kuchibhatia M, Lad SP, Bagley CA, Gottfried ON (2014) Preoperative serum albumin level as a predictor of postoperative complication after spine fusion. Spine (Phila Pa 1976) 39(18):1513–1519
45. Lapp MA, Bridwell KH, Lenke LG, Baldus C, Blanke K, Iffrig TM (2001) Prospective randomization of parenteral hyperalimentation for long fusions with spinal deformity: its effect on complications and recovery from postoperative malnutrition. Spine (Phila Pa 1976) 26(7):809–817
46. Gherini S, Vaughn BK, Lombardi AV Jr, Mallory TH (1993) Delayed wound healing and nutritional deficiencies after total hip arthroplasty. Clin Orthop Relat Res 293:188–195
47. Guo JJ, Yang H, Qian H, Huang L, Guo Z, Tang T (2010) The effects of different nutritional measurements on delayed wound healing after hip fracture in the elderly. J Surg Res 159(1):503–508
48. Jaberi FM, Parvizi J, Haytmanek CT, Joshi A, Purtill J (2008) Procrastination of wound drainage and malnutrition affect the outcome of joint arthroplasty. Clin Orthop Relat Res 466(6):1368–1371
49. Seibert DJ (1999) Pathophysiology of surgical site infection in total hip arthroplasty. Am J Infect Control 27(6):536–542
50. Reynolds JV, Redmond HP, Ueno N, Steigman C, Ziegler MM, Daly JM, Johnston RB Jr (1992) Impairment of macrophage activation and granuloma formation by protein deprivation in mice. Cell Immunol 139(2):493–504
51. Rivadeneira DE, Grobmyer SR, Naama HA, Mackrell PJ, Mestre JR, Stapleton PP, Daly JM (2001) Malnutrition-induced macrophage apoptosis. Surgery 129(5):617–625
52. Stambough JL, Beringer D (1992) Postoperative wound infections complicating adult spine surgery. J Spinal Disord 5(3):277–285
53. Jevsevar DS, Karlin LI (1993) The relationship between preoperative nutritional status and complications after an operation for scoliosis in patients who have cerebral palsy. J Bone Joint Surg Am 75(6):880–884
54. Schoenfeld AJ, Carey PA, Cleveland AW 3rd, Bader JO, Bono CM (2013) Patient factors, comorbidities, and surgical characteristics that increase mortality and complication risk after spinal arthrodesis: a prognostic study based on 5,887 patients. Spine J 13(10):1171–1179
55. Apisarnthanarak A, Jones M, Waterman BM, Carroll CM, Bernardi R, Fraser VJ (2003) Risk factors for spinal surgical-site infections in a community hospital: a case-control study. Infect Control Hosp Epidemiol 24(1):31–36
56. Klekamp J, Spengler DM, McNamara MJ, Haas DW (1999) Risk factors associated with methicillin-resistant staphylococcal wound infection after spinal surgery. J Spinal Disord 12(3):187–191
57. Eneroth M, Olsson UB, Thorngren KG (2006) Nutritional supplementation decreases hip fracture-related complications. Clin Orthop Relat Res 451:212–217
58. Hu SS, Fontaine F, Kelly B, Bradford DS (1998) Nutritional depletion in staged spinal reconstructive

surgery. The effect of total parenteral nutrition. Spine (Phila Pa 1976) 23(12):1401–1405
59. Vellas B, Villars H, Abellan G, Soto ME, Rolland Y, Guigoz Y, Morley JE, Chumlea W, Salva A, Rubenstein LZ, Garry P (2006) Overview of the MNA—Its history and challenges. J Nutr Health Aging 10(6):456–463
60. Guigoz Y (2006) The Mini Nutritional Assessment (MNA) review of the literature—What does it tell us? J Nutr Health Aging 10(6):466–485
61. Société_des_Produits_Nestlé_S.A.,_Vevey, Switzerland, Trademark owners
62. Nestlé, 1994, Revision 2009. N67200 12/99 10M

Deep Wound and Organ-Space Infection After Surgery for Degenerative Spine Disease

Seba Ramhmdani and Ali Bydon

1 Introduction

Postoperative wound infection may occur following any surgical procedure. Fortunately, it is a rare event in spinal surgery. Patients with wound infection may require prolonged hospitalization, long-term intravenous antibiotic administration, and multiple washout and revision procedures, all of which contribute to significant morbidity and hospital-related financial burden. Wound infections contribute to substantial additional hospitalization costs, with a mean cost of $25,546 per infection and $10 billion inpatient care expenditures each year [1, 2]. In certain studies, tenfold increase in mortality rate has been associated with postoperative wound infection [3].

Surgical site infections (SSI) are classified by the US Centers for Disease Control and Prevention as:

1. Superficial incisional (involving only the skin and/or subcutaneous tissue)
2. Deep incisional (involving the fascia and/or muscular layers)
3. Organ or space

In this chapter, we present the risk factors, clinical presentation, and tools of diagnosis of the last two types of SSI, deep wound and organ-space infections, with emphasis on the preventive methods and surgical management.

2 Incidence and Risk Factors

The incidence of SSI secondary to degenerative spine disease ranges between 1 and 5% [4], and the incidence of deep wound and organ-space infections ranges between 0.72 and 1.5% [3, 5]. Generally, there is a variation in the reported rates of wound infections as many variables have been identified to be associated with an increased risk of incidence, including surgery-related factors and patient-related factors. Additionally, variations in studies designs, population sizes, and surveillance methods used to follow patients contribute to the ensuing differences in incidence rates.

3 Surgery-Related Factors

3.1 Location and Approach

Based on the spinal location, the highest rate of postoperative deep wound infection for degenerative

S. Ramhmdani, M.D.
The Spinal Column Biomechanics and Surgical Outcomes Laboratory, The Johns Hopkins University School of Medicine, Baltimore, MD, USA

Department of Neurosurgery, The Johns Hopkins University School of Medicine, Baltimore, MD, USA
e-mail: sramhmd1@jhmi.edu

A. Bydon (✉)
Professor of Neurosurgery, The Spinal Column Biomechanics and Surgical Outcomes Laboratory, The Johns Hopkins University School of Medicine, 600 North Wolfe Street, Meyer 5-109, Baltimore, Maryland 21287, USA
e-mail: abydon1@jhmi.edu

Recent Clinical Techniques, Results, and Research in Wounds (2017)
DOI 10.1007/15695_2017_36, © Springer International Publishing AG
Published Online: 24 October 2017

disc disease is in the thoracic spine, followed by the lumbar and then the cervical spine [3]. The nature of the degenerative diseases of the thoracic spine is commonly more extensive (ossification of ligamentum flavum (OLF), ossification of posterior longitudinal ligament (OPLL)) and often requires more aggressive resection, including thoracic ribs, with instrumented arthrosis, and subsequently a longer operative time.

The rate of wound infection varies with the surgical approach, with the highest rate for combined anterior-posterior approach, followed by posterior and posterolateral approaches, and lastly anterior approach [3, 6]. Anterior spinal approach exploits the concept of blunt dissection and avascular tissue planes to expose spinal column, hence avoiding direct muscular tissue trauma. Anterior spine has an extensive lymphatic drainage that is crucial for bacterial clearance. On the contrary, posterior approach encompasses a wider dissection laterally to expose the transverse processes and vertically through the fascia and muscles. It also involves a prolonged retraction and extensive use of cautery, both associated with tissue ischemia and necrosis. In a retrospective study of 452 patients undergoing spinal decompression and instrumented fusion, Levi and colleagues found a 3.8% infection rate in posterior instrumentation cases and 0% rate in anterior instrumentation cases [7].

3.2 Noninstrumented Spinal Procedures

Lumbar discectomy is one of the most common spinal procedures and is associated with a low rate of infection with a reported incidence range between 0.6 and 1% [5, 8]. With a more extensive surgery, such as laminectomy, this risk increases to 2% [4]. Noninstrumented posterior spinal fusion procedures are associated with a higher rate of infection than laminectomy as they require longer operating hours, increased blood loss, greater soft tissue destruction, and placement of allograft [4].

3.3 Instrumented Spinal Procedures

As expected, surgeries incorporating instrumented arthrodesis carry a relatively higher rate of deep wound infection. This is attributed to two major factors: first, the complexity of the cases that require fusion and, second, the role of the implants as vulnerable products to organisms [3]. In a study of over 100,000 cases from the Scoliosis Research Society Morbidity and Mortality Committee Database, the incidence of deep wound infection was significantly greater in procedures with spinal fusion and/or implants compared to decompression-alone procedures (1.5 vs. 1.0%, $p < 0.001$) [3]. In the lumbar spine, anterior-only approach, TLIF (transforaminal lumbar interbody fusion) and PLIF (posterior lumbar interbody fusion) procedures are associated with a decrease in deep wound infection [3, 5].

3.4 Cervical Spine

The incidence of overall surgical site infection following a posterior cervical decompression and fusion reported as 1.02% and deep wound infection 1.47% [5, 9]. Anterior cervical spine discectomy and fusion and cervical disc replacement procedures demonstrate extremely low postoperative infection rates of 0.1% and 0.0%, respectively [5]. An iatrogenic esophageal injury, albeit very rare, can lead to infection often requiring multidisciplinary treatment approach.

3.5 Minimally Invasive Spine Surgical (MISS) Techniques

Some may claim the MISS leads to less infection than open approaches [3, 10, 11]. In one of the most frequently performed minimally invasive procedures, transforaminal lumbar interbody fusion (TLIF), the rate of deep wound infection was less than traditional open approach [3].

Minimally invasive approach restricts surgical field and leads to less exposure to potential pathogens and reduces disturbances of the skin and skin flora as they are guarded by tubes. Patients sometimes have a shorter postoperative hospital stay and less exposure to hospital-acquired pathogenic organism. MISS techniques also claim to reduce tissue destruction and blood loss [12]. This issue remains controversial and definite studies are lacking.

3.6 Graft

Similar rates of postoperative surgical site infections have been reported with the use of allograft (irradiated and nonirradiated) compared with autograft in spinal surgery. However, the use of cadaveric allografts avoids host structure sacrifice and donor-site morbidity (chronic harvest site pain, sensory changes, and infection). More importantly, allografts decrease operative time and blood loss [13].

3.7 Other Risk Factors

More extensive surgeries, surgeries with longer operative times, excessive blood loss, high volume of moving operating room personnel, revision surgeries, and other variables are commonly associated with an elevated risk for infection (Table 1). Increased operative time for more than 4 h and a delay for more than an hour in the operating room before incision might increase exposure time of the sterile field to contact and airborne contaminants [16]. Operations longer than 5 h are correlated with a surgeon's hands recontamination at levels equal to or exceed prescrub levels [17].

Prolonged surgeries are also associated with a hematoma formation, a good medium for bacterial growth, necessitating the use of closed suction drainage in the postoperative period. In fact, any collection of fluid or blood in a closed space predisposes to wound dehiscence that can progress to either superficial or deep wound infection. Moreover, excessive use of retractors, without intermittent release during surgery, and extensive use of cautery increase tissue ischemia and necrosis.

Previous studies have shown that resident physician and/or fellow physician involvement in surgical care was not associated with an increase in the incidence of perioperative wound infection. However, there is a seasonal variation of spinal wound infections with peaks during the summer (July) and winter (January). This variation is more attributable to environmental factors rather than the resident's effect, especially that this pattern was noted in both academic and nonacademic environments [18, 19].

Table 1 Surgery-related risk factors

Surgical location	Thoracic > lumbar > cervical
Surgical approach	Combined anterior-posterior procedures
Instrumentation	
Length of surgery	>4 h >1 h anesthesia ready time
Number of levels	≥7 [14]
Estimated blood loss	>1 L
Insufficient saline irrigation	<2 L/h [15]
Increased operating room traffic	
Preoperative hospital stay	
Staged procedure	
Revision surgery	

4 Patient-Related Factors

There is a strong correlation between specific medical risk factors and spinal wound infections (Table 2) [6]. Understanding these factors will help to decrease the rate of postoperative infection. Diabetes mellitus (DM) is an important factor as it considered a prevalent comorbidity in spinal surgery patients' population. Hikata et al. reported that diabetics have a fivefold increase in SSI compared with nondiabetics. They also reported that hemoglobin A1c level > 7% was correlated with 35.3% increase in SSI [20]. Diabetes impairs the wound healing process through altered collagen synthesis, diminished vascular perfusion, impaired lymphocyte chemotaxis, and, subsequently, delayed wound reepithelialization [27].

Obesity was found to be an independent risk factor for wound infection reference, although it is usually concurrent with diabetes. Obese patients require a longer operative time and are subject to a deeper incision and prolonged retraction due to increased thickness of subcutaneous fat. A relatively lower vascularity of adipose tissue facilitates forming pockets of dead space during wound disclosure. The overall effect is increased surgical wound dead space and tissue trauma and necrosis.

Table 2 Patient-related risk factors

Advanced age	>60
Diabetes mellitus	HbA1C > 7 [20]
Prolonged steroid use	
Malnutrition	Albumin <3.5 mg/dL Total lymphocyte count <1500/mL Serum protein <6 g/dL [21]
Obesity	Increased thickness of subcutaneous fat [22] BMI > 30 [23]
Smoking [24]	
Decreased immunity	Rheumatoid arthritis
Chronic alcoholism	
Concurrent infections	
Previous surgical infection	
Perioperative glucose level	>150 mg/dL (8.3 mmol/L) [25]
American Society of Anesthesiologists score	≥2 [26]
Length of postoperative stay in an intensive care unit	≥7 d [26]
Preoperative hospital stay	

Adequate preoperative nutrition is essential for a proper immune response and rapid wound healing. Malnutrition specifically affects the elderly and patients with malignancies or trauma. Malnutrition may develop during the hospital stay in patients with postoperative complications (pulmonary embolism) and patients undergoing staged procedures [28].

Serologic parameters such as total lymphocyte count, albumin level, and transferrin level have all been used as markers for nutrition status. Other measurements, such as calf and arm muscle circumference or triceps skinfold, and standardized scoring systems, such as the Rainey-MacDonald nutritional index, are useful to determine the nutritional status of a patient undergoing spinal surgery [29]. Normalization of these parameters may reduce the risk of infection.

Tobacco smoking has a direct toxic effect on wound healing process, as smoking toxins, such as nicotine, nitric oxide, and carbon monoxide, deprives body tissue of oxygen, decreases collagen production, and causes endothelial cellular dysfunction. Smokers have impaired systemic immune response due to suppressed immunoglobulin levels, an altered CD4 to CD8 cell ratio, and reduced phagocyte activity [30].

Chronic steroid use may increase the risk of wound infection by two to three times as it has numerous adverse effects on the immune system [5]. Steroids are known to inhibit leukocyte adhesion, phagocytosis, and chemotaxis, all of which are important for wound healing process.

5 Etiology and Microbiology

Oftentimes, bacteria directly contaminate surgical wounds during the operative procedure. Skin flora is the most common source of contaminants, as gram-positive bacteria, predominantly

Staphylococcus aureus and *Staphylococcus epidermidis*, are the most commonly detected [31]. Gram-negative bacteria (*Enterococcus*, *Escherichia coli*, and *Peptostreptococcus*) are more common in sacral surgical site infections which may be attributable to urine and fecal contamination and in the setting of trauma. Methicillin-resistant strains are more common in revision cases and in MRSA nasal carriers [31].

The source of bacteria could be a remote systemic infection with a hematogenous spread or direct inoculations from local extension or another spinal procedure. Hematogenous infections typically involve highly virulent or gram-negative organisms that are able to surpass host defenses. Polymicrobial infections generally are caused by contamination with common skin flora inoculated during surgery, via a drain, or directly from dressing contamination [32].

In delayed infections, patients usually present 3 months, sometimes years, after surgery with increased back or neck pain after a normal recovery period. Patients may not have intense systemic symptoms, such as high fever, chills, and night sweats, and wound appearance is often normal due to the deep location of the infection. Delayed infections are mostly related to a low-virulence organism such as *Propionibacterium acnes* and *Staphylococcus epidermidis*. Isolation of *Propionibacterium acnes* often requires prolonged incubation periods to produce positive cultures.

A WBC within the normal range does not exclude "delayed wound infection"; therefore, comprehensive imaging studies, including CT scan and MRI images with contrast, should be requested to confirm the diagnosis and determine the site of infection.

6 Clinical Symptoms

Deep wound infections have an indolent nature, requiring a high index of suspicion for an early diagnosis. Unlike superficial wound infections that manifest early in the course, symptoms of deep wound infections take 1–4 weeks to become apparent. The hallmark of deep spinal infection is axial spine pain out of proportion to the usual course or pain that returns after an initial period of improvement. However, most of patients postoperatively have an incisional pain due to muscle dissection, which may pose a diagnostic challenge in differentiating between active infections. Local tenderness with paraspinal muscles spasms is common in both cases as well.

The wound may appear well healed in most cases, and accompanying signs of superficial wound infections such as erythema and drainage can be absent. However, it is important to observe the surgical site starting 24–48 h after the surgery because if drainage develops, culture may be useful to isolate the causative agent and modify the antibiotic treatment accordingly (Fig. 1).

The severity of the symptoms depends on the depth of infection, the involvement of neural structures, the offending organism, and the host response. Neurological symptoms are usually

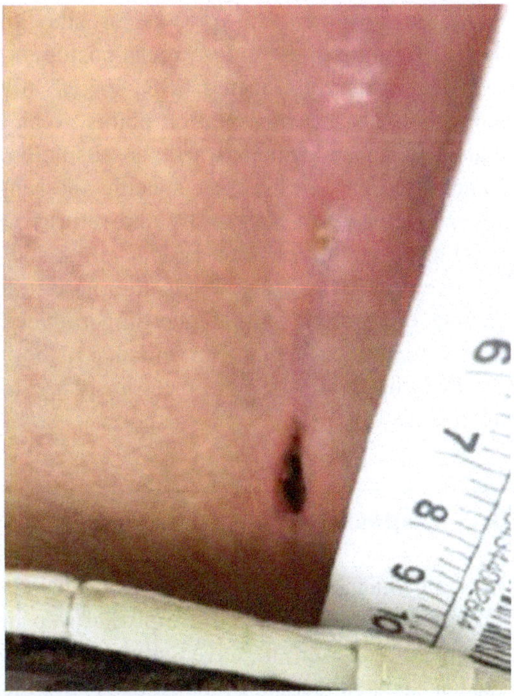

Fig. 1 Postoperative infection of a lumbar wound demonstrating dehiscence, surrounding erythema, and purulence

absent, unless a spinal epidural abscess and spinal collapse secondary to osteomyelitis develop, both of which are differentiated with delayed onset and exquisite radiological signs. Epidural abscesses arise with intense pain and with nerve root signs (limb pain or numbness) or spinal cord signs (bowel or bladder symptoms), depending on the location and the size of the abscess.

7 Laboratory Studies

When suspecting wound infection, complete blood count, ESR, and CRP are usually requested. However, these traditional inflammation markers are commonly increased during the postoperative period in the absence of infection. Therefore, it is important to observe the trend of the increase/decrease of these markers by comparing them with the preoperative baseline and the postoperative changes for each patient. ESR values typically rise maximally on postoperative day 4 and start to decline to normal levels 2–4 weeks postoperatively. Persistently elevated ESR, specifically more than 2 standard deviation points greater than the mean value, warrants suspicion. Generally, CRP level is more specific and sensitive: it elevates more rapidly and returns to baseline more quickly than ESR level. A sudden rise of CRP and ESR levels after an initial decline, or failure to normalize postoperatively, is sensitive for infection. Surveillance of both values is important in monitoring response to treatment [33].

8 Specimen Culture

Accurate diagnosis of bacterial pathogens via blood cultures and biopsies is a pivotal step in treatment; however, negative cultures do not exclude spinal infection. Blood cultures have the lowest yield in proven infection, whereas biopsy of infected tissue (open or CT-guided) is the more reliable. Specimen can also be obtained from the drain or the open wounds after sanitizing the skin surface to eliminate skin flora. During debridement, specimens should be taken from both superficial and deep parts of the wound to maximize the chances of isolating the causative agent.

9 Radiographic Images and Computer Tomography Scan

In the early stages of infection, radiological images may be normal. Paravertebral soft tissue swelling may be one of the earliest findings. Bony changes, such as end plate erosion and vertebral body destruction, need 2–3 weeks to become apparent (Fig. 2). However, radiographic images are imperative to evaluate the hardware integrity and identify pseudarthrosis or hardware failure. A radiolucent shadow around the implant or the screw indicates micromotion and potential infectious process involvement. Another important use of CT scan images is drainage of fluid or abscess collections under the CT guidance, as it improves accuracy and efficacy of the procedure [34].

9.1 Bone Scan

Although nonspecific, bone scans with technetium-99 or nuclear scintigraphy with gallium-labeled bone scan can diagnose infection earlier than plain radiographs. In the presence of infection, technetium-99 m-labeled methylene diphosphonate (Tc-99 m MDP) often identifies an area of increased uptake in two adjacent vertebrae. These modalities, in addition to indium 111-labeled WBC scans, are rarely used today to diagnose spinal infection

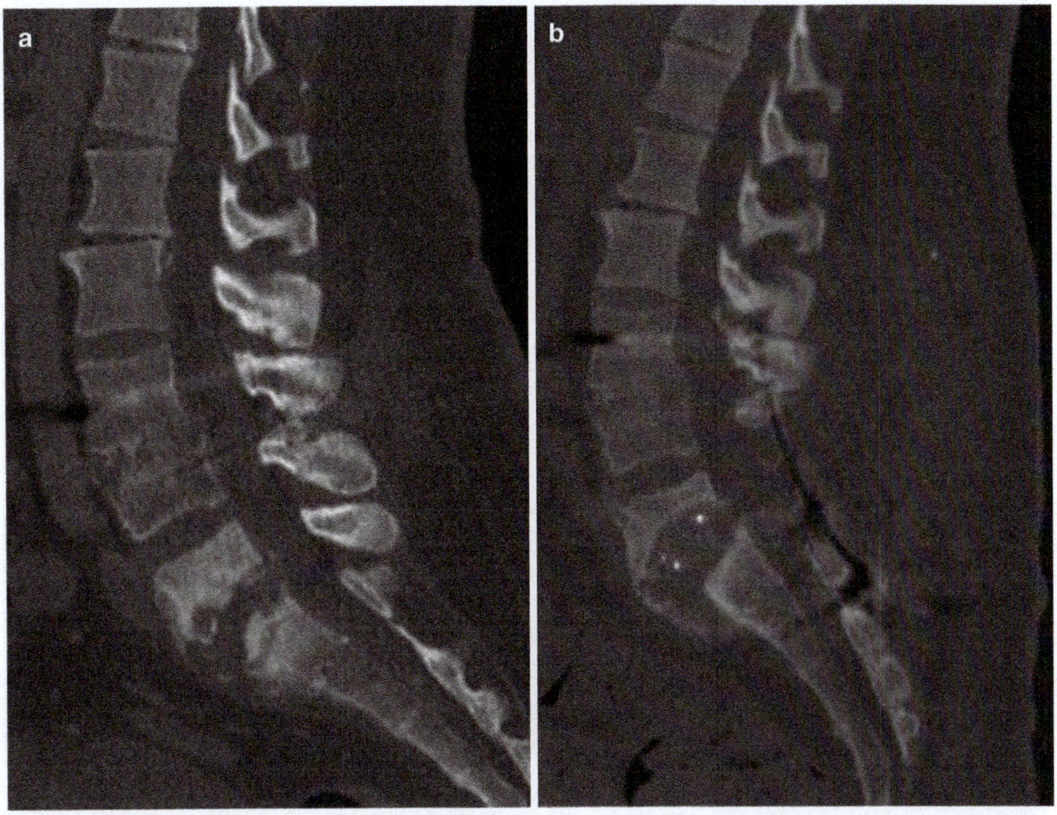

Fig. 2 Sagittal CT scans of lumbar spine show discitis and osteomyelitis at L5-S1 resulting in deformity. (**a**) Note end-plate sclerosis, vertebral body collapse. (**b**) Receding edema and end-plate changes after a successful treatment

and are only indicated if MRI is not available or contraindicated and the diagnosis was not confirmed.

9.2 Magnetic Resonance Imaging

MRI is the gold standard modality to diagnose and monitor spinal infections, as it has a higher sensitivity and specificity than the other modalities. MR images can show evidence of infection (i.e., edema) early in the course, and T2 and STIR sequences are very important for detecting early changes. MR can help to exclude other possible differential diagnoses (tumor, degeneration). Hence, it is considered the best imaging tool to differentiate between inflammatory postoperative changes, such as annular enhancement on T2-weighted images, and postoperative infection. In acute spinal infection, there is an increase in fluid signal due to marrow edema, and the signal pattern is typically signal decrease in T1-weighted and signal increase in T2- weighted sequences (Fig. 3). Enhancement with contrast medium is more specific as it can be positive when no signal change related to edema is seen yet. Erosion of the vertebral end plates, with loss of the low signal intensity line, has been shown to have a sensitivity of 84% for an infectious process

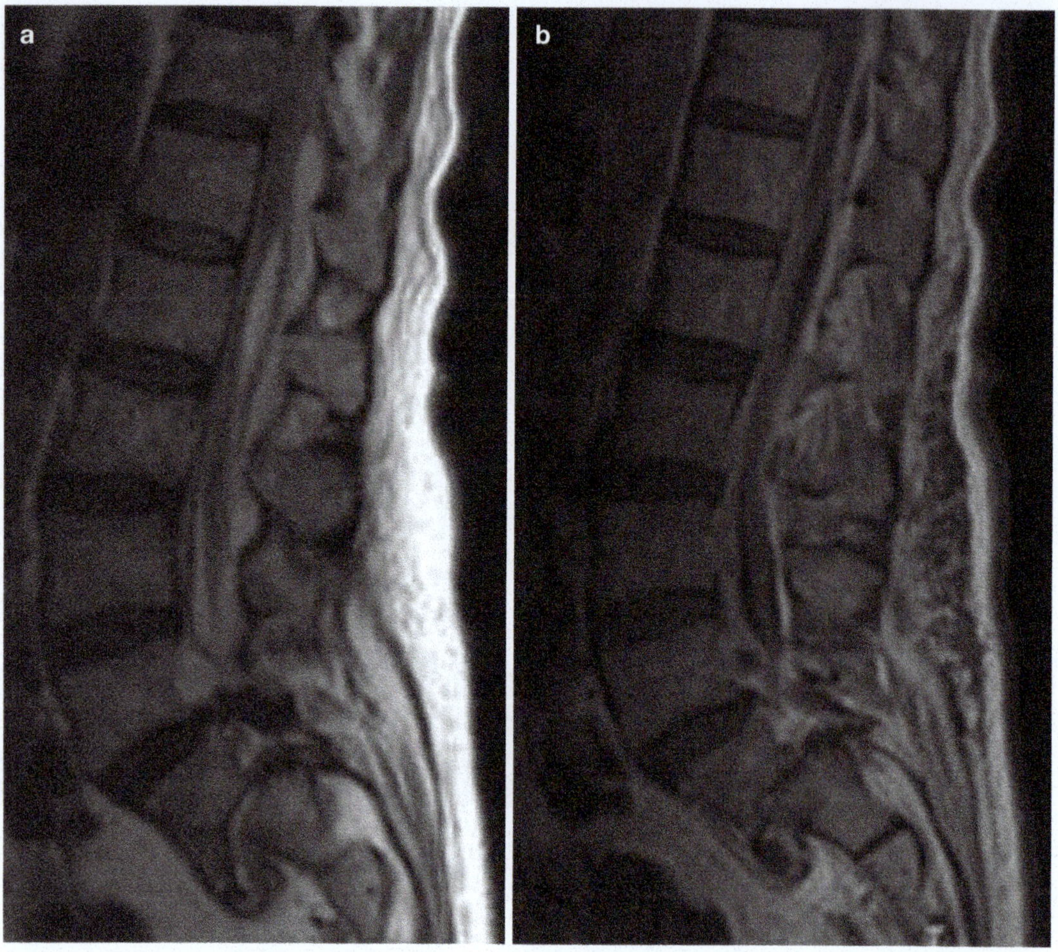

Fig. 3 (**a**) T2-weighted and (**b**) T1-weighted with contrast magnetic resonance images of the lumbar spine demonstrate pockets of spinal epidural abscesses with arachnoid adhesions and enhancement of the cauda equina nerve roots

[35]. MR images become crucial in the diagnosis of epidural abscesses, as it is the only noninvasive imaging method for the assessment of the contents of the spinal canal [36].

10 Prevention

10.1 Preoperative Approach

Preoperative evaluation of patient's immunological and nutritional status is important. This is accomplished by identifying any possible source of infection, most commonly urinary tract infection, via a thorough laboratory blood workup, chest radiographs, urinalysis, and other appropriate tests. Controlling diabetes and blood glucose level and providing malnourished patients with sufficient nutritional support are important as well [32].

Most surgeons routinely administer prophylactic antibiotic therapy 1 h prior to incision and during the procedure (50% of the initial dose). Although there is a controversy about this practice, prophylactic antibiotic treatment is warranted in complex and prolonged spinal procedures. Barker et al. performed a meta-analysis of six prospective randomized clinical trials of prophylactic antibiotic therapy during spinal surgery. They found that the use of antibiotic prophylaxis has significantly decreased infection rates (OR = 0.37, $P < 0.001$) [37].

First-or second-generation cephalosporins provide adequate coverage of gram-positive organisms, including *Staphylococcus aureus* and *Staphylococcus epidermidis*, and a combination of vancomycin and gentamycin can be administered in patients colonized with methicillin-resistant *S. aureus* (MRSA) and patients with cephalosporin allergy. MRSA screening in the preoperative period is recommended for patients undergoing high-risk procedures. Continuing prophylactic antibiotics for an extended period after surgery is not recommended. Previous studies showed that patients who received antibiotics only after surgery had a higher rate of infection than patients who received antibiotics preoperatively [38]. Additionally, extending the period of postoperative antibiotic increases the risk for secondary infections with antibiotic-resistant organisms.

10.2 Intraoperative Approach

The American Institute of Architects' design of the operating room, including the size, layout, and air handling system, has dramatically minimized the exposure to environmental microbes and decreased rate of wound infections. The role of the operating team is to apply hygiene protocols including proper handwashing and scrubbing, the use of double gloves, and adequate skin preparation and reduce operating room traffic, sterile administration, and removal of Foley catheter [39]. Intraoperatively, it is important to release soft tissue traction regularly to decrease tissue ischemia. Limiting the use of monopolar cautery with adequate and frequent saline irrigation to dissipate electrically induced heat and lessen the likelihood of tissue necrosis. Familiarity with the surgical instruments and unique technical skills may reduce the operative time and decrease the risk of infection.

Another strategy to decrease contamination of surgical wound in spinal procedures is regular, frequent saline irrigation. Supplcmenting irrigation solutions with iodine or antibiotics is a common practice for many surgeons. Theologis and colleagues found that intra-wound vancomycin powder application intraoperatively is cost-effective and resulted in significant decrease in wound infection [40]. The use of closed wound suction drain (Jackson-Pratt) for the treatment of infections is standard of care in spine surgery as it reduces surgical site hematoma and infection, especially in prolonged extensive procedures. Although it has been assumed that the drain itself could be a source of contamination, because it creates a direct access of bacteria into the normal postoperative hematoma, there is a little evidence to support this hypothesis in the literature. In fact, previous studies have shown that there is no difference in infection rate, epidural hematoma incidence, or wound healing process between patients who did receive closed wound suction and those who did not after a single-level and multilevel lumbar spine surgeries [41, 42]. Therefore, the decision to use a drain following spine surgery is at the surgeon's discretion.

11 Treatment

Treatment target is to eradicate the infection, reduce the pain, prevent neurological injury, and maintain spinal stability. Superficial wound infections can be treated initially with antibiotics only, with surgical treatment being required in certain conditions (Table 3). Conversely, the mainstay treatment of deep wound infection is surgical intervention and debridement of nonviable tissue. Debridement should be extensive and involves reopening the complete length and depth of the incision and removing all sutures and dead tissue, including the superficial and subfascial

Table 3 Indications for surgical intervention in postoperative wound infection

Ongoing infection refractory to medical treatment
Pain not responding to conservative therapy
Wound dehiscence, purulent discharge, and fluctuant
Pus on needle aspiration
Compressive large fluid collection or epidural abscess
Neurological deficit
Spinal instability or worsening of deformity

compartments and deeper muscle layers. Irrigation with antibiotic solution and pulsatile lavage system is essential for mechanical and chemical removal of the bacteria. Wide wound reopening would allow adequate inspection of bone fragments, necrotic muscles, Gelfoam or fibrin sealant remnants, and instrumentation and bone graft materials. Wound sample for culture and sensitivity test should be collected prior to debridement and irrigation.

The spinal instrumentation and bone graft materials could be left in place, and removal is indicated in certain cases, for example, in the case of pseudarthrosis due to active infection and in the case of delayed infection with solid fusion. If possible, leaving the instrumentation in place is a viable option as this can prevent instability either due to the initial spinal pathology or caused by the ensuing infection [43].

Upon wound closure, the skin edges should be sanitary and viable. If this was not possible, delayed wound closure can be performed after serial irrigation and debridement, until there is no evidence of infection. Obtaining a tight, layered closure is important to minimize dead space. Thalgott et al. [44] developed a classification system to predict high-risk patient population for wound infection following a spinal surgery and proposed a treatment guide prognostic for the number of debridement required in accordance. This system was based on two main variables: the infection and the host (Table 4). The authors proposed that healthy patients with less virulent bacteria might require a single debridement, whereas immunocompromised hosts, multiple and/or more virulent organisms, and polymicrobial infections often require multiple debridements.

If wounds fail to respond to irrigation, drainage, debridement, and delayed closure, they may require a closure with myocutaneous or fasciocutaneous flaps. Vacuum-assisted closure (VAC) systems have been proposed as an alternative, especially in cases of exposed hardware and in patients with significant comorbidities [45].

Broad-spectrum antibiotics are typically initiated after surgery and modified to sensitive agents upon intraoperative wound cultures. Consultation with an infectious disease specialist is necessary for selecting the appropriate antibiotic treatment, following up with the patient, and monitoring undesired side effects. Typically, the duration of antibiotic treatment ranges from 8 to 12 weeks intravenously followed by 6 to 8 weeks orally. Antibiotic treatment of *Staphylococcus aureus*, the most common causative agent, is mainly beta-lactam penicillinase or second-generation cephalosporin (Table 5). The decision of antibiotic discontinuation should be based on the patient's clinical response to treatment, inflammatory markers values (ESR and CRP), CBC levels, and finally imaging findings. Patients usually start to improve clinically before significant radiological signs of improvement become apparent (such as T2-signal normalization). Patients with ongoing or delayed-onset infection may require lifelong antibiotic treatment, especially in the setting of low-virulence microorganism agent, and retained instrumentation. This decision is determined with a collaborative consultation of infectious disease specialist.

Table 4 Clinical staging system for spinal wound infections [44]

Severity of wound infection		Host immune characteristics	
Group 1	Infection with a single organism (either superficial or deep)	Group A	A patient with normal systemic defenses
Group 2	A deep infection with multiple organisms	Group B	A patient with local or multiple systemic disease, smoking
Group 3	Myonecrosis with multiple organisms	Group C	Immunocompromised or severely malnourished

Table 5 Antibiotic treatment of *Staphylococcus* infection in adults [46]

Infections	Drugs
Serious infection, unlikely to be MRSA	Nafcillin or oxacillin 1 to 2 g IV q 4 to 6 h or cefazolin 1 g IV 8 h
Penicillin-allergic patients	Clindamycin 600 mg IV q 8 h or vancomycin 15 mg/kg q 12 h
Serious infection, likely to be MRSA	Vancomycin 15 mg/kg q 12 h or linezolid 600 mg IV q 12 h
Vancomycin-resistant staphylococci	Linezolid 600 mg IV q 12 h; daptomycin 4 mg/kg q 24 h; quinupristin plus dalfopristin 7 to 5 mg/kg q 8 h

Conclusions

Postoperative spinal infections are uncommon but are the source of significant morbidity. Patients undergoing prolonged, complex spinal producers are at higher risk of developing wound infection. Several patient-related risk factors, such as concurrent infections, diabetes mellitus, and malnutrition, can be identified and treated or optimized during the preoperative period. Magnetic resonance imaging is the diagnostic examination of choice in the early stages of infection, as other imaging modalities show nonspecific findings. Prophylactic antibiotic administration before and during the surgical procedure, especially with more complex and prolonged procedures, is highly recommended. Several measurements can be undertaken to decrease contamination intraoperatively including copious and frequent irrigation, decreasing room traffic, and tight fascial closure. When infection is suspected, obtaining necessary imaging studies and laboratory tests is important for early diagnosis of infection and for monitoring response to treatment. Debridement of the wound and deeper layers (muscle fascia and bone) is the gold standard of treatment when infection sets in, as well as antibiotics, IV followed by oral. Despite our best efforts, we have been unable to completely eradicate SSI in spine surgery.

References

1. Kirkland KB, Briggs JP, Trivette SL, Wilkinson WE, Sexton DJ (1999) The impact of surgical-site infections in the 1990s: attributable mortality, excess length of hospitalization, and extra costs. Infect Control Hosp Epidemiol 20(11):725–730
2. Stone PW, Braccia D, Larson E (2005) Systematic review of economic analyses of health care-associated infections. Am J Infect Control 33(9):501–509
3. Smith JS, Shaffrey CI, Sansur CA, Berven SH, Fu KM, Broadstone PA, Choma TJ, Goytan MJ, Noordeen HH, Knapp DR Jr, Hart RA, Donaldson WF 3rd, Polly DW Jr, Perra JH, Boachie-Adjei O, Scoliosis Research Society Morbidity and Mortality Committee (2011) Rates of infection after spine surgery based on 108,419 procedures: a report from the Scoliosis Research Society Morbidity and Mortality Committee. Spine (Phila Pa 1976) 36(7):556–563
4. Weinstein MA, McCabe JP, Cammisa FP Jr (2000) Postoperative spinal wound infection: a review of 2,391 consecutive index procedures. J Spinal Disord 13(5):422–426
5. De la Garza-Ramos R, Abt NB, Kerezoudis P, McCutcheon BA, Bydon A, Gokaslan Z, Bydon M (2016) Deep-wound and organ-space infection after surgery for degenerative spine disease: an analysis from 2006 to 2012. Neurol Res 38(2):117–123
6. Pull ter Gunne AF, Cohen DB (2009) Incidence, prevalence, and analysis of risk factors for surgical site infection following adult spinal surgery. Spine (Phila Pa 1976) 34(13):1422–1428
7. Levi AD, Dickman CA, Sonntag VK (1997) Management of postoperative infections after spinal instrumentation. J Neurosurg 86(6):975–980
8. Keller RB, Pappas AM (1972) Infection after spinal fusion using internal fixation instrumentation. Orthop Clin North Am 3(1):99–111
9. Sebastian A, Huddleston P 3rd, Kakar S, Habermann E, Wagie A, Nassr A (2016) Risk factors for surgical site infection after posterior cervical spine surgery: an analysis of 5,441 patients from the ACS NSQIP 2005-2012. Spine J 16(4):504–509
10. O'Toole JE, Eichholz KM, Fessler RG (2009) Surgical site infection rates after minimally invasive spinal surgery. J Neurosurg Spine 11(4):471–476
11. Pereira P, Buzek D, Franke J, Senker W, Kosmala A, Hubbe U, Manson N, Rosenberg W, Assietti R, Martens F, Barbanti Brodano G, Scheufler KM (2015) Surgical data and early postoperative outcomes after minimally invasive lumbar interbody fusion: results of a prospective, multicenter, observational data-monitored study. PLoS One 10(3):e0122312
12. Shousha M, Cirovic D, Boehm H (2015) Infection rate after minimally invasive noninstrumented spinal surgery based on 4350 procedures. Spine (Phila Pa 1976) 40(3):201–205
13. Mikhael MM, Huddleston PM, Nassr A (2009) Postoperative culture positive surgical site infections

after the use of irradiated allograft, nonirradiated allograft, or autograft for spinal fusion. Spine (Phila Pa 1976) 34(22):2466–2468
14. Fei Q, Li J, Lin J, Li D, Wang B, Meng H, Wang Q, Su N, Yang Y (2016) Risk factors for surgical site infection after spinal surgery: a meta-analysis. World Neurosurg 95:507–515
15. Watanabe M, Sakai D, Matsuyama D, Yamamoto Y, Sato M, Mochida J (2010) Risk factors for surgical site infection following spine surgery: efficacy of intraoperative saline irrigation. J Neurosurg Spine 12(5):540–546
16. Radcliff KE, Rasouli MR, Neusner A, Kepler CK, Albert TJ, Rihn JA, Hilibrand AS, Vaccaro AR (2013) Preoperative delay of more than 1 hour increases the risk of surgical site infection. Spine (Phila Pa 1976) 38(15):1318–1323
17. Hosseini P, Mundis GM Jr, Eastlack R, Nourian A, Pawelek J, Nguyen S, Akbarnia BA (2016) Do longer surgical procedures result in greater contamination of surgeons' hands? Clin Orthop Relat Res 474(7):1707–1713
18. Banco SP, Vaccaro AR, Blam O, Eck JC, Cotler JM, Hilibrand AS, Albert TJ, Murphey S (2002) Spine infections: variations in incidence during the academic year. Spine (Phila Pa 1976) 27(9):962–965
19. Durkin MJ, Dicks KV, Baker AW, Moehring RW, Chen LF, Sexton DJ, Lewis SS, Anderson DJ (2015) Postoperative infection in spine surgery: does the month matter? J Neurosurg Spine 23(1):128–134
20. Hikata T, Iwanami A, Hosogane N, Watanabe K, Ishii K, Nakamura M, Kamata M, Toyama Y, Matsumoto M (2014) High preoperative hemoglobin A1c is a risk factor for surgical site infection after posterior thoracic and lumbar spinal instrumentation surgery. J Orthop Sci 19(2):223–228
21. McPhee IB, Williams RP, Swanson CE (1998) Factors influencing wound healing after surgery for metastatic disease of the spine. Spine (Phila Pa 1976) 23(6):726–732
22. Mehta AI, Babu R, Sharma R, Karikari IO, Grunch BH, Owens TR, Agarwal VJ, Sampson JH, Lad SP, Friedman AH, Kuchibhatla M, Bagley CA, Gottfried ON (2013) Thickness of subcutaneous fat as a risk factor for infection in cervical spine fusion surgery. J Bone Joint Surg Am 95(4):323–328
23. Rihn JA, Radcliff K, Hilibrand AS, Anderson DT, Zhao W, Lurie J, Vaccaro AR, Freedman MK, Albert TJ, Weinstein JN (2012) Does obesity affect outcomes of treatment for lumbar stenosis and degenerative spondylolisthesis? Analysis of the Spine Patient Outcomes Research Trial (SPORT). Spine (Phila Pa 1976) 37(23):1933–1946
24. Durand F, Berthelot P, Cazorla C, Farizon F, Lucht F (2013) Smoking is a risk factor of organ/space surgical site infection in orthopaedic surgery with implant materials. Int Orthop 37(4):723–727
25. de Vries FE, Gans SL, Solomkin JS, Allegranzi B, Egger M, Dellinger EP, Boermeester MA (2016) Meta-analysis of lower perioperative blood glucose target levels for reduction of surgical-site infection. Br J Surg 104(2):e95–e105
26. Cassir N, De La Rosa S, Melot A, Touta A, Troude L, Loundou A, Richet H, Roche PH (2015) Risk factors for surgical site infections after neurosurgery: a focus on the postoperative period. Am J Infect Control 43(12):1288–1291
27. Blakytny R, Jude E (2006) The molecular biology of chronic wounds and delayed healing in diabetes. Diabet Med 23(6):594–608
28. Mandelbaum BR, Tolo VT, McAfee PC, Burest P (1988) Nutritional deficiencies after staged anterior and posterior spinal reconstructive surgery. Clin Orthop Relat Res 234:5–11
29. Cross MB, Yi PH, Thomas CF, Garcia J, Della Valle CJ (2014) Evaluation of malnutrition in orthopaedic surgery. J Am Acad Orthop Surg 22(3):193–199
30. Jorgensen LN, Kallehave F, Christensen E, Siana JE, Gottrup F (1998) Less collagen production in smokers. Surgery 123(4):450–455
31. Abdul-Jabbar A, Berven SH, Hu SS, Chou D, Mummaneni PV, Takemoto S, Ames C, Deviren V, Tay B, Weinstein P, Burch S, Liu C (2013) Surgical site infections in spine surgery: identification of microbiologic and surgical characteristics in 239 cases. Spine (Phila Pa 1976) 38(22):E1425–E1431
32. Klein JD, Hey LA, CS Y, Klein BB, Coufal FJ, Young EP, Marshall LF, Garfin SR (1996) Perioperative nutrition and postoperative complications in patients undergoing spinal surgery. Spine (Phila Pa 1976) 21(22):2676–2682
33. Mok JM, Pekmezci M, Piper SL, Boyd E, Berven SH, Burch S, Deviren V, Tay B, Hu SS (2008) Use of C-reactive protein after spinal surgery: comparison with erythrocyte sedimentation rate as predictor of early postoperative infectious complications. Spine (Phila Pa 1976) 33(4):415–421
34. James SL, Davies AM (2006) Imaging of infectious spinal disorders in children and adults. Eur J Radiol 58(1):27–40
35. Ledermann HP, Schweitzer ME, Morrison WB, Carrino JA (2003) MR imaging findings in spinal infections: rules or myths? Radiology 228(2):506–514
36. Tins BJ, Cassar-Pullicino VN (2004) MR imaging of spinal infection. Semin Musculoskelet Radiol 8(3):215–229
37. Barker FG 2nd (2002) Efficacy of prophylactic antibiotic therapy in spinal surgery: a meta-analysis. Neurosurgery 51(2):391–400
38. Takahashi H, Wada A, Iida Y, Yokoyama Y, Katori S, Hasegawa K, Shintaro T, Suguro T (2009) Antimicrobial prophylaxis for spinal surgery. J Orthop Sci 14(1):40–44
39. Anderson DJ, Kaye KS, Classen D, Arias KM, Podgorny K, Burstin H, Calfee DP, Coffin SE, Dubberke ER, Fraser V, Gerding DN, Griffin FA, Gross P, Klompas M, Lo E, Marschall J, Mermel LA et al (2008) Strategies to prevent surgical site infections in acute care hospitals. Infect Control Hosp Epidemiol 29(Suppl 1):S51–S61

40. Theologis AA, Demirkiran G, Callahan M, Pekmezci M, Ames C, Deviren V (2014) Local intrawound vancomycin powder decreases the risk of surgical site infections in complex adult deformity reconstruction: a cost analysis. Spine (Phila Pa 1976) 39(22):1875–1880
41. Choi HS, Lee SG, Kim WK, Son S, Jeong TS (2016) Is surgical drain useful for lumbar disc surgery? Korean J Spine 13(1):20–23
42. Brown MD, Brookfield KF (2004) A randomized study of closed wound suction drainage for extensive lumbar spine surgery. Spine (Phila Pa 1976) 29(10):1066–1068
43. Rohmiller MT, Akbarnia BA, Raiszadeh K, Canale S (2010) Closed suction irrigation for the treatment of postoperative wound infections following posterior spinal fusion and instrumentation. Spine (Phila Pa 1976) 35(6):642–646
44. Thalgott JS, Cotler HB, Sasso RC, LaRocca H, Gardner V (1991) Postoperative infections in spinal implants. Classification and analysis--a multicenter study. Spine (Phila Pa 1976) 16(8):981–984
45. Yuan-Innes MJ, Temple CL, Lacey MS (2001) Vacuum-assisted wound closure: a new approach to spinal wounds with exposed hardware. Spine (Phila Pa 1976) 26(3):E30–E33
46. Berkow R, Fletcher AJ, Beers MH (1992) Merck manual of diagnosis and therapy, 16th edn. Merck Research Laboratories, Division of Merck & Co. Inc., Rahway, NJ

Wound Infection Following Stoma Reversal: A Prospective Comparative Study

Zubaidah Nor Hanipah, Soo Jia Ying, Nik Qisti Fathi, Ong Kheng Wah, and Tikfu Gee

1 Introduction

Gastrointestinal tract stoma closure is a clean-contaminated procedure that is associated with a high incidence of surgical site infection (SSI). The nature of the enteric contents in these stomas increase the bioburden, and therefore stoma closure is likely to have wound contamination. This higher risk of wound infection invariably leads to either delayed primary closure or healing by secondary intention (SH) as opposed to primary closure (PC) [1].

Few studies have shown that PC is as good as, if not better than other methods in term of SSI rate. On the other hand, other methods of closure have frequently been reported to have better SSI rates compared to PC. Van de Pavoordt et al. [2] compared PC, partial PC and SH for loop ileostomy closure. The SSI rate for PC, partial PC and SH were 8%, 4% and 2%, respectively. Hackam et al. [3] reported that the SSI rate of PC could be as high as 41%. However, methods of stoma closure with the least SSI rate is still debatable, and no consensus has yet to be established.

As a consequence, a few modified wound closure methods for stoma reversal have been evolved in comparison to the PC. Partial closure of the wound with interrupted sutures interspersed with dressings was an alternative method of the stoma wound closure. An open wound provides a favorable environment for the growth of microorganisms by being moist, warm and nutritious [3]. This environment is conducive to healing, but also has the potential of becoming a nidus of pathogenic infection. Due to the higher risk of wound contamination, dressings are placed in between sutures of the partial PC wound following stoma closure. It will not only act as a barrier to colonization by pathogens but also help to achieve an optimal moisture balance to support healing process [3].

Currently, there is an increasing trend of using silver as an antimicrobial agent for wound dressing. A silver-containing Hydrofiber dressing, Aquacel® Ag (ConvaTec), has better exudative absorption compared to the conventional absorptive fibrous dressings. It is made of sodium carboxymethylcellulose, which is designed to absorb exudate and subsequently to release ionic silver into the wound environment in a controlled manner [4–6]. The ionic silver is delivered at a sustained rate for up to 14 days. The carboxymethylcellulose and silver components in the Aquacel® Ag makes it an ideal antimicrobial

Z.N. Hanipah, M.D. (✉) • S.J. Ying, M.B., B.Ch., B.A.O.
N.Q. Fathi, BMedSci, B.M.B.S. • Q.K. Wah, M.B.B.S.
T. Gee, M.B.B.S.
Department of Surgery, Faculty of Medicine and Health Science, University Putra Malaysia, 43400 UPM-Serdang, Selangor, Malaysia
e-mail: dr.zubaidahnh@gmail.com; soojy2003@yahoo.com; qisti@yahoo.com; ongkhengwah@gmail.com; tikfug@yahoo.com

Recent Clinical Techniques, Results, and Research in Wounds (2017)
DOI 10.1007/15695_2017_37, © Springer International Publishing AG
Published Online: 23 December 2017

dressing for contaminated wounds such as wound after stoma closures.

The aim of this study is to describe and evaluate a new method of wound closure using a partial closure with intervening silver dressings after stoma reversals. A comparison of the new method is made with a PC; the SSI and healing rates among both these groups were studied. Although the method of using a partial closure with intervening dressings has been described, the use of silver-containing dressings has yet to be elucidated.

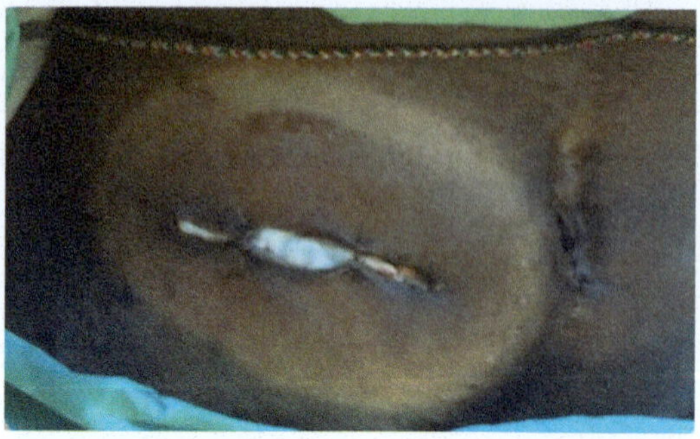

Fig. 1 Partial closure with intervening silver dressing using Aquacel® Ag

2 Methodology

A prospective study was conducted after institutional research board approval. All patients with a gastrointestinal tract stoma (ileostomy or colostomy) closure from January 2011 to April 2015 at a single academic unit based at two institutions were included. Patients with allergies to any components of the dressings or metallic silver, on antibiotics or long-term antibiotic treatment, or with history of previously complicated attempts of stoma closure were excluded from the study.

This study is a randomized prospective comparative study incorporating two groups of patients, according to the methods of wound closure following stoma reversal. All patients were randomized. Each consecutive case referred alternately without any selection. Control subjects were patients who underwent routine primary closure as the method of reversal of stoma. The study group consists of patients who had closure of the stoma via partial primary closure with intervening silver dressing using Aquacel® Ag (Fig. 1). Both types of skin closure were performed at both institutions. The entry point of the study is on the operation day itself. Patients will be assessed preoperatively, during the admission for operation, at 2 weeks for SSI and 6 weeks for wound healing.

The outcome of the study is SSI as defined by the CDC guidelines [7]. The wound will be observed for local inflammatory signs such as redness, warmness, swelling, or pain around the stoma wound closure site. Wound infection and wound healing were confirmed by one of the four general surgeons in the team. The wounds will be laid open depending on the state, i.e., purulent discharge or induration. For wounds that exhibit signs of infection, laboratory tests will be used to confirm the diagnosis. Wound inspection was done every other day during admission. Upon discharge, dressings were done, and the wound is inspected every other day in the outpatient clinic until 6 weeks.

The silver dressings used in this study incorporate ionic silver-containing Hydrofiber dressing (Aquacel® Ag) provided by ConvaTec. The investigators declare no conflict of interest.

3 Study Outcome

The primary study outcome is the wound infection and wound healing of both the PC and partial closure with intervening Aquacel Ag dressing of the stoma closure.

3.1 Statistical Analysis

Data was summarized as the mean and standard deviation (SD) for continuous variables and as counts and percentages for categorical variables. The rate of surgical site infection and wound healing in relation to both study and control groups was analyzed by the chi-square test. Statistical significance was set at p-value <0.05.

Statistical analysis was carried out using the Statistical Package for Social Sciences software (SPSS®, version 22.0).

3.2 Results

A total of 44 patients who underwent a reversal of the stoma were included in this study. Twenty-four patients were sampled into the control group (primary closure) and 20 patients in the study group (dressing with Aquacel Ag). The mean age for both control and study groups is 54 years old (SD ± 13). The type of stoma in both groups was predominantly colostomy. The demographic data between both the groups is summarized in Table 1.

At 2 weeks, SSI was seen in two patients in the primary closure group but none in the Aquacel Ag group (Fig. 2). The healing rate at 6 weeks was 100% in the Aquacel Ag group as compared to 92% in the primary closure group. However, the SSI and healing rate in both the groups were not statistically significant (Table 2).

Table 1 Demographic data between the groups

	Primary closure $N = 24$	Aquacel Ag $N = 20$
Gender		
Male	16 (67%)	10 (50%)
Female	8 (33%)	10 (50%)
Type of stoma		
Ileostomy	9 (37%)	5 (25%)
Colostomy	15 (63%)	15 (75%)

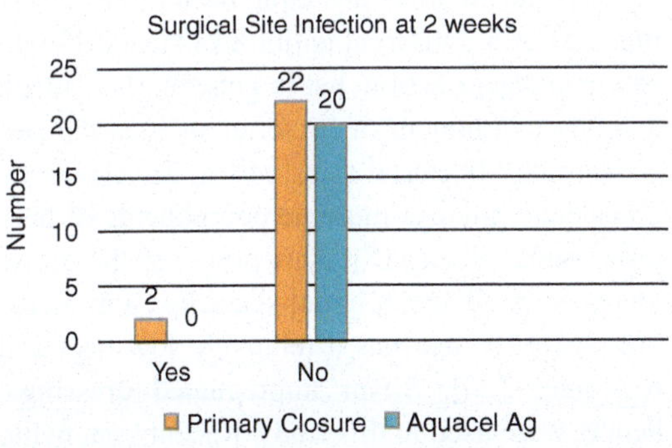

Fig. 2 Distribution of the presence of surgical site infection among the control and study group

Table 2 Surgical site infection and healing rates

	Primary closure $N = 24$	Aquacel Ag $N = 20$	*P*-value
Presence of SSI at 2 weeks			
Yes	2 (8%)	0 (0%)	0.493
No	22 (92%)	20 (100%)	
Healing by 6 weeks			
Yes	22 (92%)	20 (100%)	0.493
No	2 (8%)	0 (0%)	

SSI surgical site infection, *N* total number

4 Discussion

Wound care following stoma reversal requires an exquisite balance of optimal healing with minimal infection due to its high bioburden content. Primary closure has been a routine practice for the closure of stoma wounds. Studies have demonstrated higher surgical site infection in primary closure. Phang et al. [8] studied 339 patients who underwent ileostomy closures and reported a 15% of SSI rate. Berry et al. [9] reported SSI rate of 6% among 16 patients who had primary closure of ileostomy. Similarly, in one of the largest series in stoma closure, Wong et al. [10] reviewed 1504 cases who underwent loop ileostomy closures and found a 9.3% SSI rate in PC compared to 0.4% in both partial PC and SH.

Therefore, several wound closure techniques have been developed to take on the events of high bioburden in stoma wounds which were likewise reported to have lower infection rates. Benarjee et al. [11] in 1997 proposed a method that involves a skin-approximating closure with a subcuticular purse string of the stoma site. It is claimed that this method has the advantages of better cosmesis and arguably less SSI rate. A retrospective cohort study conducted by Klink et al. [12] reported significantly lower SSI rate in purse-string approximation wound closure as compared to the primary closure (5 vs. 17%). Suh et al. [13] and Lee et al. [14] conducted similar

Table 3 Comparison between other studies on wound infection rate after stoma closure

Studies	Study design	Total number	Primary closure (%)	Partial PC (%)	Delayed closure or healing by secondary intention (%)	Purse string (%)	Partial closure with intervening dressing (%)
Van de Pavoordt et al. [3]	Retrospective	293	7.7	4	2.1		
Hackam et al. [4]	Retrospective	95	41		15		
Berry et al. [9]	Prospective[a]	16	6.3				
Phang et al. [8]	Retrospective[b]	339	14.2				
Wong et al. [10]	Retrospective	1,504	9	0.4	0.4		
Lee et al. [14]	Retrospective	48	16.7 (linear closure)			5.6	
Klink et al. [12]	Retrospective	140	17 (linear closure)			5	
Suh et al. [13]	Retrospective	157	11.4 (linear closure)			0	
Zubaidah et al. [15]	Prospective	44	8				0

[a]All patients had primary closure
[b]Majority of the patients had primary closure (90%)

studies on the skin closure after ileostomy reversals in Korea and found similar results. Despite having a lower SSI rate in purse-string wound closure, the SSI rate was still higher as compared to SH. Table 3 summarizes the comparison studies on wound infection after stoma closure.

There were no standard methods of wound closure following stoma reversals. Even though SH has lower infection rates, it has its own disadvantages. The trade-off with leaving wounds opened or partially opened, however, is a prolonged time for final closure and increased local wound care requirements [1]. When the hosts' immune response is unable to cope with the opportunistic colonization, this wound may become infected. Subsequently, the healing process will be delayed [5]. Health-care costs will increase not forgetting the impact on patients themselves, i.e., pain, inconvenience, and risk of further systemic illnesses.

The best possible wound dressing is something that can provide a moist environment for healing, causes the least discomfort for patients, and has antimicrobial property [2]. Not all dressings have all this ideal property. Traditional gauze dressing which keeps the wound dry causes more fluid depletion through evaporation, which in turn reduces the local tissue temperature at a wound site. Dry gauze dressings are also often painful and adherent to the wound. It also lacks antimicrobial properties to suppress bacterial growth, especially in highly bioburden wounds such as stoma wounds [5]. This process depresses host immunity and wound healing function and, therefore, increases the chances of wound infection [16, 17].

For centuries, metallic silver exhibited some antimicrobial properties, hence its use in the past in sanitation of water, complementary health care, and food preservation [18, 19]. In vitro studies have shown that silver-impregnated dressing exhibits effective and rapid bactericidal activities [20, 21]. Different antibiotics have different mechanisms of action, but in general, they attack a single component of bacteria, such as the cell wall, to halt bacterial metabolism. Silver, on the other hand, attacks multiple components of bacterial metabolism [18]. This property, therefore, makes it an effective, broad-spectrum, antimicrobial agent. It also has a relatively low bacterial resistance [20]. Silver impregnated dressings, hence, were used in this study. Recent systematic review and meta-analysis reported that silver-impregnated dressings improved the short-term healing of wounds and ulcers in terms of wound size [22]. For this reason, silver-impregnated dressings were chosen in this current study.

In our study [15], we compared stoma wound closure with PC to partial closure with interrupted sutures and intervening silver dressings. Our study showed a higher incidence of SSI in the PC group (8%) as compared to zero in partial closure with the intervening dressing group; however, the surgical site infection and healing rate between the two groups were not statistically significant. The higher incidence of SSI in the PC group results in the need for regular wound dressing and antibiotic usage. As consequences, these patients resulted in delayed wound healing following stoma reversal, resulting in an indirect financial burden to the patients and to the hospital in the PC group as compared to the study group. In the partial closure with the intervening dressing group, there was zero wound infection and complete healing at 6 weeks post closure. However, the cost-effectiveness and cosmetic effect between both the groups were not studied.

The advantage of our study is this study is a randomized control study on stoma wound closure. A combination of both colostomy and ileostomy closures were studied with more than 60% in both the groups had colostomy closures. One of the major limitation of many of the available studies reported is the retrospective design of the study. Our small sample size is not sufficient to represent the population.

Conclusions

Reversal of stoma with partial primary closure with intervening silver dressings is a feasible method with less SSI and good wound healing outcome.

Funding Research grant from University Putra Malaysia.
Conflict of Interest None.

References

1. Harold DM, Johnson EK, Rizzo JA, Steele SR (2010) Primary closure of stoma site wounds after ostomy takedown. Am J Surg 199:621–624
2. Van de Pavoordt H, Fazio V, Jagelman D (1987) The outcome of loop ileostomy closure in 293 cases. Int J Colorect 2:214–217
3. Hackam DJ, Rotstein OD (1995) Stoma closure and wound infection: an evaluation of risk factors. Can J Surg 38:144–148
4. Jones SA, Bower PG, Walker M, Parsons D (2004) Controlling wound bioburden with a novel silver-containing Hydrofiber dressing. Wound Repair Regen 12:288–294
5. Vanscheidt W, Lazareth I, Routkovsky-Norval C (2003) Safety evaluation of a new ionic silver dressing in the management of chronic ulcers. Wounds 15(11):371–378
6. Coutts P, Sibbald RG (2005) The effect of a silver-containing Hydrofiber dressing on superficial wound bed and bacterial balance of chronic wounds. Int Wound J 2:348–356
7. Mangram AJ, Horan TC, Pearson ML, Silver LC, Jarvis WR (1999) Hospital Infection Control Practices Advisory Committee. Guideline for prevention of surgical site infection. American journal of infection control. 30;27(2):97–134
8. Phang P, Hain J, Perez-Ramirez J (1999) Techniques and complications of ileostomy takedown. Am J Surg 177:463–466
9. Berry DP, Scholefield JH (1997) Closure of loop ileostomy. Br J Surg 84(4):524
10. Wong KS, Remzi FH, Gorgun E, Arrigain S, Church JM, Preen M, Fazio VW (2005) Loop ileostomy closure after restorative proctocolectomy: outcome in 1,504 patients. Dis Colon Rectum 48:243–250
11. Benarjee A (1997) Purse-string skin closure after stoma reversal. Dis Colon Rectum 40:993–994
12. Klink CD et al (2013) Influence of skin closure technique on surgical site infection after loop ileostomy reversal: retrospective cohort study. Int J Surg 11:1123–1125
13. Suh YJ, Park JW, Kim YS, Park SC, JH O (2014) A beneficial effect of purse-string skin closure after ileostomy takedown: a retrospective cohort study. Int J Surg 12(6):615–620
14. Lee JR, Kim YW, Sung JJ, Song OP, Kim HC, Lim CW, Cho GS, Jung JC, Shin EJ (2011) Conventional linear versus purse-string skin closure after loop ileostomy reversal: comparison of wound infection rates and operative outcomes. J Korean Soc Coloproctol 27(2):58–63
15. Zubaidah NH, Soo JY, Qisti N, Ong KW, Gee T (2016) Wound infection following stoma reversal: a prospective comparative study between primary closure and partial closure with intervening silver dressings. Int J Colorectal Dis 31(7):1381–1382
16. Ovington LG (2001) Hanging wet to dry dressings out to dry. Home Healthc Nurse 19:477–483
17. White RJ (2001) New developments in the use of dressings on surgical wounds. Br J Nurs 10(6 suppl):S70
18. Leaper DJ (2006) Silver dressings: their role in wound management. Int Wound J 3:282–294
19. White RJ (2001) An historical overview of the use of silver in wound management. Br J Nurs 10(suppl):3–8
20. Ip M, Sau LL, Poon VKM, Lung I, Burd A (2006) Antimicrobial activities of silver dressings: an in vitro comparison. J Med Microbiol 55:59–63

21. Fraser JF, Bodman J, Sturgess R, Faoagali J, Kimble RM (2004) An in vitro study of the anti-microbial efficacy of a 1% silver sulphadiazine and 0.2% chlorhexidine digluconate cream, 1% silver sulphadiazine cream and a silver coated dressing. Burns 30:35–41
22. Carter MJ, Tingley-Kelley K, Warriner RA (2010) Silver treatments and silver- impregnated dressings for the healing of leg wounds and ulcers: a systematic review and meta-analysis. J Am Acad Dermatol 63(4):668–679

Primary Necrotizing Fasciitis of the Breast: Combined Use of Hyperbaric Oxygen and Negative-Pressure Wound Therapy to Conserve the Breast

Francesco Marongiu, Andrea Giurdanella, Federico Buggi, Francesca Fiorentini, Daniele Alfio Vecchio, Matteo Mingozzi, Secondo Folli, and Annalisa Curcio

1 Introduction

The term necrotizing fasciitis (NF) describes a group of soft tissue infection spreading along fascial planes causing gradual destruction of the fascia at the rate reaching 2–3 cm/h. Developing in the lower or upper extremities, perineum and genital area, and abdominal wall, its swift clinical course is correlated with polymicrobial infection and synergy, which usually coexists [1]. NF has been historically reported from almost all parts of the world and is now understood to be caused by either a single organism or more frequently by a variety of microbes, aerobic and anaerobic.

Necrotizing infections of the soft tissue have been known since ancient times when Hippocrates, in 500 BC, reported a clinical description of a complication of erysipelas disease, resembling the current description of NF [2, 3]. In 1783 Colles described a condition that was very similar to the modern description of NF. In 1871 a military surgeon in the Confederate Army of United States, Joseph Jones, made the first description of modern NF when he reported 2642 cases of gas gangrene treated in hospital during the American Civil War, with a mortality rate of 46%. Since his description, it has been variously named as "necrotizing erysipelas," "hemolytic streptococcal gangrene," "suppurative fasciitis," and "acute dermal gangrene" [4–9]. In 1883, Fournier described a syndrome with necrosis of the perineum, and this type of NF was subsequently given his name and is currently known as Fournier's gangrene. The current term "NF" was coined by Wilson in 1952, for he observed that cutaneous gangrene is not invariably present, yet fascial necrosis is a constant feature of the syndrome [6, 10].

F. Marongiu, M.D. (✉) • F. Buggi • D.A. Vecchio
M. Mingozzi • A. Curcio
Breast Surgical Unit, Morgagni-Pierantoni Hospital
Forlì, Forlì-Cesena, Italy
e-mail: marongiufra@gmail.com

A. Giurdanella
Department of Surgery, University of Sassari, University Hospital Trust, Microsurgery and Medical nd Surgical specialties, Plastic Surgery Unit, Forlì, Italy

F. Fiorentini
Division of Oncology and Diagnostics, Morgagni-Pierantoni Hospital, Forlì, Italy

S. Folli
Breast Surgery Unit, IRCCS-Arcispedale Santa Maria Nuova, Reggio Emilia, Italy

Department of Breast Surgery, Plastic and Reconstructive Surgery Unit, Fondazione IRCCS Istituto Nazionale Tumori Milano, Milan, Italy

Recent Clinical Techniques, Results, and Research in Wounds (2017)
DOI 10.1007/15695_2017_33, © Springer International Publishing AG
Published Online: 24 October 2017

The annual incidence of NF is estimated at 500–1000 cases annually, and its prevalence globally has been reported to be 0.40 per 100.000 population. The disease affects all age groups; it is seen to have a predilection for men which correlated an increased incidence of Fournier's gangrene. The mortality rate has not changed in the last 30 years and remains 25–35%; the rate is directly proportional to the time of the intervention [11].

NF is even more unusual as a primary disease of the breast, with no previous invasive procedure or other conditions. In literature only 11 cases of spontaneous necrotizing infection of the breast have been reported, and five of these were otherwise healthy women. In the treatment of NF in the breast, mastectomy has been reported to be the main treatment [12]. Usually patients with NF experience severe pain and tenderness; the skin might have normal appearance in the early stages of the disease because the infection tracks the subcutaneous tissue. Skin changes will become evident with resulting skin ischemia, as a late feature of the disease [13]. We present a first case of healthy patient exhibiting necrotizing fasciitis of the breast (PNFB), treated by combining conservative surgery with hyperbaric oxygen (HO) and negative-pressure wound therapy (NPWT) (Table 1).

2 Case Report

A 39-year-old woman presented to the emergency department with fever and swelling of her right breast. Patient's history showed no previous use of drugs nor oral contraceptives, no recent pregnancy, no trauma, and no thromboembolic disease or other comorbidities. She was nonobese and non-smoker. Her family history was negative for breast cancer or other malignancies. She had never undergone surgery or any other invasive procedure of the breast. She reported having only fever during the night and noting once awake a redness on the superior pole of her right breast. 12 h later this area occupied the whole breast surface. Upon admission to the emergency unit, she was febrile. On examination the right breast showed swelling with erythema and edema and ecchymosis and bluish bulla on the lower quadrant (Fig. 1). The left breast was normal, and there was no axillary lymphadenopathy bilaterally. Blood pressure was normal and the ECG showed sinus tachycardia only. Blood test results were normal. Ultrasound examination showed diffuse edema of the entire right breast, with few subdermal gas bubbles in the outer lower quadrant and several undefined hypoechoic areas. The provisional diagnosis was "breast mastitis," and

Table 1 Summary of cases of primary necrotizing fasciitis of the breast

Author	Country	Year	Comorbidity	Culture	Treatment
Shah	India	2001	Diabetes	Polymicrobial	Mastectomy
Nizami	Pakistan	2006	Steroid treatment	Polymicrobial	Mastectomy + skin graft
Rajakannu	India	2006	None	Polymicrobial	Mastectomy + skin graft
Wong	Singapore	2008	None	Unknown	Quadrantectomy + secondary suture
Keune	U.S.A	2008	None	Polymicrobial	Mastectomy
Venkatramani	India	2009	HIV positive	Polymicrobial	Mastectomy
Vishwanath	India	2011	Lactating	Unknown	Mastectomy
Soliman	Kuwait	2011	None	Polymicrobial	Multiple selective debridements + skin graft
Yaji	India	2014	Diabetes	Polymicrobial	Wide debridement
Lee	Korea	2015	Pregnant	Monomicrobial	Wide debridement + VAC therapy and secondary suture
Yang	Europe	2015	None	Polymicrobial	Selective debridement + skin graft
Present case	Europe	2015	None	Monomicrobial	Selective debridement + hyperbaric oxygen + VAC therapy and skin graft

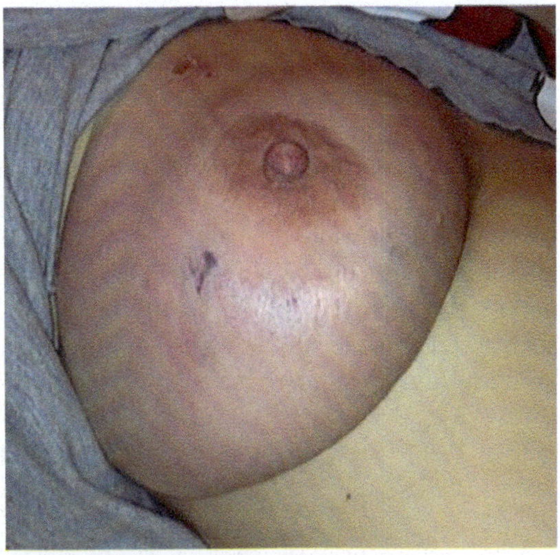

Fig. 1 The appearance of the breast on initial examination

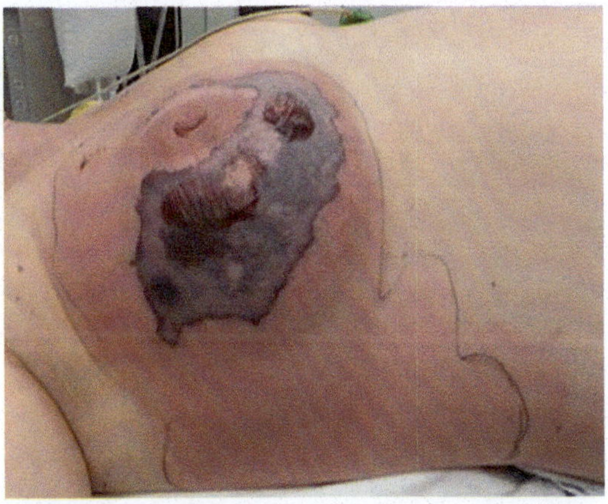

Fig. 2 New area of necrosis with rapid extension of the skin redness to the ipsilateral hemithorax

antibiotic therapy (ceftriaxone) was started. Several hours later the patient showed high fever (39.8 °C), a new area of necrosis appeared on the outer lower quadrant of the right breast, and a rapid extension of the skin redness to the ipsilateral hemithorax was evident (Fig. 2). Blood tests showed leukocytosis of 18.67 cells/mm3, with 92% neutrophils, Hb 11.3 day/dL, INR 1.50, Na + 129 mM, K+ 3.1 mM, and PCR 315.9 mg/L. Glycemia, platelet, and other results were normal. The CT scan showed skin thickening and subcutaneous gas in the deep tissues of the breast and beneath the skin surface, extending down the pectoral and latissimus dorsi fascial planes until the second lumbar vertebra (Fig. 3). The patient was prepared for emergency surgery. In the operating room, following incision, necrosis and purulent infiltrate of the breast tissue was noted, involving mainly the lower outer quadrant, extending to the lower inner quadrant but sparing the nipple areola complex; the infection appeared to reach the fascial planes of the pectoralis major and latissimus dorsi muscles until the second lumber vertebra, confirming the CT report. We performed a selective debridement, and apparently, all breast necrotic tissue was removed. Several drains were left in place and in the ipsilateral hemithorax (Figs. 4 and 5). After surgery, the patient was admitted to the intensive care unit and remained intubated. The HO was immediately started and continued every day (once/day 2.8 Bar × 120 min). Culture results demon-

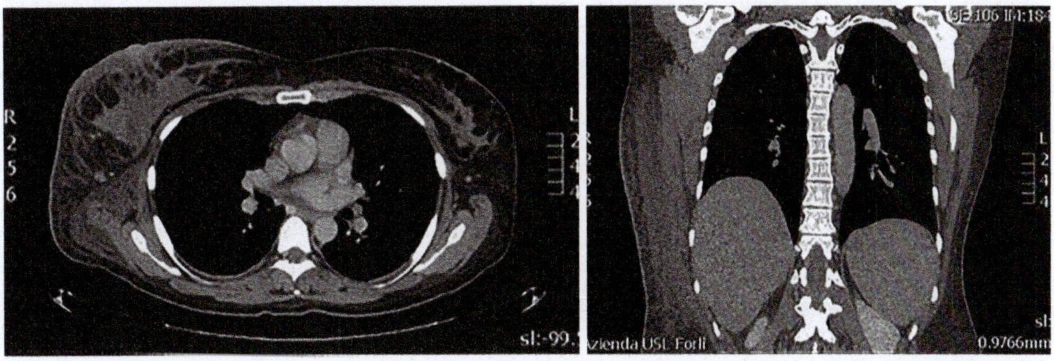

Fig. 3 (*Left*) CT scan revealing skin thickening and subcutaneous gas of the breast and beneath the skin surface, extending down the pectoral and (*right*) latissimus dorsi fascial planes until the second lumbar vertebra

strated Group A *Streptococcus pyogenes*, and adequate antibiotic treatment was initiated with Vancomicina-Meropenem-Clindamicina. The wound dressing was changed every other day. After 3 days, the patient's condition stabilized, the fever dropped down, and white blood cell count began to normalize. She was extubated with no further complications and was transferred to our surgical department. The pathology reports indicated acute necrotizing inflammation of the dermis and breast tissue, with bacterial colonies in the areas of necrosis and no evidence of malignancy. A week later, we made a second selective debridement under general anesthesia. Former overtly necrotic areas in the breast were maintained open to heal secondarily, while counter incisions were surrounded by healthy granulation tissue and were approxi-

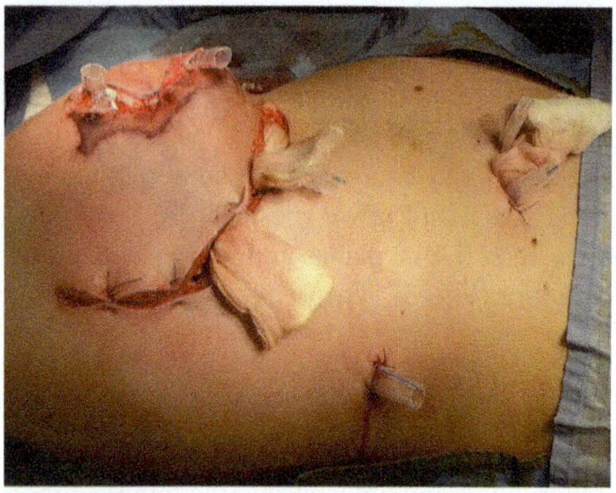

Fig. 4 Wounds partially sutured after selective debridement of breast necrotic tissue. Several drains were left in place in the breast and in the ipsilateral hemithorax. The hyperbaric therapy was immediately started and continued every day (once/day 2.8 Bar × 120 min)

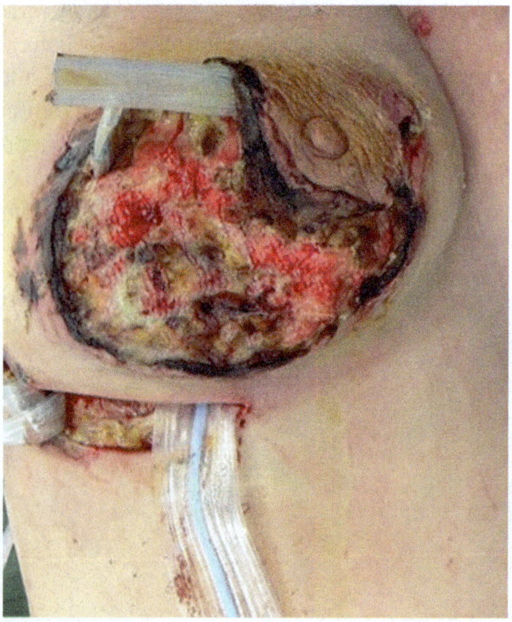

Fig. 5 The breast after 10 days showed only superficial marginal skin loss with small residual islands of necrosis, but the deep tissue appeared healthy

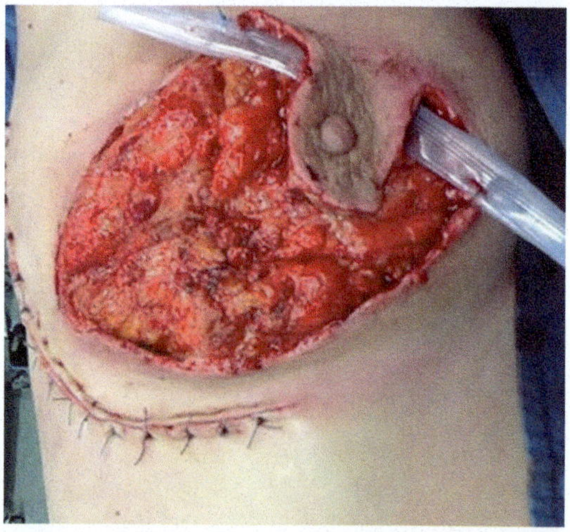

Fig. 6 Postoperative demonstrating the vitality of the wound tissue after second selective debridement under general anesthesia

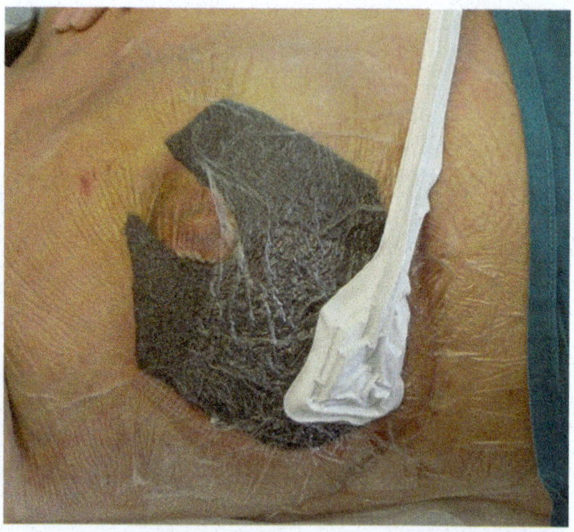

Fig. 7 After 18 days the hyperbaric oxygen therapy was suspended and the wound defect closed with negative-pressure wound therapy (120–135 mmHg)

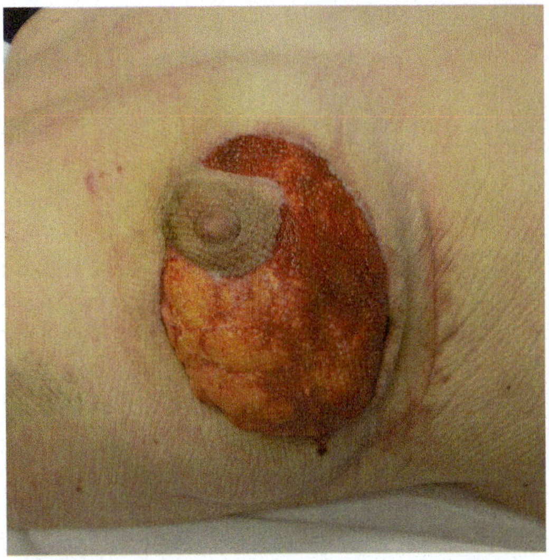

Fig. 8 45 days after the last debridement. No further tissue necrosis was seen and the breast began to exhibit signs of healing so we removed the negative-pressure wound therapy and performed a new operation to cover the wound

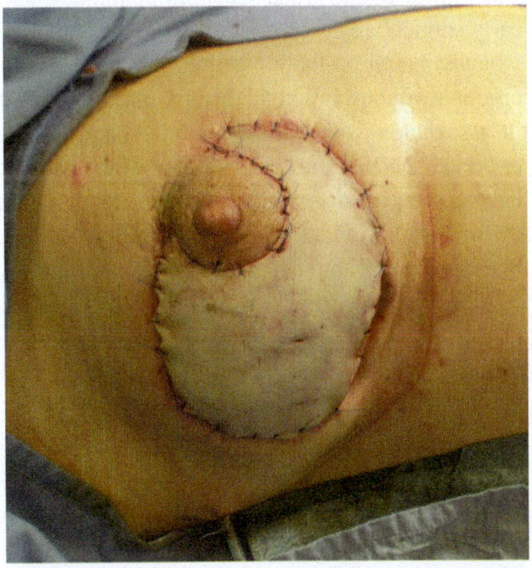

Fig. 9 Postoperative showing full-thickness skin graft reconstruction taken from the abdomen region

mated, and new drains were positioned (Fig. 6). After 18 days, the HO was suspended, and an NPWT that provided a continuous negative pressure to the wound (120–135 mmHg) was applied (Fig. 7). Following that, the patient's condition continued to improve. We progressively removed the drains; the wound started to granulate nicely; no further tissue necrosis was seen; and the breast began to exhibit signs of healing (Fig. 8), so 45 days after the last debridement, we removed the PNWT and performed a new operation to cover the breast wound using a full-thickness skin graft taken from the abdomen region (Fig. 9). After 5 days, no complication occurred, so the drain was removed and the patient was discharged. Several months later, an excellent cosmetic result was observed (Fig. 10).

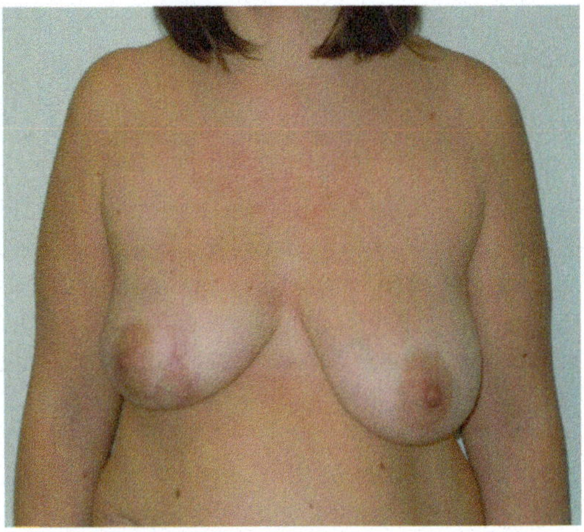

Fig. 10 Cosmetic result after 4 months

3 Discussion

NF is a rare disease but is associated with systemic toxicity and a high death rate despite aggressive treatment [11]. Patients with NF usually present with the classic triad of symptoms: local pain, swelling, and erythema [14]. Tachycardia and fever are the most common vital sign abnormalities, followed by hypotension and tachypnea. These vital sign abnormalities, with the skin erythema, are most useful in securing the diagnosis of NF from other soft tissue infections [15]. The infected site displays tenderness, sclerosis, skin necrosis, and hemorrhagic bullae [16].

Standard NF risk factors include chronic debilitating comorbidities (diabetes mellitus, peripheral vascular disease, smoking, alcohol abuse, liver disease, obesity, and immunosuppression) and condition compromising skin integrity (surgery, trauma, burns, intravenous drug use, biopsy, pressure ulcers, and chronic skin disease). Breast cancer, operation, wound dehiscence, and previous biopsies are other possible risk factors that could facilitate the development of NF in the breast [12, 17–19]. Recent studies have concluded that NF can be classified into four types, depending on the pathogen. Type 1 infections are the most common, also known as the polymicrobial type. Type 2 comprises monomicrobial infections caused by beta-hemolytic *Streptococcus* A (*S. pyogenes*). Type 3 is less common and includes monomicrobial infection involving the *Clostridium* species or Gram-negative bacteria. Finally, type 4 is the result of fungal infection, mainly *Candida* spp. and Zygomycetes [1, 18, 20]. Bacteria quickly reproduce, spread rapidly along tissue planes, and give off toxins and enzymes that destroy the soft tissues and fascias, which quickly become gangrenous. Furthermore, because of the systemic toxicity, the bacteria may cause multi-organ failure and death. For this reason, the timeliness of diagnosis and treatment is crucial to save the patients' lives [21]. Meleney recognized the importance of early surgical intervention [22].

Intraoperatively, an incision should be made down the pectoralis muscle over the area of maximal tenderness and most obvious skin involvement [13]. The first case of NF of the breast was described by Shah in 2001, and only 11 cases of PNFB have been reported in literature so far; among these, only five cases without any associated comorbidity are reported [13, 23–32]. The current case is the first described Italian case of PNFB in otherwise healthy patients, the second in Europe, and the sixth reported in the English literature. The diagnosis of NF is mainly clinical; however, clinical suspicion may not be enough; the use of imaging (ultrasound, CT scan, or MRI) may help in this context because findings such as irregularity of the fascias, abnormal fluid collections or gas tracking along fascial planes, fat stranding, and diffuse thickening of the fascias outline the presence of necrosis that demands aggressive surgical management [21, 33, 34]. Blood tests also proved useful, and Wong [26] proposed the use of the "laboratory risk indicator for necrotizing fasciitis' score may help in suspicious cases, as a score >6 of 13 indicates that NF should be seriously considered, and they also showed that the positive predictive value for NF increases as the score rises above 7 [21]. In our case, clinical signs showed fever but no associated pain, swelling, erythema, or edema, with an ecchymosis and bluish bulla on the patient's right breast. The laboratory risk indicator score was 8 and indicated the use of CT scan that suggested a surgical exploration. As a different radiological method to diagnose NF, MRI has a high sensitivity of 80–100% but a low specificity of 46–86%. MRI may not be readily available in an emergency setting and can be time-consuming [13, 35].

Unfortunately, as no signs, imaging, or tests are pathognomonic, today, the mortality rate is still 25–35% because time is the most important factor in survival [11, 21]. Standard management includes fluid resuscitation, intensive care support if indicated, intravenous broad-spectrum antibiotics, and early surgical aggressive debridement leaving open wounds; based on the blood culture results, a specific intravenous antibiotic therapy must be started in association with multiple debridement if indicated [11, 21]. For the NF of the breast, mastectomy has been reported in the published literature to be the most common surgical procedure [11, 12, 21], but the most effective treatment is not well established because of the lack of a large case series. Some authors have suggested breast conservative treatment [30, 32], and only one paper reported about wound management using NPWT [13].

NPWT has become a common method of treating large wounds once infection is controlled, although there have been no well-designed studies evaluating the role of NPWT in patients with large wounds following infection [11]. NPWT increases local oxygenation by enhancement of dermal perfusion and accelerates formation of granulation tissue by stimulating fibroblasts [36]. NPWT has been used for lesions in the breast such as chest wall defects following bilateral NF and salvage of infected breast implants [12].

HO is widely used in the treatment of acute and chronic infections because of numerous profitable actions: direct antimicrobial effect, increase antibiotic drug's efficacy, reduction of edema, enhanced angiogenesis, and fibroblasts proliferation [37]. These benefits may theoretically impact positively on all the phases in the treatment of NF, synergistically improving both infection control and wound healing [37]. However, nobody reported so far about the use of HO in the management of PNFB: on the basis of this consideration, we performed a selective surgical debridement, and the HO was immediately associated to exploit its additional effect of infection control and enhanced wound healing. This allowed us to obtain an excellent clearance of the infection from the breast tissue in association with a healthy, lively growing surrounding tissue sustained by NPWT; thus, the number of debridement procedures was minimal. Once the main goal of survival was granted, some room for pursuing an aesthetic outcome was created; when the clinical condition was stable and the breast tissue was definitively healthy, the NPWT could be removed and the wound was covered with a split skin graft. We decided to take the skin from the abdomen region because the patient had a skin excess, thus optimizing the cosmetic results.

Conclusions

Early diagnosis and timely treatment are crucial to save the patients' life. The multimodal approach is necessary in all phases of the treatment and may also allow the balancing of surgical aggressiveness to conserve the breast. This is the first case of PNFB case successfully treated conservatively, associating HO with selective surgical debridement and NPWT. This association resulted in a complete recovery and breast conservation, with the additional benefit of facilitated reconstruction and satisfactory cosmetic result. We recommend more prospective clinical studies to be conducted to analyze this kind of approach to such life-threatening diseases.

References

1. Misiakos EP, Bagias G, Patapis P, Sotiropoulos D, Kanavidis P, Machairas A (2014) Current concepts in the management of necrotizing fasciitis. Front Surg 36(1):1–10
2. Descamps V, Aitken J, Lee MG (1994) Hippocrates on necrotising fasciitis. Lancet 334:556
3. Giuliano A, Lewis F Jr, Hadley K, Blaksdell FW (1977) Bacteriology of necrotising fasciitis. Am J Surg 134:52–57
4. Hammar H, Wanger L (1977) Erysipelas and necrotising faciitis. Br J Dermatol 96:409–419
5. Ledingham IM, Tehrani MA (1975) Diagnosis, clinical course and treatment of acute dermal gangrene. Br J Surg 62:364–372
6. Wilson B (1952) Necrotising fasciitis. Am Surg 18:416–431
7. Collins RN, Nadel MS (1965) Gangrene due to the hemolytic streptococcus: a rare but treatable disease. N Engl J Med 272:578–580
8. Meleney FL (1929) Hemolytic streptococcus gangrene: importance of early diagnosis and early operation. JAMA 92:2009–2012
9. Webb HE, Hoover NW, Nichols DR, Weed LA (1962) Streptococcal gangrene. Arch Surg 85:969–973
10. Fournier JA (1988) Gangrene foudroyante de la verge. Med Pract 4:589–597
11. Sarani B, Strong M, Pascual J, Schwab CW (2009) Necrotizing fasciitis: current concepts and review of the literature. J Am Coll Surg 208:279–288
12. Angarita FA, Acuna SA, Torregrosa L, Tawil M, Sanchez EF, Heilbron O, Dominguez LC (2014) Bilateral necrotizing fasciitis of the breast following quadrantectomy. Breast Cancer 21:108–114
13. Lee J, Ju Lee K, Sun WY (2015) Necrotising fasciitis of the breast in a pregnant woman successfully treated using negative-pressure wound therapy. Ann Surg Treat Res 89:102–106
14. Goh T, Goh LG, Ang CH, Wong CH (2014) Early diagnosis of necrotizing fasciitis. Br J Surg 101:119–125
15. Shimizu T, Tokuda Y (2010) Necrotizing fasciitis. Intern Med 49:1051–1057
16. Frazee BW, Fee C, Lynn J, Wang R, Bostrom A, Hargis C (2008) Community-acquired necrotizing soft tissue infections: a review of 122 cases presenting to a single emergency department over 12 years. J Emerg Med 34:139–146
17. Salcido RS (2007) Necrotizing fasciitis: reviewing the causes and treatment strategies. Adv Skin Wound Care 20:288–293
18. Cho YS, Yang HT, Yim H, Park JM, Kim D, Hur J (2010) Necrotizing fasciitis following a small burn. J Korean Surg Soc 79:71–74
19. Flandrin A, Rouleau C, Azar CC, Dubon O, Giacalone PL (2009) First report of a necrotising fasciitis of the breast following a core needle biopsy. Breast J 15:199–201
20. Morgan MS (2010) Diagnosis and management of necrotising fasciitis a multiparametric approach. J Hosp Infect 75:249–257
21. Puvanendran R, Huey JC, Pasupathy S (2009) Necrotizing fasciitis. Can Fam Physician 55:981–987
22. Meleney FL (1933) A differential diagnosis between certain types of infectious gangrene of the skin – with particular reference to hemolitic streptococcus gangrene and bacterial synergistic gangrene. Surg Gynecol Obstet 56:847–867

23. Shah J, Sharma AK, O'Donoghue JM, Mearns B, Johri A, Thomas V (2001) Necrotizing fasciitis of the breast. Br J Plast Surg 54:67–79
24. Nizami S, Mohiuddin K, Azam M, Zafar H, Memon MA (2006) Necrotizing fasciitis of the breast. Breast J 12:168–169
25. Rajakannu M, Kate V, Ananthakrishnan N (2006) Necrotizing infection of the breast mimicking carcinoma. Breast J 12:266–267
26. Wong CH, Tan BK (2008) Necrotizing fasciitis of the breast. Plast Reconstr Surg 122:151e–1512
27. Keune J, Melby S, Kirby J, Aft R (2009) Shared management of a rare necrotizing soft tissue infection of the breast. Breast J 15:321–323
28. Venkatramani V, Pillai S, Marathe S, Rege SA, Hardikar JV (2009) Breast gangrene in an HIV-positive patient. Ann R Coll Surg Engl 91:W13–W14
29. Vishwanath G, Basarkod SI, Katageri GM, Mirji P, Mallapur AS (2011) Necrotizing fasciitis of the breast with shock and postpartum psychosis. J Clin Diagn Res 5:1117–1119
30. Soliman MO, Ayyash EH, Aldahham A, Asfar S (2011) Necrotizing fasciitis of the breast: a case managed without mastectomy. Med Princ Pract 20:567–569
31. Yaji P, Bhat B, Harish E (2014) Primary necrotizing fasciitis of the breast: case report and brief review of literature. J Clin Diagn Res 8:ND01–ND02
32. Yang B, Connolly S, Ball W (2015) Necrotizing fasciitis of the breast: a rare primary case with conservation of the nipple and literature review. J Plast Reconstr Aesth Surg Open 6:15e19
33. Brothers TE, Tagge DU, Stutley JE, Conway WF, Del Schutte H Jr, Byrne TK (1988) Magnetic Resonance imaging differentiates between necrotizing and non-necrotizing fasciitis of the lower extremity. J Am Coll Surg 187:416–421
34. Tsai CC, Lai CS, Yu ML, Chou CK, Lin SD (1996) Early diagnosis of necrotizing fasciitis by utilization of ultrasonography. Kaohsiung J Med Sci 12:235–240
35. Hanif MA, Bradley MJ (2008) Sonographic findings of necrotizing fasciitis in the breast. J Clin Ultrasound 36:517–519
36. Liao EC, Breuing KH (2007) Breast mound salvage using vacuum-assisted closure device as bridge to reconstruction with inferolateral AlloDerm hammock. Ann Plast Surg 59:218–224
37. Bhutani S, Vishwanath G (2012) Hyperbaric oxygen and wound healing. Indian J Plast Surg 45:316–324

Novel Antimicrobial Peptides: Targeting Wound Infections Caused by 'Superbugs' Resistant to All Current Antibiotics

Tony Velkov, Chongyu Zhu, David M. Haddleton, and Jian Li

1 Introduction

The annual costs of wound care in Australia ($2.6 billion AUD), the UK (£2.3–3.1 billion) and the USA ($50 billion USD) are staggering. The cost of chronic wound infections is often due to lengthy hospitalisations because of infections caused by multidrug-resistant (MDR) bacterial pathogens [1]. There is an urgent unmet medical need for new antibiotics for wound and burn infections caused by MDR Gram-negative 'superbugs' *Pseudomonas aeruginosa*, *Acinetobacter baumannii* and *Klebsiella pneumoniae*. Resistance to the last-line therapy polymyxins (polymyxin B and colistin) has been increasingly reported, which virtually means no antibiotic will be available for treatment of wound and burn infections. Considering potential systemic toxicity and suboptimal pharmacokinetic/pharmacodynamic attainment, the topical use of antibiotics often remains a superior approach for wound infections than parenteral administration.

The present chapter covers the development of novel broad-spectrum lipopeptides that are very active against not only polymyxin-resistant Gram-negative pathogens but also MDR Gram-positive *Staphylococcus aureus* and *Enterococcus faecium* that also commonly cause serious wound infections. Furthermore, we have developed a chitosan-based colistin self-healable hydrogel that provides high localised release of colistin for the treatment of burn wound infections. The development of these novel topical lipopeptide agents could slash the billion-dollar annual cost of wound treatment and result in improved healthcare on a global scale.

2 MDR Bacterial Wound Infections

Wound and burn infections are a major medical challenge worldwide and represent a considerable healthcare burden [2–4]. They are a common risk for patients with chronic non-healing wounds which cause high morbidity and mortality. As a poignant

T. Velkov, Ph.D. (✉)
Department of Pharmacology and Therapeutics, School of Biomedical Sciences, Faculty of Medicine, Dentistry and Health Sciences, The University of Melbourne, Parkville, VIC 3010, Australia
e-mail: tony.velkov@unimelb.edu.au

C. Zhu
Department of Chemistry, University of Warwick, Coventry, CV4 7AL, UK
e-mail: chongyu.zhu@warwick.ac.uk

D.M. Haddleton
Department of Chemistry, University of Warwick, Coventry, CV4 7AL, UK
e-mail: d.m.haddleton@warwick.ac.uk

J. Li
Monash Biomedicine Discovery Institute, Department of Microbiology, Monash University, Clayton, Victoria 3800, Australia
e-mail: jian.li@monash.edu

Recent Clinical Techniques, Results, and Research in Wounds (2017)
DOI 10.1007/15695_2017_34, © Springer International Publishing AG
Published Online: 24 October 2017

example, ~75% of all deaths following major burn injuries are related to bacterial infections [3, 4]. Wound and burn infections caused by the aforementioned Gram-negative 'superbugs' are immensely concerning [5]. Burns are particularly susceptible to infections due to the disruption of the epidermal barrier, the systemic apoptotic response and immunosuppression that disrupts self-defence mechanisms to fight infection [3, 6]. Even though systemic antibiotic treatment is usually the most common therapeutic option, the significant difficulties are adverse effects and the risk of an insufficient tissue penetration due to impaired blood circulation. The use of topical chemotherapy has been fundamental and helped to improve the survival of patients with major burns and to minimise the incidence of life-threatening burn wound sepsis [7]. The topical use of antibiotics plays a significant role in the management of serious wound infections caused by Gram-negative bacteria *P. aeruginosa*, *A. baumannii* and *K. pneumoniae* and Gram-positive *S. aureus* and *E. faecium* [3, 4]. Very worryingly, these bacteria are increasingly resistant to almost all current topical antibiotics [8, 9]. These bacterial 'superbugs' have been identified by the Infectious Diseases Society of America (IDSA) and Centre for Disease Control and Prevention (CDC) as the top-priority dangerous 'superbugs' that require urgent attention for discovery of novel antibiotics [10–13].

Polymyxins are an important last-line therapy against Gram-negative 'superbugs'.

Polymyxins consist of a linear tripeptide fragment having an N-terminal fatty acyl tail attached to a cyclic heptapeptide (Fig. 24.1). They are polycations at pH 7.4 owing to the five diaminobutyric acid (Dab) residues. Polymyxins were discovered more than 60 years ago. Because the early experience in the 1960s with parenteral polymyxins led to some cases of nephrotoxicity and neurotoxicity, their clinical use waned [14–17]. Since the mid-1990s, there has been a greatly renewed interest in polymyxins because of the increasing prevalence of MDR *P. aeruginosa*, *A. baumannii* and *K. pneumoniae* [14–17]. Polymyxin B and colistin (polymyxin E) are the two clinically available polymyxins that are most commonly administered parenterally in patients as a last-line therapy for serious infections, when all other available antibiotics are inactive. Our in vitro studies have shown that resistance can rapidly emerge in *P. aeruginosa*, *A. baumannii* and *K. pneumoniae* [18–20], and polymyxin resistance in hospitalised patients has been increasingly reported [10, 21, 22]. Even more worrying is the recent reports in the *Lancet Infect Dis* of the emergence of plasmid-mediated colistin resistance [23, 24], which implies resistance to these important last-line antibiotics can now rapidly spread. Resistance to polymyxins implies a total lack of antibiotics for treatment of life-threatening Gram-negative infections.

The majority of the modern pharmacological data of polymyxins are obtained by our group [18, 20, 25–43]. We were the first to characterise the modern pharmacokinetics of colistin and polymyxin B in patients [25, 30, 39, 40] and demonstrate that polymyxins exhibit rapid, concentration-dependent killing of susceptible strains of *P. aeruginosa*, *A. baumannii* and *K. pneumoniae* [20, 34, 41]. Our studies in both in vitro and animal infection models have, for the first time, elucidated that fAUC/MIC (i.e. ratio of the area under the free plasma concentration—time curve to minimal inhibitory concentration [MIC]) is the pharmacokinetic/pharmacodynamic (PK/PD) index best correlating with colistin activity [44]. Our findings are led to the first scientifically based dosage regimens in patients. Our recent data suggest that intravenous polymyxins are not ideal for treatment of lung infections and wound infections due to suboptimal PK/PD exposure at infection sites. We first reported colistin heteroresistance (i.e. colistin-resistant subpopulations in an isolate susceptible based upon MIC) in the Gram-negative pathogens [20, 31, 36] and the potential for resistant subpopulations to rapidly amplify upon exposure to colistin in an in vitro PK/PD model that mimics clinical dosing regimens in humans [18–20]. The latter highlights the urgency to develop new antibiotics active against isolates which are resistant to polymyxins and all other current antibiotics.

3 Mechanisms of Polymyxin Activity and Resistance

The initial cellular target of polymyxins is the lipid A component of lipopolysaccharide (LPS) in the outer membrane (OM). The purported primary mechanism of polymyxin activity involves an initial electrostatic interaction of the cationic Dab residues of the polymyxin molecule with the negatively charged phosphate groups of lipid A [45]. This initial polar interaction is followed by insertion of the fatty acyl tail of the polymyxin into the lipid A fatty acyl layer in the outer membrane. Many of the Gram-negative bacterial mechanisms of resistance to polymyxins are based on modifications to lipid A which reduce or abolish this initial electrostatic interaction. Modification of the phosphates of lipid A with positively charged moieties such as 4-amino-4-deoxy-L-arabinose or phosphoethanolamine reduces the net negative charge of lipid A, thereby increasing resistance to polymyxins [46–53].

4 Discovery of New Polymyxin-Like Lipopeptides Targeting MDR 'Superbugs'

We were invited by the *Journal of Medicinal Chemistry* to review the current state of development of polymyxin analogues [54]. Previous medicinal chemistry strategies for improving the antibacterial activity of polymyxins have been empirical and limited to modifications of the Dab residues, the heptapeptide ring and the length of the N-terminal fatty acyl chain (Fig. 1) [55–60]. Notably, numerous attempts have been made to modify the N-terminus with polar and lipophilic groups but with little success [54]. One such notable N-terminal analogue (CB-182804) came from Cubist; unfortunately this analogue failed in a Phase 1 clinical trial. Importantly, CB-182804 was not active against any polymyxin-resistant isolates [61]. None of the previous discovery programmes were specifically driven by an SAR approach nor was polymyxin resistance targeted. These major shortcomings led to the failure of the novel polymyxin discovery programmes by Cubist, AstraZeneca and Pfizer. To the best of our knowledge, we are the first to apply an SAR-based mechanistic model (Fig. 2) to discover novel lipopeptides against polymyxin-resistant Gram-negative 'superbugs' [62]. The SAR model has allowed us to identify key structural properties of polymyxins that confer antibacterial activity. In our model, the polymyxin-lipid A complex is stabilised by a combination of polar and hydrophobic interactions (Fig. 2). The positive charges on Dab1

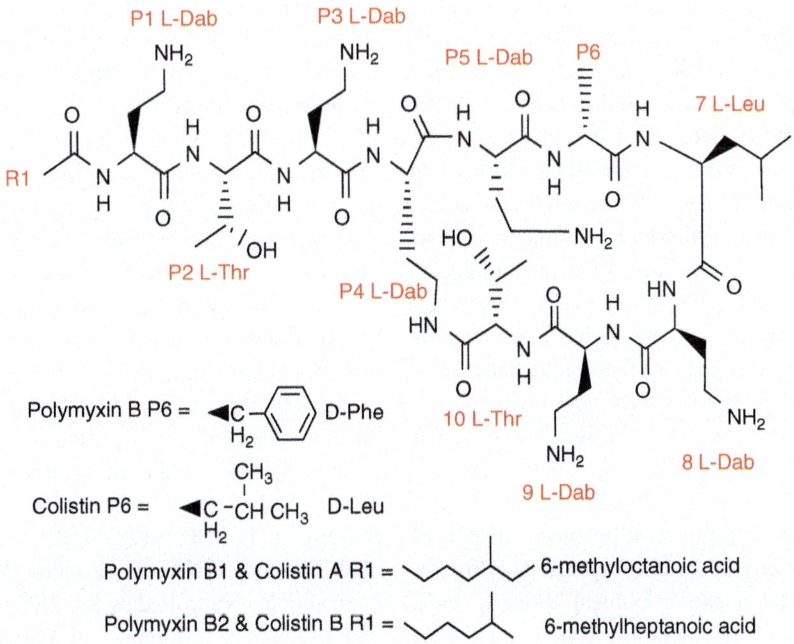

Fig. 1 Structures of colistin and polymyxin B. *Thr* threonine, *Leu* leucine, *Phe* phenylalanine, *Dab* α,γ-diaminobutyric acid

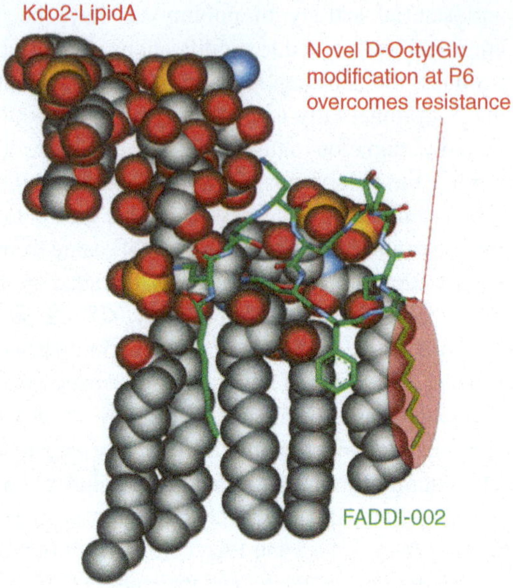

Fig. 2 SAR model of novel lipopeptide FADDI-002 in complex with *E. coli* Kdo2-lipid A

and Dab5 of polymyxin B interact with the negatively charged 4′-phosphate group of lipid A, and Dab8 and Dab9 similarly interact with the 1-phosphate of lipid A. The polymyxin-lipid A complex is further stabilised by hydrophobic contacts between the N-terminal fatty acyl chain and position 6/7 D-Phe-L-Leu segment of the polymyxin molecule, with the fatty acyl chains of lipid A. Evidently, the SAR model indicates that the polymyxin-lipid A interaction in both polymyxin-susceptible and polymyxin-resistant strains can be significantly accentuated through the introduction of additional hydrophobic contacts. To circumvent bacterial resistance mechanisms due to modifications of lipid A, in one series of our novel FADDI lipopeptides, hydrophobic modifications were introduced at position 6 or 7 to enhance penetration into the lipid A fatty acyl layer as suggested by the SAR model (Fig. 2). The SAR model was validated when our first generation lipopeptides (e.g. FADDI-002) (Table 1) with L-octylglycine substituted at position 7 displayed potent antimicrobial activity against polymyxin-resistant Gram-negative clinical isolates [62]. Subsequently, expansion of our SAR-based design strategy to include compounds incorporating lipidic groups at position 6 and the N-terminus

Table 1 Structures of representative lipopeptides

Lipopeptide	Structure
FADDI-002	Octanoyl-Dab-Thr-Dab-Dab*-Dab-D-Phe-OctGly-Dab-Dab-Thr*
FADDI-003	Biphenyl-Dab-Thr-Dab-Dab*-Dab-D-Phe-OctGly-Dab-Dab-Thr*
FADDI-019	Octanoyl-Dab-Thr-Dab-Dab*-Dab-D-OctGly-Leu-Dab-Dab-Thr*
FADDI-043	Dansylgly-OctGly-Dab-Thr-Dab-Dab*-Dab-D-Phe-Leu-Dab-Dab-Thr*
FADDI-052	Biphenyl-Dab-Thr-Dab-Dab*-Dab-D-Cys(6F3-Hex)-Leu-Dab-Dab-Thr*

*Cyclisation point of the peptide

also generated potent lipopeptides active against polymyxin-resistant Gram-negative ‘superbugs’ (Table 1). Notably, FADDI-019 and FADDI-020 which have the same or very similar MICs (1–4 mg/L) as colistin against colistin-susceptible *P. aeruginosa* isolates displayed significant activity (MICs 1–4 mg/L) against colistin-resistant *P. aeruginosa* (colistin MICs 32 or >128 mg/L). In static time-killing studies, FADDI-019 (MIC 1 mg/L) at 4 × MIC achieved ~6 $\log_{10}$ kill against a polymyxin-resistant MDR clinical *P. aeruginosa* isolate (colistin MIC >128 mg/L) with no viable cells detected even at 2 h; no killing was observed with colistin even at 32 mg/L. Against polymyxin-susceptible *P. aeruginosa* ATCC 27853 (colistin MIC 1 mg/L), FADDI-019 (MIC 1 mg/L) had comparable bacterial time-kill to colistin. For most of our lipopeptides, the ratios of MBCs (minimal bactericidal concentrations) to MICs were ≤4 indicating a low potential for development of resistance. Isothermal titration calorimetry studies confirmed that the hydrophobic contribution from the N-terminal fatty acyl chain is the predominant driving force for polymyxin-lipid A complexation [63, 64].

Serendipitously, a series of our lipopeptides have unexpected activity against MDR Gram-positive *S. aureus* and *E. faecium* which are intrinsically resistant to polymyxins (colistin and polymyxin B MIC >128 mg/L). Transcriptome analysis using RNA-seq revealed that virulence determinants controlled by SaeRS and the expression of enterotoxins yent2, sei, sem and seo were all significantly downregulated by FADDI-019 [65]. Clearly, our SAR-based mechanistic model has led to unique opportunities to optimise the polymyxin structure to overcome both adaptive and intrinsic resistance to current polymyxins. There was no haemolysis in human red blood cells treated with the tested FADDI lipopeptides or polymyxins at 128 mg/L (the highest concentration examined). After administration of FADDI-002, FADDI-003, FADDI-019 or FADDI-020 to rats (intravenous, 0.75 mg/kg) and mice (subcutaneous, 40 mg/kg), no adverse effects were observed.

Preliminary in vitro studies to examine the impact of the lipopeptides on human keratinocytes and murine fibroblast cells, polymyxin B, FADDI-019 and FADDI-073 at 1.5, 5, 15 and 50 mg/L had little effect over 48 h on the morphology of fibroblasts (3 T3) and keratinocytes (HaCaT). FADDI-019, FADDI-073 and polymyxin B stimulated metabolic activity above mock-treated cultures in 3T3 cells in a dose-dependent manner at 24 and 48 h. However, similar responses were not observed in HaCaT cells; neither FADDI-019 nor FADDI-073 affected the cellular metabolic activity at any of the four concentrations at 24 or 48 h, while only 1.5 and 5 mg/L polymyxin B slightly decreased the cellular metabolic activity at both time points. It is noteworthy that for many years a topical formulation containing polymyxin B has been used for treating skin infections, with negligible toxicity [66]. Our results suggest that our lipopeptides have at least similar tolerability to colistin and polymyxin B.

5 Synthesis of a Chitosan-Colistin Hydrogel and Testing in a Mouse Burn Infection Model

We have synthesised a chitosan-colistin hydrogel and assessed its efficacy in a mouse burn infection model (Fig. 3) [67]. The chitosan-colistin hydrogel is an inexpensive, self-healable and highly biocompatible material which provides up to 95% colistin release within 24 h and showed excellent in vitro activity against *P. aeruginosa* in a disc diffusion assay. The physical properties of the hydrogel were unaffected by colistin; this allowed us to load a wide range of colistin concentrations into the hydrogel matrix without impacting its size. Serendipitously, the hydrogel formation process was accelerated in the presence of colistin. Excitingly, the chitosan-colistin hydrogel dressing (containing 0.3 mg colistin) displayed excellent in vivo activity, producing a ~4 log reduction in the bacterial load in a burn wound (1 cm^2) infection, established in mice by inoculating 100 μL 10^8 CFU/mL of *P. aeruginosa* ATCC 27853. We are currently exploring lipopeptide-hydrogel dressing systems using the superior FADDI lipopeptides, for which formulation characteristics (e.g. lipopeptide loading and mechanical properties) will be investigated and optimised.

Silk proteins serve as excellent scaffolds for wound healing and in tissue engineering [68].

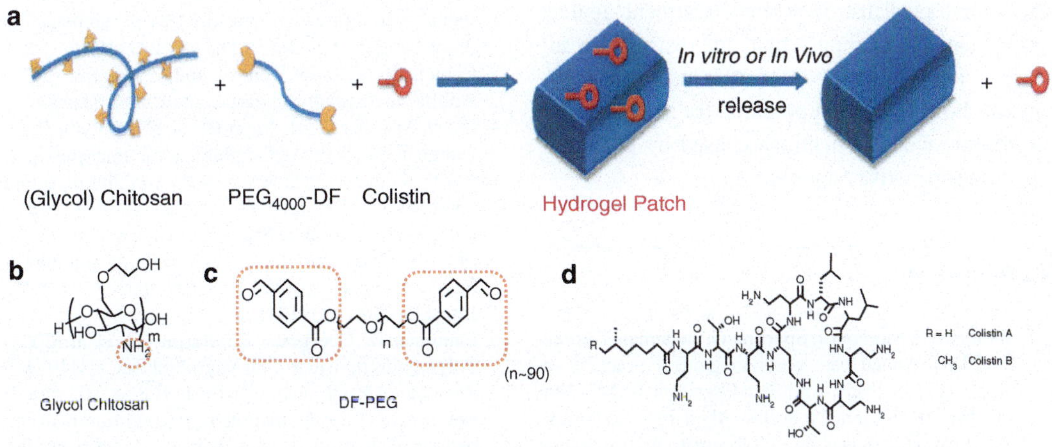

Fig. 3 (**a**) Synthesis of chitosan-colistin hydrogel. (**b**) Glycol chitosan. (**c**) DF-PEG. (**d**) Colistins A and B

Steinstraesser et al. [68] loaded ST-silk protein membranes (thickness, 100 μm; pore size, <100 nm) with colistin (0.027–270 mg/mL) and examined their efficacy against *P. aeruginosa* in animal wound infection models. The ST-silk membranes loaded with 270 mg/mL colistin demonstrated *a* > 3 log reduction in colony-forming units of *P. aeruginosa* ATCC 27853 after 4 days (~25-fold decrease from the carrier control). Similarly, in a porcine wound infection model, the ST-silk membranes loaded with 270 mg/mL colistin demonstrated an almost complete clearance of the infection after the entire follow-up of 6 days.

6 Perspective

The World Health Organization has identified antimicrobial resistance as one of the three greatest threats to human health. The last-line therapy polymyxins are losing their activity; however, no new antibiotic will be available for many years to come. The prevalence of wound infections caused by the bacterial 'superbugs' highlights the urgency of discovering novel antibiotics for topical treatment of serious wound infections. As the Infectious Diseases Society of America highlighted, 'as antibiotic discovery stagnates, a public health crisis brews', the recent emergence of plasmid-borne resistance to the last-line polymyxins highlights the urgency to develop novel antibiotics to combat these very problematic pathogens. This chapter details the development of novel polymyxin lipopeptides and hydrogel formulations as new antibiotics for topical use in wound treatment against problematic 'superbugs' that are resistant to all current antibiotics. These next-generation polymyxins hold significant potential for the treatment of chronic wound infections caused by problematic Gram-negative 'superbugs'.

References

1. Whitlock E, Morcom J, Spurling G, Janamian T, Ryan S (2014) Wound care costs in general practice—a cross-sectional study. Aust Fam Physician 43:143–146
2. Jacobsen F, Fisahn C, Sorkin M, Thiele I, Hirsch T, Stricker I, Klaassen T, Roemer A, Fugmann B, Steinstraesser L (2011) Efficacy of topically delivered moxifloxacin against wound infection by Pseudomonas aeruginosa and methicillin-resistant Staphylococcus aureus. Antimicrob Agents Chemother 55:2325–2334
3. Church D, Elsayed S, Reid O, Winston B, Lindsay R (2006) Burn wound infections. Clin Microbiol Rev 19:403–434
4. Vindenes H, Bjerknes R (1995) Microbial colonization of large wounds. Burns 21:575–579
5. Bad bugs, no drugs. https://www.idsociety.org/uploadedFiles/IDSA/Policy_and_Advocacy/Current_Topics_and_Issues/Advancing_Product_Research_and_Development/Bad_Bugs_No_Drugs/Statements/As%20Antibiotic%20Discovery%20Stagnates%20A%20Public%20Health%20Crisis%20Brews.pdf. Accessed 21 Mar 2017
6. Gravante G, Delogu D, Sconocchia G (2007) "Systemic apoptotic response" after thermal burns. Apoptosis 12:259–270
7. Honari S (2004) Topical therapies and antimicrobials in the management of burn wounds. Crit Care Nurs Clin North Am 16:1–11
8. Thomas CM, Hothersall J, Willis CL, Simpson TJ (2010) Resistance to and synthesis of the antibiotic mupirocin. Nat Rev Microbiol 8:281–289
9. Sevgi M, Toklu A, Vecchio D et al (2013) Topical antimicrobials for burn infections – an update. Recent Pat Antiinfect Drug Discov 8:161–197
10. Talbot GH, Bradley J, Edwards JE Jr, Gilbert D, Scheld M, Bartlett JG, Antimicrobial availability task force of the infectious diseases society of America (2006) Bad bugs need drugs: an update on the development pipeline from the Antimicrobial Availability Task Force of the Infectious Diseases Society of America. Clin Infect Dis 42:657–668
11. Boucher HW, Talbot GH, Bradley JS, Edwards JE, Gilbert D, Rice LB, Scheld M, Spellberg B, Bartlett J (2009) Bad bugs, no drugs: no ESKAPE! An update from the Infectious Diseases Society of America. Clin Infect Dis 48:1–12
12. Gilbert DN, Guidos RJ, Boucher HW, Talbot GH, Spellberg B, Edwards JE Jr, Scheld WM, Bradley JS, Bartlett JG (2010) The 10 × 20 Initiative: Pursuing a global commitment to develop 10 new antibacterial drugs by 2020. Clin Infect Dis 50:1081–1083
13. Centers for Disease Control and Prevention (2013) Antibiotic resistance threats in the United States
14. Evans ME, Feola DJ, Rapp RP (1999) Polymyxin B sulfate and colistin: old antibiotics for emerging multiresistant gram-negative bacteria. Ann Pharmacother 33:960–967
15. Falagas ME, Kasiakou SK (2005) Colistin: the revival of polymyxins for the management of multidrug-resistant gram-negative bacterial infections. Clin Infect Dis 40:1333–1341
16. Landman D, Georgescu C, Martin DA et al (2008) Polymyxins revisited. Clin Microbiol Rev 21:449–465
17. Zavascki AP, Goldani LZ, Li J, Nation RL (2007) Polymyxin B for the treatment of multidrug-resistant pathogens: a critical review. J Antimicrob Chemother 60:1206–1215

18. Bergen PJ, Tsuji BT, Bulitta JB, Forrest A, Jacob J, Sidjabat HE, Paterson DL, Nation RL, Li J (2011) Synergistic killing of multidrug-resistant Pseudomonas aeruginosa at multiple inocula by colistin combined with doripenem in an in vitro pharmacokinetic/pharmacodynamic model. Antimicrob Agents Chemother 55:5685–5695
19. Tan CH, Li J, Nation RL (2007) Activity of colistin against heteroresistant Acinetobacter baumannii and emergence of resistance in an in vitro pharmacokinetic/pharmacodynamic model. Antimicrob Agents Chemother 51:3413–3415
20. Poudyal A, Howden BP, Bell JM, Gao W, Owen RJ, Turnidge JD, Nation RL, Li J (2008) In vitro pharmacodynamics of colistin against multidrug-resistant Klebsiella pneumoniae. J Antimicrob Chemother 62:1311–1318
21. Gales AC, Jones RN, Sader HS (2011) Contemporary activity of colistin and polymyxin B against a worldwide collection of Gram-negative pathogens: results from the SENTRY Antimicrobial Surveillance Program (2006–09). J Antimicrob Chemother 66:2070–2074
22. Paterson DL, Lipman J (2007) Returning to the pre-antibiotic era in the critically ill: the XDR problem. Crit Care Med 35:1789–1791
23. Liu YY, Wang Y, Walsh TR, Yi LX, Zhang R, Spencer J, Doi Y, Tian G, Dong B, Huang X, Yu LF, Gu D, Ren H, Chen X, Lv L, He D, Zhou H, Liang Z, Liu JH, Shen J (2016) Emergence of plasmid-mediated colistin resistance mechanism MCR-1 in animals and human beings in China: a microbiological and molecular biological study. Lancet Infect Dis 16(2):161–168
24. Webb HE, Granier SA, Marault M, Millemann Y, den Bakker HC, Nightingale KK, Bugarel M, Ison SA, Scott HM, Loneragan GH (2016) Dissemination of the mcr-1 colistin resistance gene. Lancet Infect Dis 16:144–145
25. Li J, Coulthard K, Milne R, Nation RL, Conway S, Peckham D, Etherington C, Turnidge J (2003) Steady-state pharmacokinetics of intravenous colistin methanesulfonate in patients with cystic fibrosis. J Antimicrob Chemother 52:987–992
26. Li J, Milne RW, Nation RL, Turnidge JD, Smeaton TC, Coulthard K (2003) Use of high-performance liquid chromatography to study the pharmacokinetics of colistin sulfate in rats following intravenous administration. Antimicrob Agents Chemother 47:1766–1770
27. Li J, Milne RW, Nation RL, Turnidge JD, Smeaton TC, Coulthard K (2004) Pharmacokinetics of colistin methanesulphonate and colistin in rats following an intravenous dose of colistin methanesulphonate. J Antimicrob Chemother 53:837–840
28. Li J, Nation RL, Owen RJ, Wong S, Spelman D, Franklin C (2007) Antibiograms of multidrug-resistant clinical Acinetobacter baumannii: promising therapeutic options for treatment of infection with colistin-resistant strains. Clin Infect Dis 45:594–598
29. Li J, Nation RL, Turnidge JD, Milne RW, Coulthard K, Rayner CR, Paterson DL (2006) Colistin: the re-emerging antibiotic for multidrug-resistant Gram-negative bacterial infections. Lancet Infect Dis 6:589–601
30. Li J, Rayner CR, Nation RL, Deans R, Boots R, Widdecombe N, Douglas A, Lipman J (2005) Pharmacokinetics of colistin methanesulfonate and colistin in a critically ill patient receiving continuous venovenous hemodiafiltration. Antimicrob Agents Chemother 49:4814–4815
31. Li J, Rayner CR, Nation RL, Owen RJ, Spelman D, Tan KE, Liolios L (2006) Heteroresistance to colistin in multidrug-resistant Acinetobacter baumannii. Antimicrob Agents Chemother 50:2946–2950
32. Dudhani RV, Turnidge JD, Coulthard K, Milne RW, Rayner CR, Li J, Nation RL (2010) Elucidation of the pharmacokinetic/pharmacodynamic determinant of colistin activity against Pseudomonas aeruginosa in murine thigh and lung infection models. Antimicrob Agents Chemother 54:1117–1124
33. Dudhani RV, Turnidge JD, Nation RL, Li J (2010) fAUC/MIC is the most predictive pharmacokinetic/pharmacodynamic index of colistin against Acinetobacter baumannii in murine thigh and lung infection models. J Antimicrob Chemother 65:1984–1990
34. Owen RJ, Li J, Nation RL, Spelman D (2007) In vitro pharmacodynamics of colistin against Acinetobacter baumannii clinical isolates. J Antimicrob Chemother 59:473–477
35. Bergen PJ, Bulitta JB, Forrest A, Tsuji BT, Li J, Nation RL (2010) Pharmacokinetic/pharmacodynamic investigation of colistin against Pseudomonas aeruginosa using an in vitro model. Antimicrob Agents Chemother 54(9):3783
36. Bergen PJ, Forrest A, Bulitta JB, Tsuji BT, Sidjabat HE, Paterson DL, Li J, Nation RL (2011) Clinically relevant plasma concentrations of colistin in combination with imipenem enhance pharmacodynamic activity against multidrug-resistant Pseudomonas aeruginosa at multiple inocula. Antimicrob Agents Chemother 55:5134–5142
37. Bergen PJ, Li J, Nation RL, Turnidge JD, Coulthard K, Milne RW (2008) Comparison of once-, twice- and thrice-daily dosing of colistin on antibacterial effect and emergence of resistance: studies with Pseudomonas aeruginosa in an in vitro pharmacodynamic model. J Antimicrob Chemother 61:636–642
38. Bergen PJ, Li J, Rayner CR, Nation RL (2006) Colistin methanesulfonate is an inactive prodrug of colistin against Pseudomonas aeruginosa. Antimicrob Agents Chemother 50:1953–1958
39. Garonzik SM, Li J, Thamlikitkul V, Paterson DL, Shoham S, Jacob J, Silveira FP, Forrest A, Nation RL (2011) Population pharmacokinetics of colistin methanesulfonate and formed colistin in critically ill patients from a multicenter study provide dosing suggestions for various categories of patients. Antimicrob Agents Chemother 55:3284–3294
40. Zavascki AP, Goldani LZ, Cao GY, Superti SV, Lutz L, Barth AL, Ramos F, Boniatti MM, Nation RL, Li J (2008) Pharmacokinetics of intravenous polymyxin B in critically-ill patients. Clin Infect Dis 47:1298–1304

41. Li J, Turnidge J, Milne R, Coulthard K (2001) In vitro pharmacodynamic properties of colistin and colistin methanesulfonate against Pseudomonas aeruginosa isolates from patients with cystic fibrosis. Antimicrob Agents Chemother 45:781–785
42. Velkov T, Roberts KD, Nation RL, Thompson PE, Li J (2013) Pharmacology of polymyxins: new insights into an 'old' class of antibiotics. Future Microbiol 8:711–724
43. Nation RL, Velkov T, Li J (2014) Colistin and Polymyxin B: Peas in a pod, or chalk and cheese? Clin Infect Dis 59:88–94
44. Cheah SE, Li J, Nation RL, Bulitta JB (2015) Novel rate-area-shape modeling approach to quantify bacterial killing and regrowth for in vitro static time-kill studies. Antimicrob Agents Chemother 59:381–388
45. Clausell A, Garcia-Subirats M, Pujol M, Busquets MA, Rabanal F, Cajal Y (2007) Gram-negative outer and inner membrane models: insertion of cyclic cationic lipopeptides. J Phys Chem B 111:551–563
46. Helander IM, Kilpelainen I, Vaara M (1994) Increased substitution of phosphate groups in lipopolysaccharides and lipid A of the polymyxin-resistant pmrA mutants of Salmonella typhimurium: a 31P-NMR study. Mol Microbiol 11:481–487
47. Moskowitz SM, Ernst RK, Miller SI (2004) PmrAB, a two-component regulatory system of Pseudomonas aeruginosa that modulates resistance to cationic antimicrobial peptides and addition of aminoarabinose to lipid A. J Bacteriol 186:575–579
48. Helander IM, Kato Y, Kilpeläinen I, Kostiainen R, Lindner B, Nummila K, Sugiyama T, Yokochi T (1996) Characterization of lipopolysaccharides of polymyxin-resistant and polymyxin-sensitive Klebsiella pneumoniae O3. Eur J Biochem 237:272–278
49. Clements A, Tull D, Jenney AW, Farn JL, Kim SH, Bishop RE, McPhee JB, Hancock RE, Hartland EL, Pearse MJ, Wijburg OL, Jackson DC, McConville MJ, Strugnell RA (2007) Secondary acylation of Klebsiella pneumoniae lipopolysaccharide contributes to sensitivity to antibacterial peptides. J Biol Chem 282:15569–15577
50. Perez JC, Groisman EA (2007) Acid pH activation of the PmrA/PmrB two-component regulatory system of Salmonella enterica. Mol Microbiol 63:283–293
51. Adams MD, Nickel GC, Bajaksouzian S, Lavender H, Murthy AR, Jacobs MR, Bonomo RA (2009) Resistance to colistin in Acinetobacter baumannii associated with mutations in the PmrAB two-component system. Antimicrob Agents Chemother 53:3628–3634
52. Beceiro A, Llobet E, Aranda J, Bengoechea JA, Doumith M, Hornsey M, Dhanji H, Chart H, Bou G, Livermore DM, Woodford N (2011) Phosphoethanolamine modification of lipid A in colistin-resistant variants of Acinetobacter baumannii mediated by the pmrAB two-component regulatory system. Antimicrob Agents Chemother 55:3370–3379
53. Fernandez L, Gooderham WJ, Bains M, McPhee JB, Wiegand I, Hancock RE (2010) Adaptive resistance to the "last hope" antibiotics polymyxin B and colistin in Pseudomonas aeruginosa is mediated by the novel two-component regulatory system ParR-ParS. Antimicrob Agents Chemother 54:3372–3382
54. Velkov T, Thompson PE, Nation RL, Li J (2010) Structure-activity relationships of polymyxin antibiotics. J Med Chem 53:1898–1916
55. Weinstein J, Afonso A, Moss E Jr, Miller GH (1998) Selective chemical modifications of polymyxin B. Bioorg Med Chem Lett 8:3391–3396
56. Tsubery H, Ofek I, Cohen S, Fridkin M (2001) N-terminal modifications of Polymyxin B nonapeptide and their effect on antibacterial activity. Peptides 22:1675–1681
57. Tsubery H, Ofek I, Cohen S, Fridkin M (2000) Structure-function studies of polymyxin B nonapeptide: implications to sensitization of gram-negative bacteria. J Med Chem 43:3085–3092
58. Vaara M, Fox J, Loidl G, Siikanen O, Apajalahti J, Hansen F, Frimodt-Møller N, Nagai J, Takano M, Vaara T (2008) Novel polymyxin derivatives carrying only three positive charges are effective antibacterial agents. Antimicrob Agents Chemother 52:3229–3236
59. O'Dowd H, Kim B, Margolis P, Wang W, Wu C, Lopez SL, Blais J (2007) Preparation of tetra-Boc-protected polymyxin B nonapeptide. Tetrahedron Lett 48:2003–2005
60. Chihara S, Ito A, Yahata M, Tobita T, Koyama Y (1974) Chemical synthesis, isolation, and characterization of alpha-N-fattyacyl colistin nonapeptide with special reference to the correlation between antimicrobial activity and carbon number of fattyacyl moiety. Agr Biol Chem 38:521–529
61. Leese RA (2010) Antibiotic compositions for the treatment of Gram-negative infections. US Patent Number 8343912
62. Velkov T, Roberts KD, Nation RL, Wang J, Thompson PE, Li J (2014) Teaching 'old' polymyxins new tricks: new-generation lipopeptides targeting gram-negative superbugs. ACS Chem Biol 9:1172–1177
63. Srimal S, Surolia N, Balasubramanian S, Surolia A (1996) Titration calorimetric studies to elucidate the specificity of the interactions of polymyxin B with lipopolysaccharides and lipid A. Biochem J 315(Pt 2):679–686
64. Soon RL, Velkov T, Chiu F, Thompson PE, Kancharla R, Roberts K, Larson I, Nation RL, Li J (2011) Design, synthesis, and evaluation of a new fluorescent probe for measuring polymyxin-lipopolysaccharide binding interactions. Anal Biochem 409:273–283
65. Zhao J, Cheah S-E, Roberts KD, Nation RL, Thompson PE, Velkov T, Du Z, Johnson MD, Li J (2016) Transcriptomic Analysis of the Activity of a Novel Polymyxin against Staphylococcus aureus. mSphere 1(4):e00119-16
66. Bonomo RA, Van Zile PS, Li Q, Shermock KM, McCormick WG, Kohut B (2007) Topical

triple-antibiotic ointment as a novel therapeutic choice in wound management and infection prevention: a practical perspective. Expert Rev Anti-Infect Ther 5:773–782
67. Zhu C, Zhao J, Kempe K, Wilson P, Wang J, Velkov T, Li J, Davis TP, Whittaker MR, Haddleton DM (2017) A hydrogel-based localized release of colistin for antimicrobial treatment of burn wound infection. Macromol Biosci 17(2):1600320
68. Steinstraesser L, Trust G, Rittig A, Hirsch T, Kesting MR, Steinau HU, Jacobsen F (2011) Colistin-loaded silk membranes against wound infection with Pseudomonas aeruginosa. Plast Reconstr Surg 127:1838–1846

Novel Use of a Biologically Active-Prefabricated-Random-Three-Dimensional-Polymer Scaffold of Hyaluronic Acid (HYAFF) to Facilitate Complicated Wound Closure

Tammy Luttrell, Samantha Rosenberry, Nancy Estacado, and Jay Coates

1 Introduction

The focus of this chapter is the relatively new introduction of a 3D scaffolding fiber composed of HA, one of the major glycosaminoglycans (GAGs) found in the extracellular matrix (ECM) (Fig. 1). Hyaluronic acid is water loving hydrophilic and is found in the dermis of the skin (Fig. 2). Recently, it is appreciated that ECM molecules, like HA, lie between the cells and not only provide a structural framework and foundation; but also exert major effects on cellular function. Hyaluronic acid (HA) is unique among glycosaminoglycans in that it is nonsulfated; forms in the plasma membrane, instead of the Golgi apparatus; and can become very large with its weight often reaching the millions of KDa. In a stabilized form, it provides a 3D-biopolymer scaffold that promotes endothelial cell migration [1], thus supporting neovascularization, a foundation of granulation tissue and extracellular matrix revitalization.

Under light microscopy, these molecules appear amorphous; however, in vivo they form highly organized structures. The ECM is composed mainly of GAGs, proteoglycans, and structural proteins like collagen. In the ECM hyaluronic acid (HA) is known to be biologically selectively active based on the size of the molecule. Low molecular weight HA (LMWHA) is associated with inflammatory processes and cell phenotypes consistent with inflammation. High molecular weight HA (HMWHA) is associated with inflammatory resolution and proliferative cell phenotypes.

The major requirements for burn and wound healing are presented in Fig. 3. HA has a role to play in each of these types of injury because of the associated dermal loss. The effect that either LMWHA or HMWHA imparts is largely via the effect on resident macrophage phenotype. As indicated, the first step in healing is the removal of bioburden including dead and decaying cells or senescent cells. This process can be expedited with surgical sharp selective debridement. Control of swelling is imperative so as to avoid collateral damage to the peri-wound. Granulation tissue is promoted via the infiltration of fibroblasts, keratinocytes, and neoangiogenesis. Mobilization of soft tissue prevents adhesions and improves interstitial and laminar flow, further contributing to the decreasing of edema while simultaneously promoting epithelial cell migration and ultimately resurfacing. The replacement of dermal tissue either through biologically engineered tissues or through biologically active molecules responsible for cell signaling and

T. Luttrell (✉) · S. Rosenberry · N. Estacado
J. Coates
Las Vegas, NV, USA
e-mail: Tammy_luttrell@msn.com

Recent Clinical Techniques, Results, and Research in Wounds (2018)
https://doi.org/10.1007/15695_2018_114, © Springer International Publishing AG
Published Online: 22 August 2018

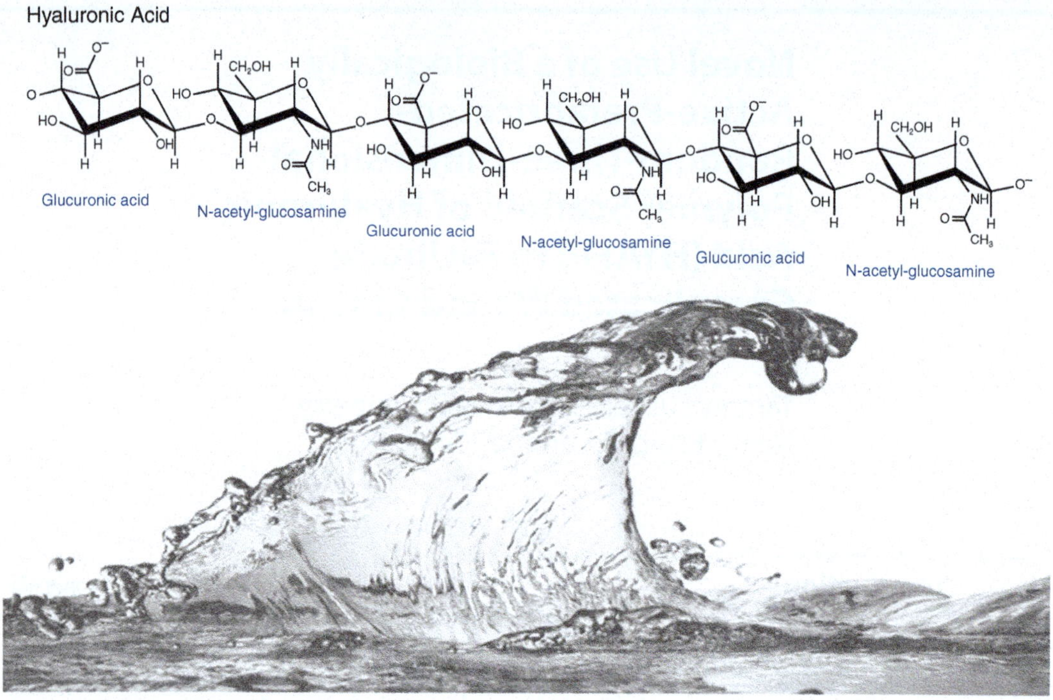

Fig. 1 Structure of hyaluronic acid (HA). HA is a long-chained glycosaminoglycan composed of D-glucuronic acid and *N*-acetyl-D-glucosamine bound with β-glycosidic linkages. This simple molecular unit is repeated thousands of times and forms a structure of a very long linear polymer with molecular weight reaching 5×10^6 kDa. Hyaluronic acid has a very high affinity for water

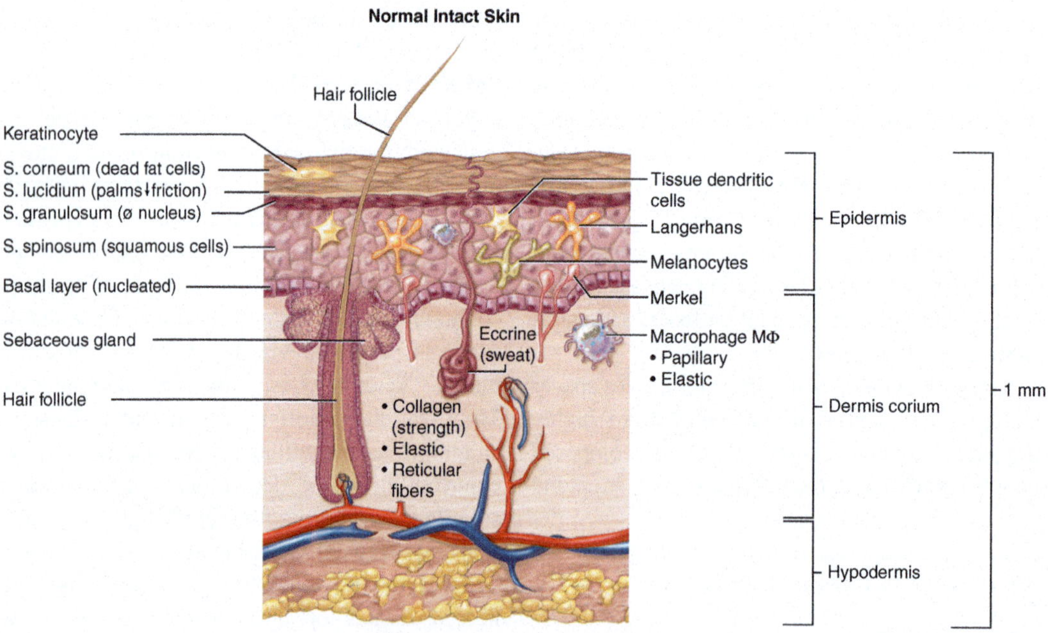

Fig. 2 Layers of the skin including the epidermis and dermis. Fifty percent of the human body's HA is found in the dermis and interconnects with many other proteins, collagen, elastin, and versican, to name a few, as well as resident cells of the extracellular matrix (ECM). Reproduced with permission [31]

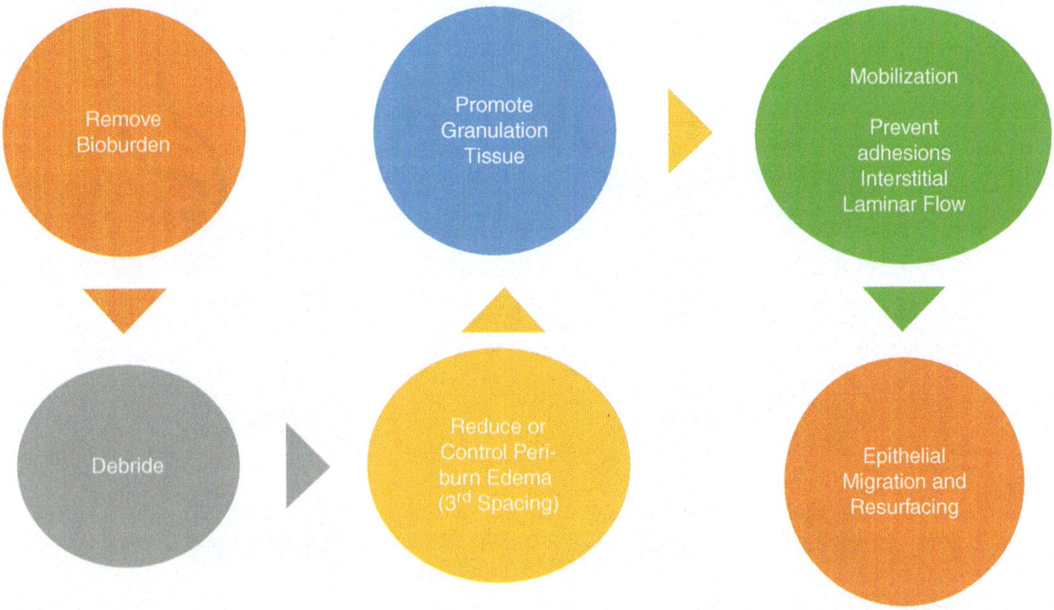

Fig. 3 Steps involved in burn or wound bed granulation

orchestration of EMC replacement bias the wounded area to resolve and continue the healing process moving toward resurfacing.

2 HA Background

As a nonsulfated GAG, HA is composed of repeating polymeric disaccharides of D-glucuronic acid and *N*-acetyl-D-glucosamine linked by a glucuroradic $\beta 1 \rightarrow 3$ bond [2–4]. Despite the molecular simplicity of the composition of HA, HA has a variety of physicochemical properties. Polymers of HA occur in a multitude of configurations and shapes depending on their size, salt concentration, pH, and associated cations. In addition, HA is not covalently bonded to a protein core, but aggregates with proteoglycans [5, 6]. Functions of HA include hydration, lubrication of joints, and delineation and support of the foundational framework through which cells aggregate and migrate in the ECM. HA synthesis increases during wound healing and is imperative in directing many aspects of tissue repair [7, 8]. The size of HA appears to be critical for the delineation of its function, either as a pro-inflammatory mediator (LMWHA) or a proliferative (HMWHA) influence. HMWHA (usually in excess of 1000 KDa) is present in intact tissues and exerts anti-angiogenic and immune suppressive bias. Smaller polymers of HA are potent distress signals and induce both inflammation and angiogenesis. Biosynthesis of HA occurs via specific enzymes, HA synthases (HAS) [8–10]. HAS are membrane-bound enzymes that synthesize HA on the inner surface of cell plasma membranes, and then the HA is extruded through pore-like structures into the extracellular space. There are three mammalian enzymes HAS-1, HAS-2, and HAS-3 which all synthesize HA polymeric chains of various lengths [11].

3 HA Receptors

A variety of proteins that bind to HA are termed hyaladherins, which are widely distributed in the ECM and in and on the surfaces, cytoplasm, and nucleus of cells (Figs. 4 and 5) [1, 12]. The most prominent among these receptors is the transmembrane glycoprotein "cluster of differentiation 44" (CD44) (Fig. 5). CD44 occurs in many isoforms, products of a single gene with variable exon expression [13]. CD44 is found on virtually all mammalian cells with the primary exception being red blood cells. Cell adhesion, migration,

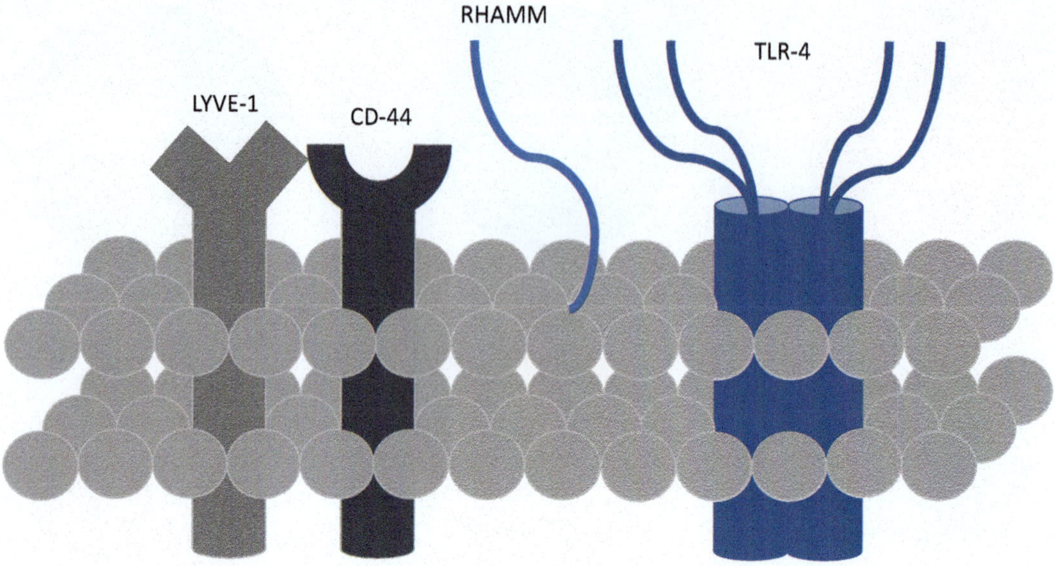

Fig. 4 Receptor cell signaling for HMWHA and LMWHA. These are the major receptors for HA signaling as localized in cell membranes. Lymphatic vessel endothelial receptor 1; cluster of differentiation 44 (CD44) antigen, a type of transmembrane glycoprotein. RHAMM is the receptor for hyaluronan-mediated motility and Toll-like receptor (TLR) 4

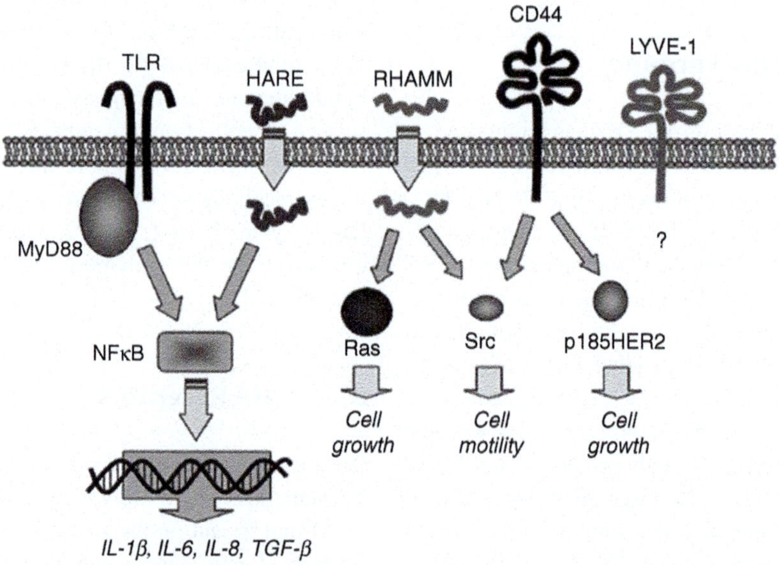

Fig. 5 Receptor signaling pathways. Symbolic representations of the major signaling pathways, including downstream effects, that are activated by hyaluronic acid. TLR; hyaluronan receptor for endocytosis (HARE); receptor for hyaluronan-mediated motility (RHAMM); cluster of differentiation 44 (CD44) antigen, a type 1 transmembrane receptor; lymphatic vessel endothelial receptor 1 (LYVE-1); myeloid differentiation primary response gene 88 (MyD88); nuclear factor kappa-light-chain-enhancer of activated B cells (NF-kβ); Src kinase p185HER@ tyrosine kinase p185 human epidermal growth factor receptor 2; interleukin 2 (IL-2); transforming growth factor beta (TGF-β)

lymphocyte activation, homing, and cancer metastasis are all regulated to varying degrees through CD44 [8, 14–16] receptors. The receptor for HA-mediated motility (RHAMM) is another primary receptor for HA and also occurs in several isoforms [17, 18]. RHAMM is a functional receptor for endothelial cells and smooth muscle cells in pulmonary arteries and airways. The interaction of HA with RHAMM influences and controls cell growth and migration through a complex network of signal transduction events and interactions with the cytoskeleton [19]. Through these interactions, HA is a potent stimulator of cell motility and transforming growth factor β-1 (TGF-β1) [20–27]. TGF-β1 elicits the synthesis and expression of RHAMM and HA. HA in conjunction with TGF-β1 initiates cell locomotion [19, 28, 29]. These interactions are depicted in Fig. 5.

Hyalomatrix is now commercially available as a benzyl-esterified hyaluronic acid three-dimensional fiber known as HYAFF. The benzyl ester stabilizes the HA so that degradation is slowed. HYAFF is appropriate as a choice in wounds or burns where there is a significant soft tissue or integumentary defect. The soft tissue defect may be a result of debridement, the removal of necrotic/nonviable tissue. In addition, often the mechanism of injury will predispose the individual to a large integumentary defect. Necrotizing fasciitis (NF) and degloving injuries are known for large defects. The soft tissue defect in the case of NF frequently is a result of the surgical debridements to remove the infected tissues. In the instance of degloving injuries, the delamination that occurs destroys the anchors and connections between the integumentary layers.

4 Wound Healing Background

The complex interactions that occur between the components of the extracellular matrix (ECM) at a fiber level (Fig. 6) and at a cellular level (Fig. 7)

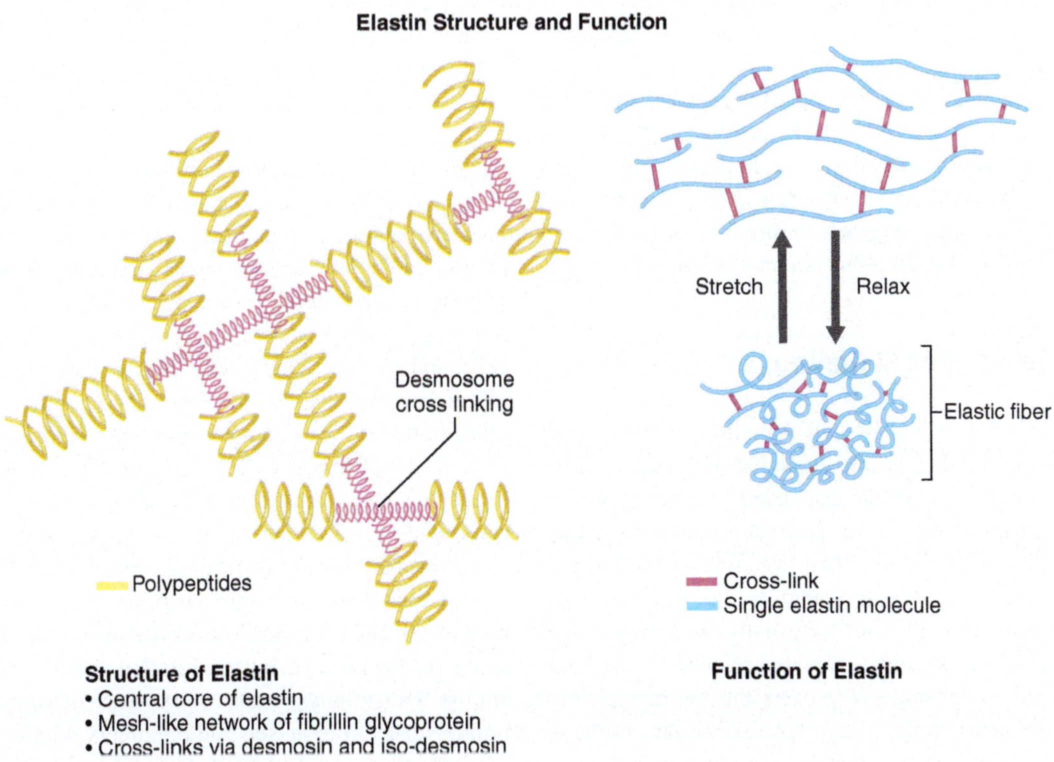

Fig. 6 Elastin structure. Reproduced with permission [31]

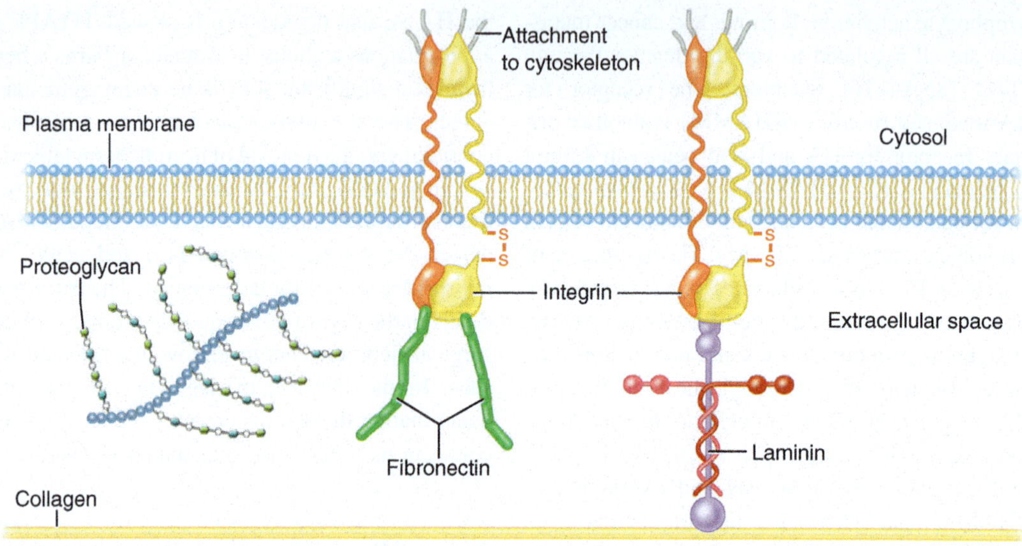

Fig. 7 Components of the extracellular matrix. Reproduced with permission [31]

are shown. The ECM is a very complex environment that is constantly remodeling. In the ECM cell signaling occurs constantly supporting the changing ECM functions and in response to wounding. HA as a molecule is intimately involved and responsible for altering cell phenotype and the resulting environmental changes that occur by virtue of the chemokines and cytokines that are produced in the important cells. The ECM is a dynamic structure consuming 4% of an individual's oxygen as a direct result of the constant remodeling that occurs [9, 30].

5 Cell Signaling

A brief review of cell signaling in the healing response is presented to assist in the understanding of the clinical response observed in wound healing when using HA scaffolding fiber, here HYAFF. Concert of cell signaling and cell migration as it occurs in wound healing is presented in brief (Figs. 8 and 9). Perhaps the hamartia, the flaw, in the study of wound resolution and healing is the tendency to oversimplify the truly elegant system that aims to ensure healing, complete healing, both anatomically and functionally. However, what causes marvel is the multitude of redundant though not repetitive processes which ensure success, wound closure [31].

The following serves to introduce the clinician, novice and experienced alike, to the interplay of cellular signaling, molecular signaling, and vascular events that occur in concert during the healing process. First the figures demonstrate how cells central to the repair process are directed based on global and local stimuli, which may be cytokine, chemokine, pH, or galvanically driven [32–34]. If invaders/pathogens (e.g., bacteria, fungi, virus, or debris) are present, key innate immune cells migrate and proliferate to the site of injury [33, 34]. These include macrophage, neutrophils, NK cells, and gamma delta T cells. If the invader is a repeat offender, one that the host has successfully fended off previously, adaptive immune responses (B cell clonal expansion) are triggered [33–35]. Simultaneously, debris (necrotic and/or injured cells) is removed and a "new" wound bed excavated via proteases and extracellular matrix (ECM) degradation. This serves two purposes: the clearance of cell and invader refuse and the provision of pathways for (new) cellular migration and proliferation constituting repair [36]. The delivery timing, concentration, scaffold binding (via heparin activation or other mechanisms), target cell receptor availability, active form after cleavage,

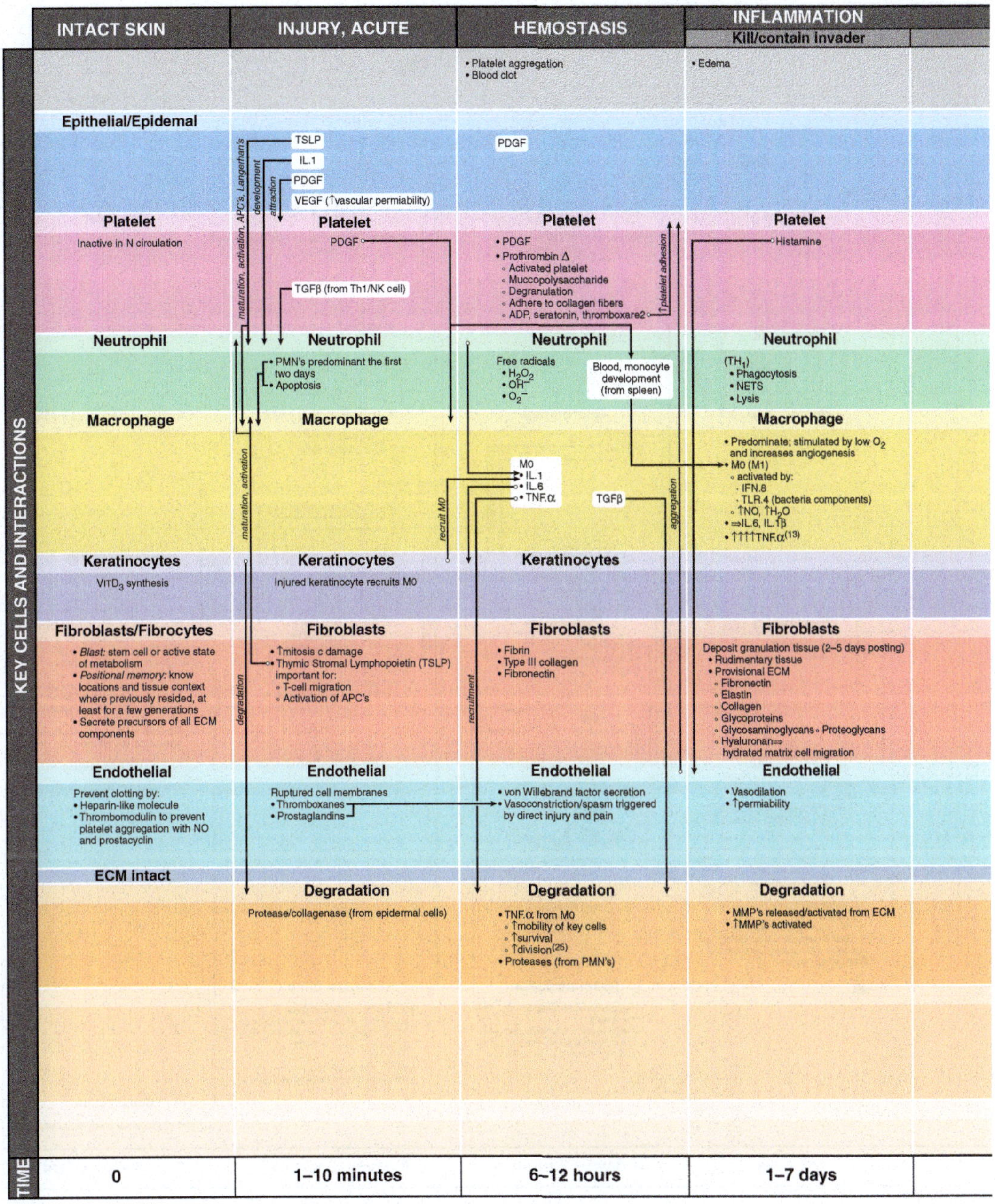

Fig. 8 The Healing Map 1 of 2 depicts the phases of wound healing and the cells responsible for many of the signaling events to move the healing process forward in detail. The inflammatory phase is subdivided into three "mini-phases" to permit clarity in discussion of the overlapping activities occurring simultaneously. Reproduced with permission [31]

degradation rate, half-life, pH and presence of enzymes (proteases, etc.) in the wound milieu, hydrophobicity, hydrophilicity, scaffold (whether fibrin, collagen, or ECM) shape, and adhesion via integrins all conspire to drive growth factor, cytokine, and chemokine bioavailability. Second, vascular changes via endothelial cell migration and capillary expansion occur in response to tissue

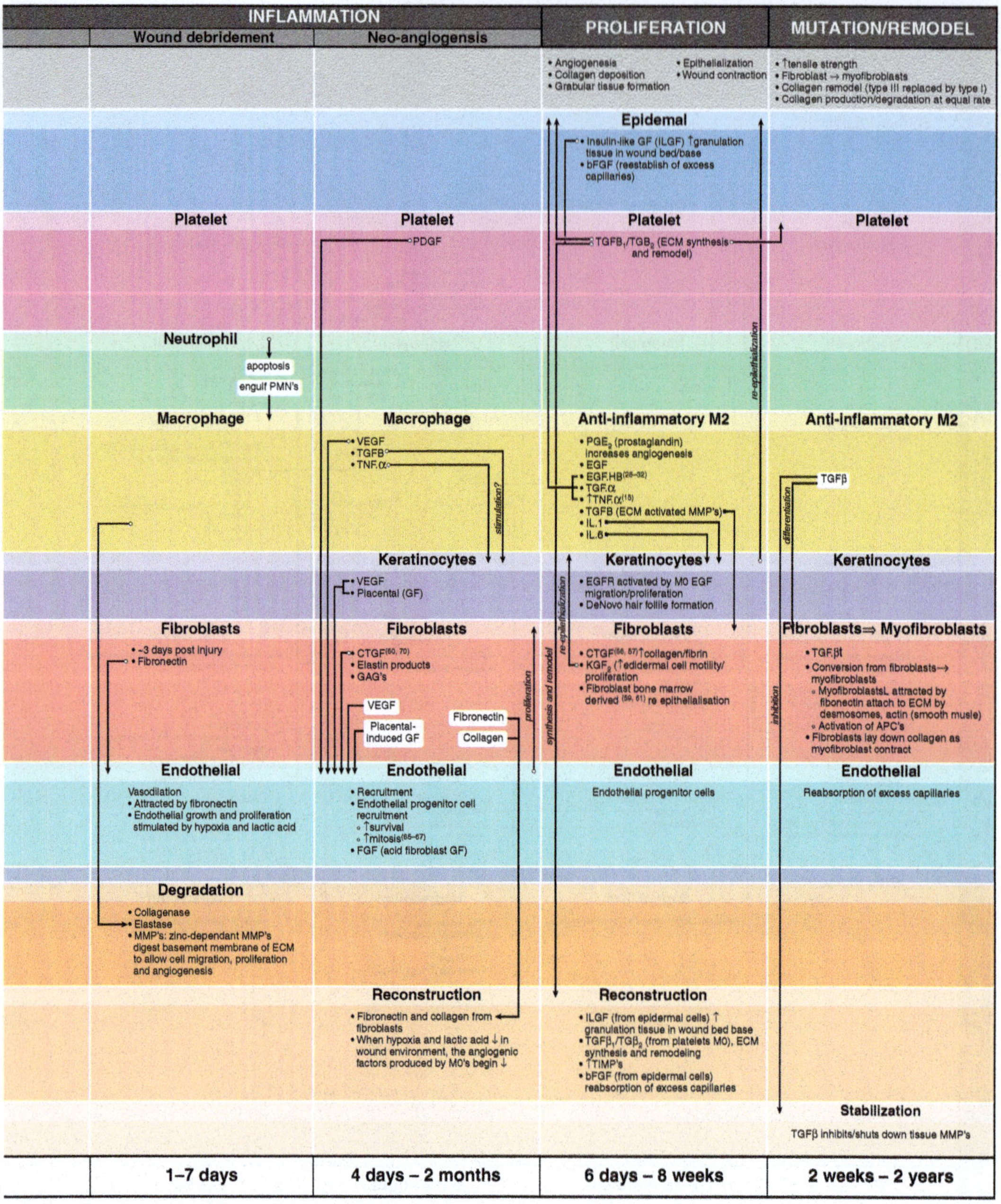

Fig. 9 The Healing Map 2 of 2 depicts the phases of wound healing and the cells responsible for many of the signaling events to move the healing process forward. The inflammatory phase is subdivided into three "mini-phases" to permit clarity in discussion of the overlapping activities occurring simultaneously. Reproduced with permission [31]

hypoxia and increased lactic acid concentration. These responses are depicted along with the appropriate cells and signaling mechanisms. Finally, prominent cells which direct and produce many of the chemical messengers have the ability to change phenotypes during the course of the healing process. The macrophages offer a pronounced display of this cellular functional metamorphosis. Macrophage have pervasive flexible and ever-changing role along with a multitude of other cells with which they communicate and effect change during the healing process.

The key cells and phases of healing are depicted in Figs. 8 and 9. These figures provide a cross-reference by "stage" of healing, key cells and signals, as well as a chronological time line, thus providing the reader an appreciation of the overlapping and essential functions directed in concert as opposed to an isolated or over-simplified view of cell function. Although exceeding complex, the elegance lies in both the redundancy and the use of paracrine, autocrine, and juxtacrine mediators to effect expedient resolution using the resources immediately available. Figures 8 and 9 also illuminate the intricate and exquisite concert of cell migration, proliferation, and signaling in the context of vascular events, joining to culminate in healing.

5.1 Cell to Matrix

Cell to wound matrix communication occurs during debridement and angiogenesis. Matricellular proteins destabilize the cell-matrix interactions, in essence creating a more fluid environment for cell migration. Proteinases, both plasminogen activators and matrix metalloproteinases (MMPs), act to dissolve the wound matrix both immediately after injury and during the proliferative and remodeling phase. In angiogenesis this is necessary for the directed migration of endothelial cells [36–38].

6 Cell Metamorphosis

Typically, a cell is thought of as having a unique phenotype and set of correlating functions. For example, a red blood cell is a myeloid cell that has differentiated and now has the phenotype of a red blood cell (RBC) whose function primarily is to transport and facilitate the exchange of dissolved gases, typically CO_2 and O_2. However, in the science of wound healing, several key cells demonstrate the ability to significantly morph in function. Three prevalent cell chameleons are reviewed here, platelets, macrophages, and fibroblasts.

Platelets, although anucleate, provide chemical messengers at the point of initial injury to achieve hemostasis. Alpha granules, contained within the platelets, release PDGF, platelet factor IV, and TGF-β1 which function during the proliferative phase of healing to accelerate granulation and connective tissue proliferation [5]. Macrophages, usually thought of as a phagocyte, transition from antigen-presenting cell (APC) to phagocyte, to chief air traffic controller, adapting their cytokine phenotype expression profile to progress the healing cascade and accelerate closure. Fibroblasts are vital early during clot construction, granulation tissue formation, and neoangiogenesis. Uniquely, during the later stages of proliferation and early remodeling, under the influence of TGF-β, fibroblasts truly change phenotype, becoming myofibroblast. The myofibroblast facilitates wound edge approximation, decreasing the size of the wound.

7 Recognized Stages of Wound Healing

The cells most affected by either LMWHA or HMWHA are the resident macrophage which undergoes distinct phenotypical changes in response to the size of the HA present. LMWHA is associated with pro-inflammatory macrophage bias and HMWHA with inflammatory resolution and proliferative cellular responses [1, 3–48].

A representation of the overall activities initiated by wounding and required for preparation of the wound bed and terminal closure is depicted in Fig. 10. Importantly, LMWHA enhances cell infiltration and increases pro-inflammatory cytokines TNF-alpha, IL1-beta, and IL-8 via a CD44-mediated mechanism (Figs. 4 and 5). The presence of LMWHA also facilitates primary adhesion of cytokine-activated lymphocytes to endothelium. The presence of LMWHA moderates the inflammatory response, free radical scavenging, and antioxidant properties as well as contributing to the destabilization of granulation tissue matrix. The inflammatory response is localized.

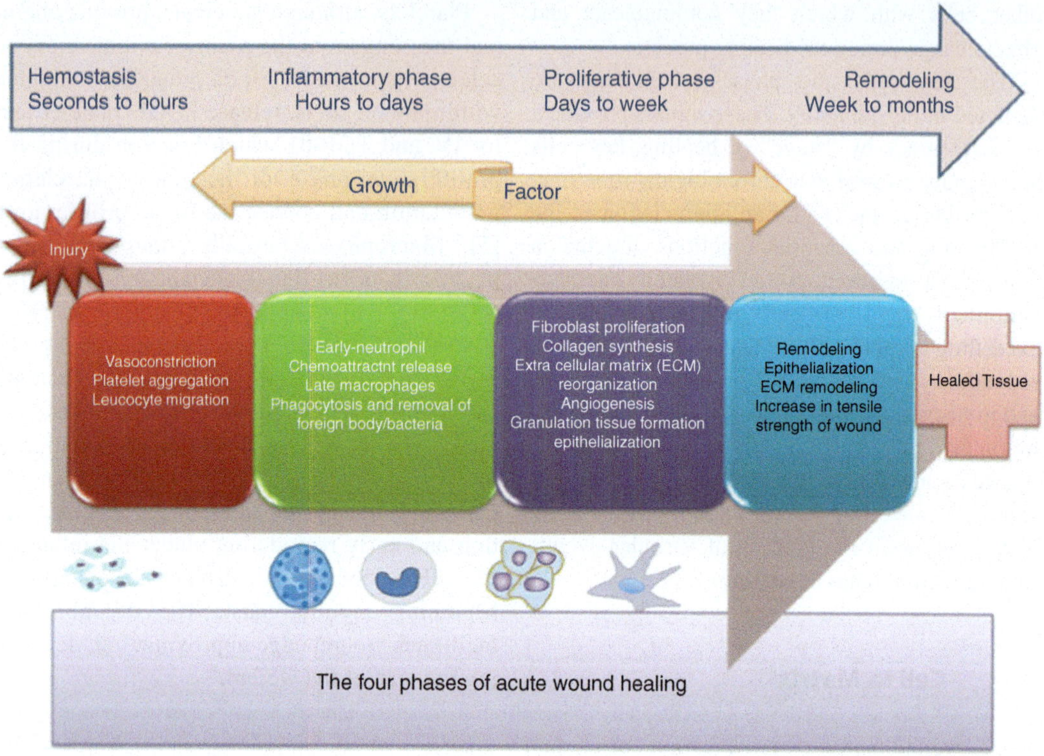

Fig. 10 Phases of wound healing. This is a 30,000 ft view of the activities involved in wound healing. They are represented as separate phases, but in fact, they all overlap and occur in concert and simultaneously

7.1 Macrophage

Macrophage is known to be one of the cells central to the directional biasing of wound healing. Macrophages demonstrate a myriad of phenotypes, level of activation, and differentiation based on the phase of wound healing (Fig. 11). Their ability to differentiate into either M1 wound-activated macrophage (WAM) or M2 repair macrophage highlights their complex plasticity and responsiveness to the wound. The phenotypic changes are not merely a result of the wound milieu or environment but are also directed and specific to advancing the healing processes. Macrophage transitions from an innate immune cell (phagocyte and APC) to a pro-inflammatory cell to an immunoregulatory (proliferation and reepithelization) and finally to a phagocytic cell aiding in the tissue remodeling state [38, 49–69].

Only a few macrophages are typically located in the dermis as surveillance macrophage. However, neutrophil apoptosis during the first 24 h after injury signals macrophage to massively infiltrate the wound. The numbers of macrophage are the greatest/most elevated beginning approximately 2 days after injury. During this phase macrophage demonstrates increased antigen presentation and phagocytic activity [43].

Macrophage is activated by microbial agents or cytokines like IFN-γ and is classified as M1 or wound-activated macrophages (WAM). The M1 macrophage produces nitric oxide (NO) and pro-inflammatory cytokines including TNF-α, IL1β, IL-6, or IL-12 (Fig. 11). These M1 macrophages also overexpress MHC class II molecules. MHC class II molecules present antigens to T cells and B cells to activate both innate and adaptive immune system responses [70]. The antigen presentation is largely via major histocompatibility complex class II (MHC class II) complex. Antigens presented by MHC class II molecules are derived from extracellular proteins of the

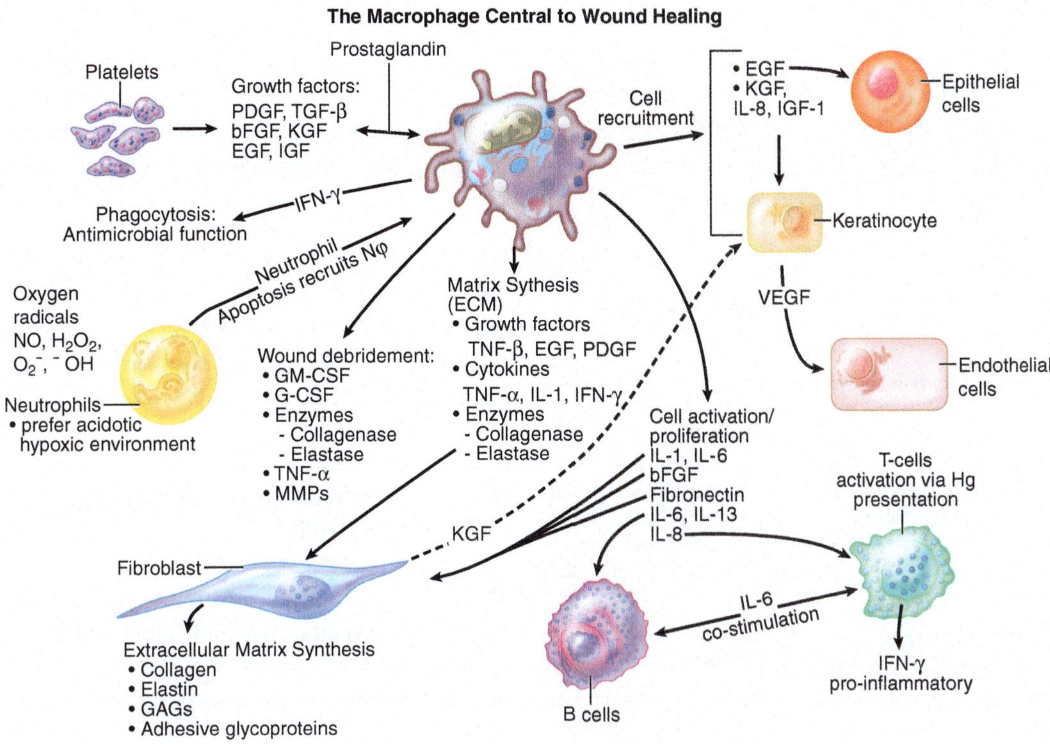

Fig. 11 Role of macrophage. Reproduced with permission [31]

pathogen, for example, a bacterium that may be infecting the wound. The loading of the MHC class II occurs after phagocytosis by the macrophage. The extracellular proteins are endocytosed and ingested by lysosomes, and signature peptides unique to the specific invader are loaded onto the MHC class II complex and then presented on the macrophage cell surface. Thus, in the early phase of healing, the macrophage is both phagocytic and important in stimulating the immune system.

During the inflammatory and proliferative phase where new tissue formation and angiogenesis are paramount, macrophage produces vaso-endothelial growth factor VEGF, stimulating the recruitment of endothelial progenitor cells and the proliferation of existing endothelium [71]. In addition, macrophages are also vital to lymphangiogenesis, as $VEGF_c$ and $VEGF_D$ modulate this process. It has been demonstrated that decreased macrophage numbers are associated with decreased lymphangiogenesis [72–74].

Remodeling begins with the gradual involution of granulation tissue and simultaneous dermal renewal. During this phase, apoptosis of a significant percentage of macrophage occurs. The remaining macrophage will facilitate the remodeling process cleaning up the cellular and matrix debris. This ECM debris is largely a result of the degradation of collagen type III by metalloproteinases produced by epidermal and endothelial cells [62].

Although the phenotype of macrophage (M0) infiltrating dermal wounds is not fully characterized, the evidence supports the changing role of the macrophage during the phases of healing. This suggests that the “same cell,” the macrophage, has different and diverse roles during the phases of skin or wound regeneration [24, 71]. Macrophages exhibit phenotypic diversity permitting wide-ranging roles in maintaining physiologic homeostasis. HA, a major glycosaminoglycan of the extracellular matrix,

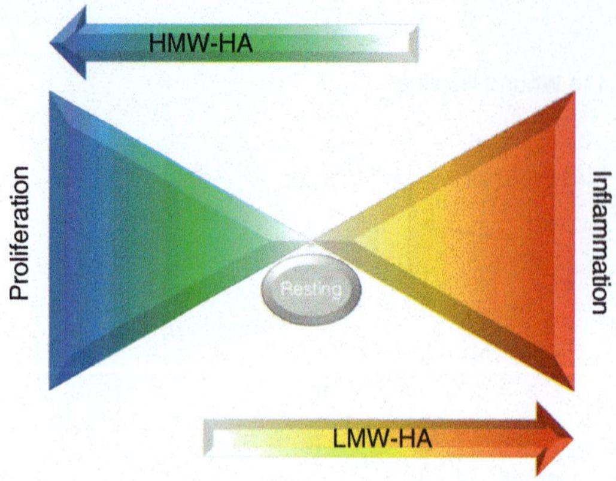

Fig. 12 Continuum relative to the size of hyaluronic acid. Pictorial representation of the continuum of activity and influence of high versus low molecular weight hyaluronic acid (HA). HA's effects occur at the cellular and molecular level with changes in local cytokine and chemokine levels that bias the wound milieu toward inflammation in the case of LMWHA or proliferation in the instance of HMWHA. The effects exist in gradation; they are not all or none

has been shown to have differential signaling based on its molecular weight (Fig. 12). This interaction with and response to HA polymeric size results in a phenotypic shift from M0 to M1 when the macrophage is exposed to LMWHA or in the case of HMWHA the phenotypic expression of an M1 or M0 will shift to a M2, the proliferative macrophage. Thus, the expressed phenotype of the macrophage drives the local production of cytokines and chemokines associated with either inflammation or proliferation. In the case of LMWHA, the pro-inflammatory M1 or wound-activated macrophage (WAM), there is an increased concentration of interferon gamma (IFN-γ) and a decrease in interleukin 4 (IL-4). In the presence of HMWHA, the macrophage phenotype is consistent with M2 and the associated cytokines including IL-4.

Figure 12 illustrates the continuum from a perspective of LMWHA biasing the wound environment toward inflammation. The role of OH and lactate in the activation of hyaf-1 hyaluronidase and the resulting enzymatic degradation of HMWHA. In the inflammatory phase -LMWHA-is associated with lactate and wound hypoxia, triggering NFK-β and the differentiation of the macrophage M0 to M1 phenotype. The result is the liquefaction and degradation of damaged ECM or portions of the ECM that are just ahead of angiogenesis (liquification). Understanding of the intricate cell signaling that occurs as a result of HMWHA or LMWHA is imperative in order to interpret the different responses in a wound after the application of polymeric HA. Frequently the peripheral aspects of the wound tend toward proliferation, while the more central areas, areas of high bioburden or necrotic tissue, will tend toward inflammation. The areas of high bioburden versus low bioburden stimulate differentiated response as the breakdown of polymeric HA occurs, here Hyalomatrix® [3].

8 Considerations for the Use of HYAFF

The synthesis and the deposition of the ECM is a critical component of wound healing when there has been a substantial loss of the dermal and epidermal matrix. Acute wounds progress through a series of events that are relatively orderly (Fig. 10). Chronic wounds on the other hand exhibit delayed and failed closure. The failed closure is often characterized by a prolonged and excessive inflammatory response.

There are vast interactions among growth factors, the ECM and glycoproteins, including GAGS, one of which is HA. HA is predominantly located in the ECM with at least 50% of the HA found in the body located in the ECM. All of these elements interact in an ongoing reciprocally and mutually influential series of events referred to as dynamic reciprocity illustrated in Fig. 12.

HA is present and has varied functions which are dependent on molecular weight. HA has recognized cellular receptors on mammalian cells; therefore, it does not set off an immune response as can be the case with other tissue substitutions or bioengineered tissue substitutions. This is one benefit of HA, the fact that there are no adverse immune responses. There are, however, differentiated responses depending on the size of the polymeric HA. Receptor cell signaling occurs via alternate cell receptors that trigger either a pro-inflammatory or proliferative response depending on whether the dominant molecule is

LMWHA or HMWHA. The receptors are elucidated in Figs. 4 and 5 and the varied reciprocal wound environment bias in Fig. 12. In Fig. 13 the seesaw representation is that of LMWHA predominating the wounded tissue along with the associated increase in versican, depletion of elastin, and increased monocyte adhesion. Many of the cellular responses generated by LMWHA or HMWHA are due in large part to the phenotypical changes of resident macrophages to either LMWHA (pro-inflammatory) or HMWHA (proliferative).

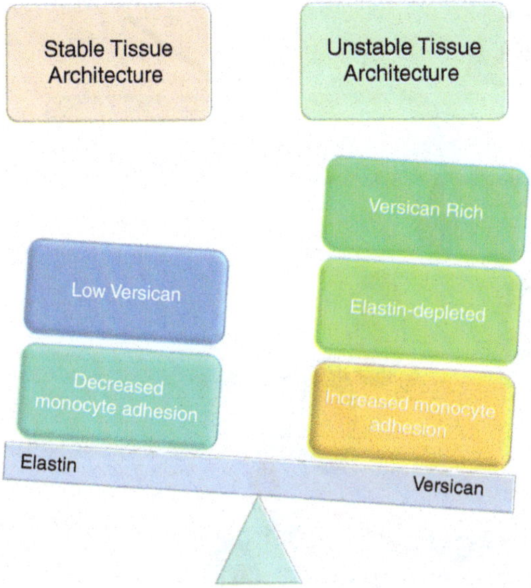

Fig. 13 Versican seesaw for inflammation and proliferation. With higher gradients of versican, the wound environment is biased toward inflammation with associated depletion in elastin and increased adhesion of monocytes

Versican belongs to the lectican protein family, with aggrecan (abundant in cartilage), brevacan, and neurocan (nervous system proteoglycans) as other members. Versican is also known as chondroitin sulfate proteoglycan core protein 2 or chondroitin sulfate proteoglycan 2 (CSPG2) and PG-M. Because of their negatively charged sulfates or carboxyl groups, chondroitin sulfate chains are attracted to various positively charged molecules such as certain growth factors, cytokines, and chemokines. This interaction in the extracellular matrix or on the cell surface is important in the formation of gradients of these factors (inflammation versus proliferation), their protection from proteolytic cleavage, and their presentation to specific cell-surface receptors. The binding of versican with leukocyte adhesion molecules L-selectin, P-selectin, and CD44 is

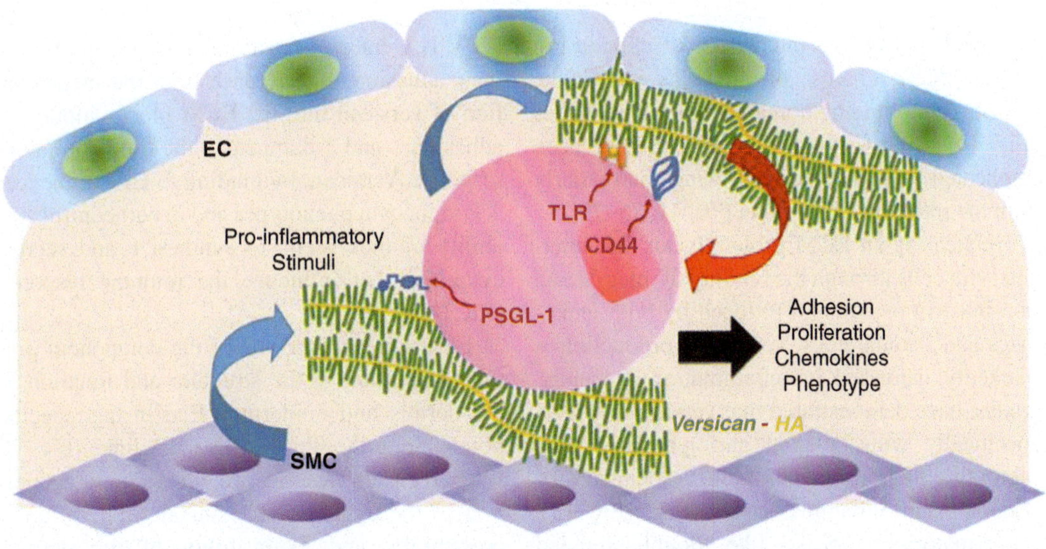

Fig. 14 Versican and hyaluronic acid bias toward or away from inflammation. The endothelium cells (EC) become more permeable in response to inflammation bias. Extracellular matrix (ECM) areas that are high in versican interact with LMWHA/hyaluronan and further stimulate pro-inflammatory responses. Stromal cells, myeloid cells, and lymphocytes all can contribute to the production of versican. The versican-enriched ECM is associated with an unstable ECM architecture

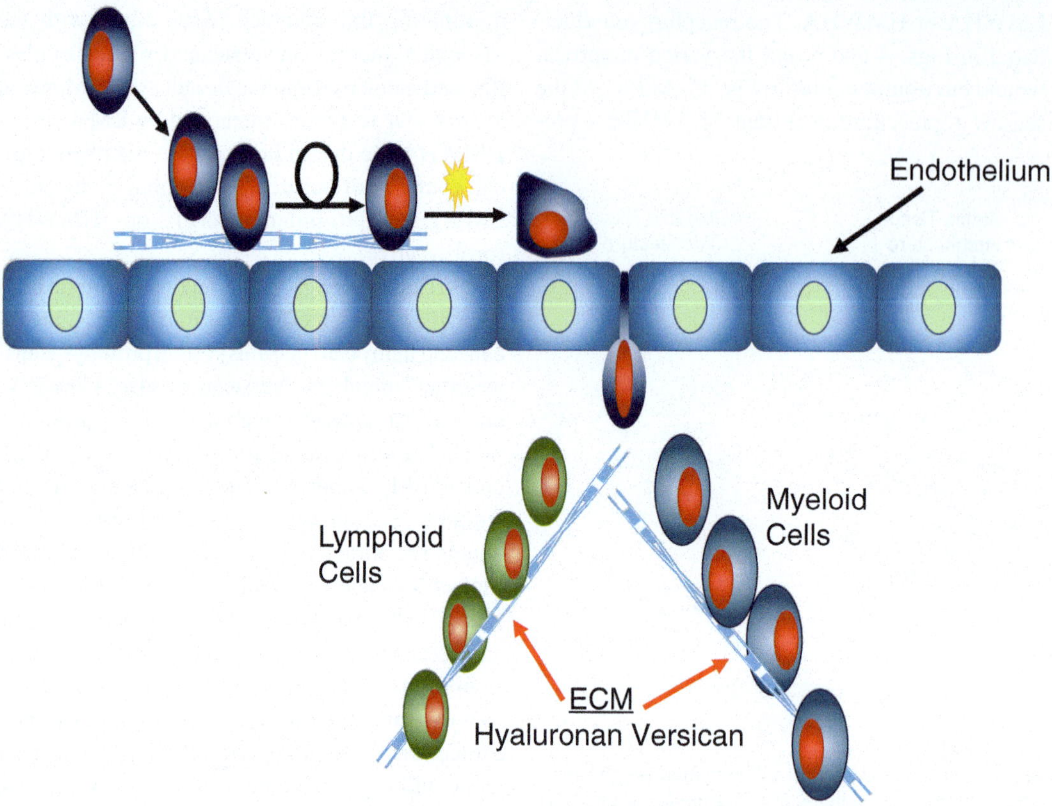

Fig. 15 Myeloid and lymphoid cells extravasate into the ECM and interact with HA and versican

also mediated by the interaction of chondroitin sulfate (CS) chains of versican with the carbohydrate-binding domain of these molecules (Fig. 14). Both CD44 and L-selectin have been implicated in leukocyte trafficking, particularly with the interplay of versican [70, 71, 75–79].

Versican is an ECM proteoglycan that interacts with cells through the binding of integrin and non-integrin receptors. Produced by both leukocytes and stromal cells, versican's production is markedly increased in inflammation. Recently, studies have demonstrated that versican interacts specifically with myeloid and lymphoid cells promoting their adhesion and an associated production of pro-inflammatory cytokines (Fig. 15). Inflammatory agonists, like double-stranded RNA, stimulate stromal cells (smooth muscle cells and fibroblasts) to produce fibrillar ECM that is enriched in versican and hyaluronan (HA). This type of ECM with elevated versican and LMWHA interacts with leukocytes promoting their adhesion. Interference with the incorporation of versican into the ECM blocks monocyte adhesion and dampens the inflammatory response. Versican, by binding to HA, influences T-lymphocyte phenotypes and in part controls the ability of these cells to synthesize and secrete cytokines that influence the immune response [71, 75–81].

Elastin is another one of the component proteins important in the structure and function of the dermis and epidermis. Elastin has specific points along the fibrils where HA links (Fig. 7). HA and elastin together provide a significant portion of the dynamic mechanical strength, compressibility, and extensibility of the dermis. Together these molecules allow the dermis to dynamically respond to mechanical loading and shear without incurring dermal or ECM damage [82–86].

As a molecule HA directs and interacts with cells and molecules throughout the phases of wound healing. Wound healing has been separated into overlapping phases of inflammation, proliferation, and remodeling; each phase is characterized by dynamic, reciprocal interactions between growth factors, cells, and the ECM, including HA one of the major GAG proteins (Fig. 14). This binding stimulates phagocytosis [87] and the liquification of the ECM fragments and local debris [87–89].

During the inflammatory phase/bias, the following occurs:

1. Increased cell infiltration (Fig. 14).
2. An increase of pro-inflammatory cytokines TNF-alpha, IL1-beta, and IL-8 all mediated via the CD44 cell receptor.
3. Adhesion to the endothelium (Fig. 14) of cytokine-activated lymphocytes occurs.
4. Moderation of the inflammatory response:
   (a) Free radical scavenging and antioxidant properties
   (b) TSG-mediated inhibition of inflammatory proteinases
   (c) stabilization of the granulation tissue matrix

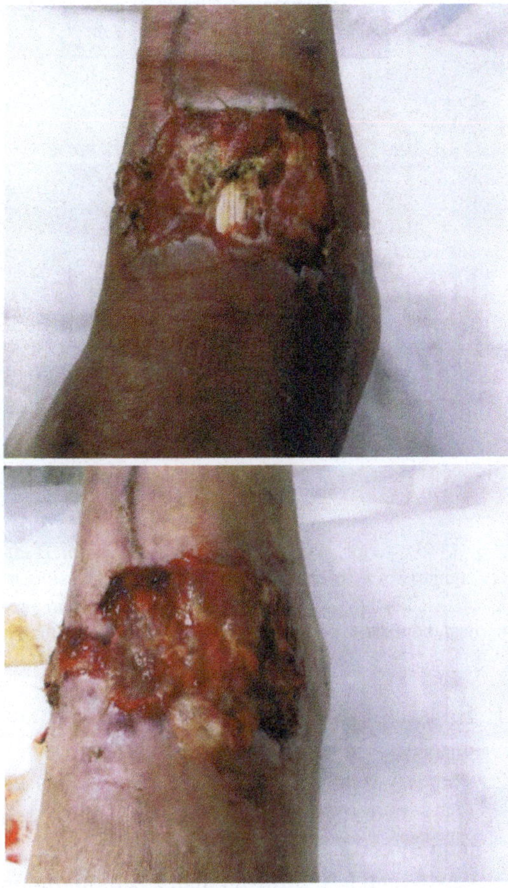

Fig. 16 Pediatric dog bite over the anterior aspect of the ankle. (Top) The patient at the wound center on January 20, 2015, with exposed anterior tibialis tendon, necrotic tissue, and decreased circulation to the distal foot. (Bottom) On February 6, 2015, after one application of HA under a pressure dressing. Note the change in the coloration of the extremity, granulation over the anterior tibialis tendon, and improved general granulation. The wound was closed the following day, on February 7, 2015, with a split-thickness skin graft (STSG) without complication

As an illustration of the inflammatory and debris removal stimulated by the application of polymeric HA, Fig. 16 has two photographs of a pediatric dog bite occurring over the anterior aspect of the ankle. The top photograph is the presentation of the patient to the wound center on January 20, 2015, with an exposed and desiccated anterior tibialis tendon, adjacent necrotic tissue, and decreased circulation to the distal foot. The bottom photograph is taken on February 6, 2015, taken after one application of HA under a pressure dressing. Note the change in the coloration of the extremity, granulation over the anterior tibialis tendon, and improved general granulation. The patient was closed the following day, on February 7, 2015, with a split-thickness skin graft (STSG) without complication and with complete function of the extremity.

In the continuum of wound healing, from inflammation to resolution and proliferation, HMWHA, the preferred and stable polymeric HA structure, accumulates. The continuum of activity and influence of high versus low molecular weight (HA) is in Fig. 12. HA's effects occur at the cellular and molecular level with changes in local cytokine and chemokine levels that bias the wound milieu toward inflammation in the case of LMWHA or proliferation in the instance of HMWHA. The effects exist in gradation; they are not all or none.

The granulation phase is intertwined with HMWHA in the following [87]:

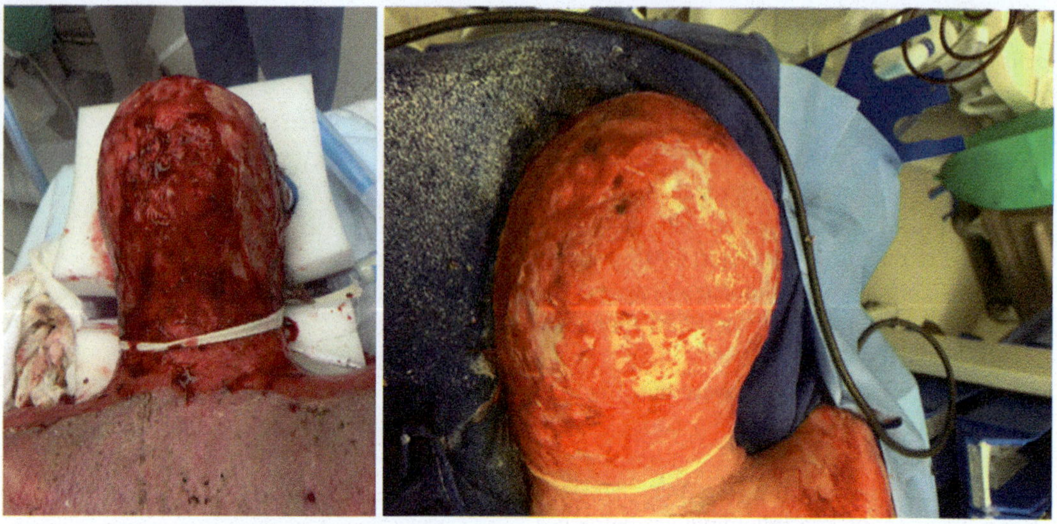

Fig. 17 Posterior skull deep third-degree burn. (Left) Hyalomatrix was placed in the OR without the silicone laver such that the 3D fibers directly contacted the damaged cortical bone and periosteum. (Right) The Hyalomatrix stimulated a proliferative response (over damaged periosteum and cortical bone), on the right-hand side, in preparation for final closure

1. HA synthesis facilitates cell detachment and mitosis.
2. The HA-rich granulation tissue provides an open hydrated matrix that facilitates cell migration.
3. CD44- and RHAMM-mediated cell migration (Fig. 5) links with protein kinases associated with cell locomotion.
4. Promotes angiogenesis.

Figure 17 demonstrates the ability of HYAFF through HMWHA to promote granulation and the proliferative phase of healing, even over exposed posterior skull void of periosteum as a result of a deep third-degree burn. Hyalomatrix was placed in the OR without the silicone laver such that the 3D fibers directly contacted the damaged cortical bone and periosteum. The Hyalomatrix stimulated a proliferative response (over damaged periosteum and cortical bone), as seen in the second photograph on the right-hand side, in preparation for final closure.

It is imperative for the clinician to understand the varied function and result of HA that are dependent on the molecular weight of HA. The general influences of low versus high molecular weight HA are:

LMWHA is associated with:

1. Pro-inflammatory response IL-1B and IL-8
2. Activates innate immune system
3. Activates B lymphocytes

HMWHA is associated with:

1. Proliferation
2. Anti-inflammatory bias
3. Cellular migration
4. Cell motility

The selective local wound response to HYAFF is in Fig. 18. In areas where the granulation tissue is more stable, HMWHA pervades, and granulation tissue and proliferation bias predominate. In areas where the wound milieu is biased toward inflammation, HYAFF responds by degrading into primarily LMWHA, evidenced by the increased cellular exudate, the accumulation of white blood cells and fluid. This is labeled in the photo as LMWHA. This liquefaction trapped under the silicone membrane is not necessarily infection but more accurately an area where the inflammatory process predominates. The leg which has had HYAFF applied as Hyalomatrix® is shown, and the areas of the wound are labeled with HMWHA and LMWHA to help the reader visualize both the proliferative and the inflammatory response occurring. In this instance the Hyalomatrix® bioactive dressing is indicating the state of the wound according to the response that HA has to the local wound milieu. Figure 18 demonstrates both ends of the spectrum, inflammation versus proliferation and continuum in between. The clinician should examine and evaluate the response of and the varied interactions of polymeric HA with a wound after each application of Hyalomatrix®. It is common for certain portions of the wound to be in a proliferative stage (HMWHA) and other areas of the wound are involved in an inflammatory response (LMWHA) as labeled in Fig. 18.

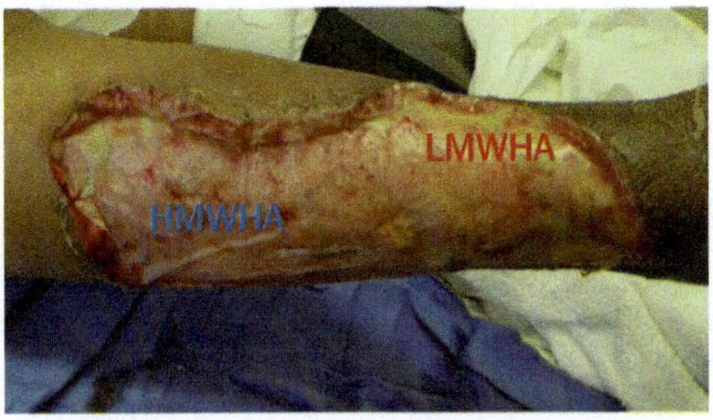

Fig. 18 Leg after one application of Hyalomatrix—HMWHA and LMWHA areas of bias are labeled

8.1 How Is HYAFF® Produced

HYAFF is a hyaluronic acid that has been stabilized through the use of a benzyl alcohol esterification (Fig. 19). This esterification of hyaluronic acid results in a biocompatible polymer that is responsive to the local wound milieu. As a result the HYAFF (Fig. 20) undergoes biodegradation to either LMWHA or HMWHA, again depending on local environment. HYAFF is a 3D scaffold that has receptor sites allowing the infiltration and migration of cell as appropriate. Cells like fibroblasts can colonize wound bed and thrive in the presence of HMWHA and the resulting proliferative bias. Cells are anchored to the 3D scaffolding by CD44 cell receptors. The result is the facilitation of an ordered reconstruction of dermal tissues. Capillary growth via the infiltration of endothelial

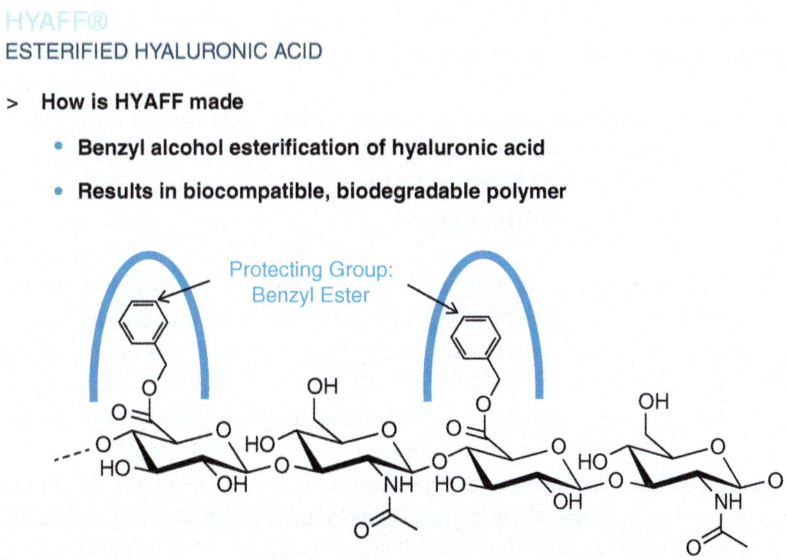

Fig. 19 HYAFF stabilization. Benzyl alcohol esterification of hyaluronic acid results in a biocompatible, biodegradable polymer that is more stable than hyaluronic acid when exposed to the wound milieu

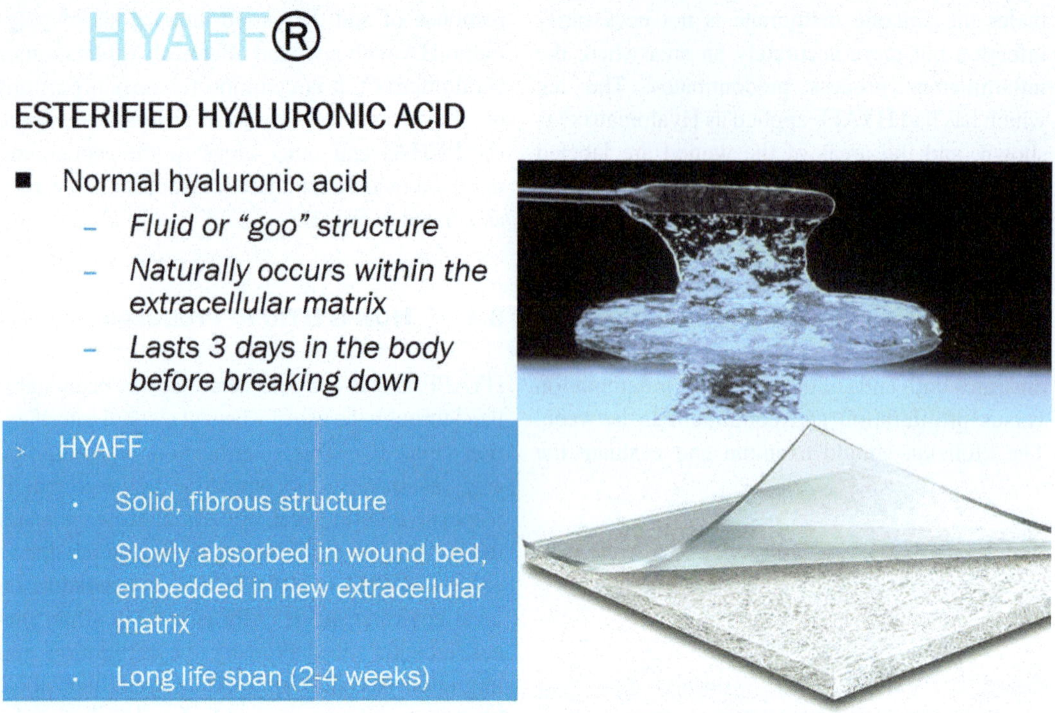

Fig. 20 HYAFF structure is that of a 3D fiber that is a fluffy-white-fibrous structure with a top layer of silicone. The silicone membrane assists with stabilization of temperature and hydration

cells occurs (RHAMM receptor), contributing to the reversal of the previously hypoxic environment and supporting cell mitosis. Pasquinelli et al. [90, 91] very clearly explain and illustrate the importance of a 3D scaffold structurally and more importantly the cell to matrix interaction.

9 Comparison Between HA and Current Biomaterials for Tissue Engineering

Skin substitutes have an important role in the treatment of deep dermal and full-thickness wounds of various etiologies. At present, there is no ideal skin substitute on the market. Skin substitutes can be divided into two main classes, namely, biological and synthetic substitutes. The biological skin substitutes are structured so that there is more of an intact extracellular matrix structure. Synthetic skin substitutes that can be synthesized on demand can be modulated for specific purposes. Placement of biological skin substitutes may allow for the construction of a more natural new dermis and allow for reepithelialization characteristics due to the presence of a basement membrane. The ultimate goal for bioengineered skin substitutes is the achievement of an ideal skin substitute that provides effective and scar-free wound healing. By placing skin substitutes early on, moisture loss is prevented and the hope is that healing can be expedited.

A well-designed skin substitute provides a barrier layer, attaches to the underlying dermis, becomes well vascularized, and provides an area for renewable keratinocytes to dwell and an elastic structure support for epidermis. Bioengineered materials and techniques are required in traumatic full-thickness wounds or deep burns (deep second or third degree). In the event that there is a full-thickness (epidermal and dermal) loss of skin greater than 4 cm in diameter, the wound will not heal well without surgical intervention.

One of the first bioengineered skin substitutes developed for the treatment of full-thickness burn injuries was Integra®. Integra is a very structurally ordered matrix, composed of bovine tendon collagen keratinically linked with glycosaminoglycan, derived from shark cartilage. A silicone membrane is sealed to the upper surface to act as a temporary epidermal substitute layer, persevering temperature and preventing water loss, as well as forming a barrier to assist with the prevention of bacterial entrance into the wound or burn. Integra® is intended for use as a foundation to promote a dermal substrate. One of the challenges with Integra® is the absence of living cells. Without living cells, it is very difficult to see how one could create a permanent artificial dermal barrier. In the best case, the Integra® serves as a template to generate a neodermis that will sustain a new epidermal layer, typically via a split-thickness skin graft (STSG) [92–98].

Dermagraft® is another type of dermal substrate. It is a bio-prepared-acellularized-cryopreserved human skin. It is a fibroblast dermal substitute for chronic, full-thickness diabetic wounds. Research has shown that Dermagraft® may increase the rates of healing but it often requires repeated application. Donor fibroblasts are then implanted in the mesh scaffold provided by the Dermagraft®. Dermagraft® has a silicon membrane that is attached to provide for an instant barrier to the wound [99–109]. All of the previously described tissue matrix, Integra® and Dermagraft® lend a scaffolding structure to the wound that is without a dermal base. These implantable scaffolds ideally resist fibrosis and promote epidermal resurfacing such that scarring and contractures are minimalized. Unless neutrophils and macrophages can successfully degrade implanted collagenous structures, they will activate lymphocyte TH2 cells, which provoke an extreme inflammatory reaction, as opposed to the induction of TH1 helper immune cells, which lead to constructive remodeling and integration of natural or bioengineered scaffolds.

HA polymers, on the other hand, do not require focused manufacture of organized 3D scaffolds which resist fibrosis, because HA polymers naturally occur in a random pattern that is a "pre-fabricated 3D scaffolding." HA occurs naturally in the body and is connected to the production and interconnection of elastin, collagen, and versican, which is the true dynamic scaffolding of skin (Figs. 6, 7, and 14). Polymeric HA then connects to versican and collagen through naturally occurring receptor site [70, 75, 76].

Challenges in tissue engineering skin include safety issues, including an inflammatory response or secondary infection, as well as a structure that permits function of the repaired area without scarring or contracture bands. An advantage of bioengineered HA polymers is that they are not derived from animals or donor human cells. As a result, there are no safety issues that often need to be addressed as with other bioengineered skin matrices. The other clinical observations with polymeric HA is an improvement in the rate of neovascularization of tissue-engineered skin and associated granulation. Polymeric HA can operate in either an oxygen-rich or oxygen-depleted environment. In either environment an appropriate liquification of the ECM occurs and allows for a more rapid development of neovascularization. This integration and continued ECM development facilitates healing and decreases the likelihood of contraction and fibrosis.

Figures 21 and 22 illustrate the steps required prior to clinical application of polymeric HA. Hyalomatrix® is illustrated in the following case studies. In the first stage of clinical preparation, a broad-spectrum, non-cytotoxic irrigation solution, like Vashe® or Prophase®. These solutions can be used in conjunction with either Misonix or Versajet. The Hyalomatrix is then applied and the silicone layer fenestrated. The HA is placed under NPWT, short stretch compression, or a total contact cast. At Days 3–4, the dressing is changed and the wound bed inspected. At the time of dressing change, the Hyalomatrix will have either broken down into LMWHA stimulating a pro-inflammatory response or HMWHA, and the HA will have integrated and stimulate an ongoing proliferative response (Fig. 18). The wound is recleansed and Hyalomatrix reapplied where necessary. The same steps are repeated until granulation is to surface and then the terminal closure method applied. Terminal closure may be a split-thickness skin graft (STSG), a full-thickness skin graft (FTSG), or an amnion/chorion.

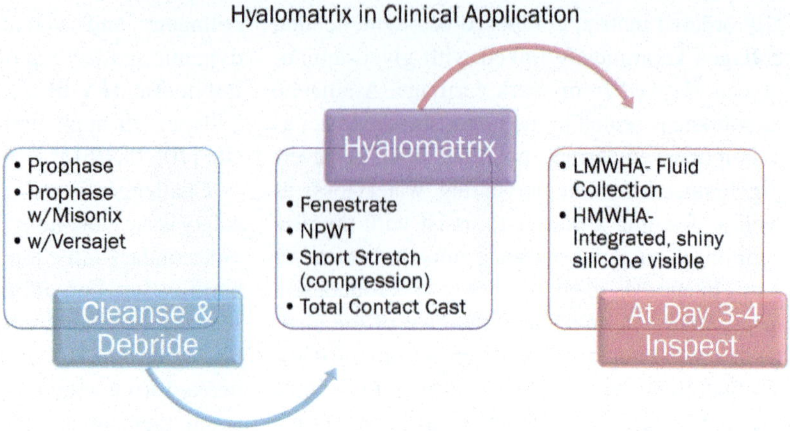

Fig. 21 Clinical Application 1 of 2

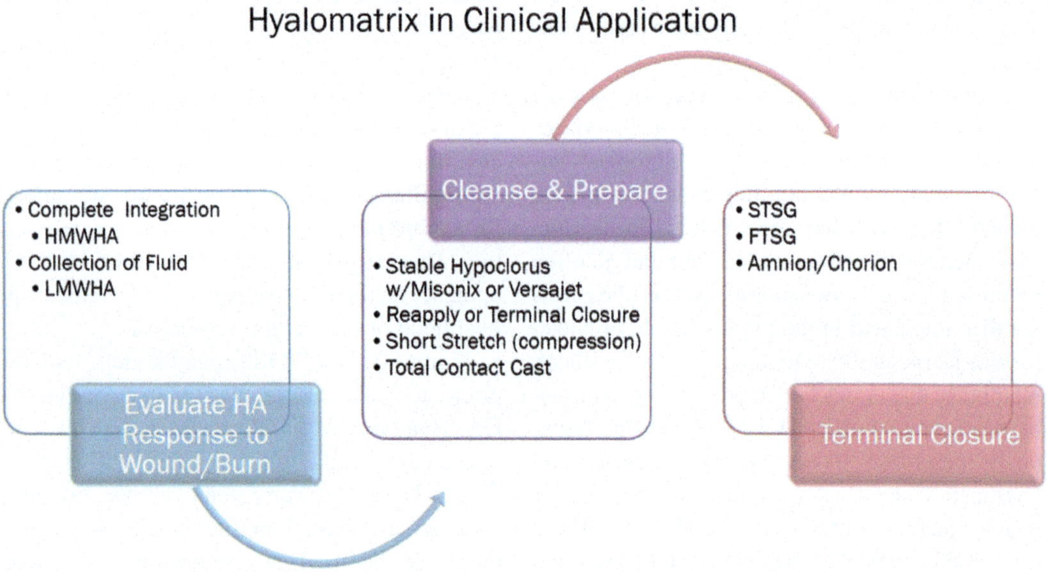

Fig. 22 Clinical Application 2 of 2

9.1 Case 1: Full-Thickness Pavement Burn with Deep Tissue Injury (Figs. 23, 24, 25, and 26)

Figure 23 is an example of a patient found down in Las Vegas in the hot summer months. The patient sustained a dual mechanism of injury, both pressure/deep tissue and a pavement/thermal full-thickness burn. The patient required substantial full-thickness debridement with compartment release. The common extensor tendons and the anterior tibialis tendon were both exposed in addition to the associated muscle bellies. Figure 24 is after one application of HA under negative pressure wound therapy (NPWT). There is already visible incorporation of the Hyalomatrix® into granulation tissue with coverage over and including the exposed tendons, one of the most challenging clinical applications. In Fig. 25, the granulation over the extensor tendon sheaths and anterior tibialis muscle belly proximally is observed at the second NPWT change. Note the decreased depth and the shiny healthy appearance of the tendon sheaths. Figures 25 and 26 document the

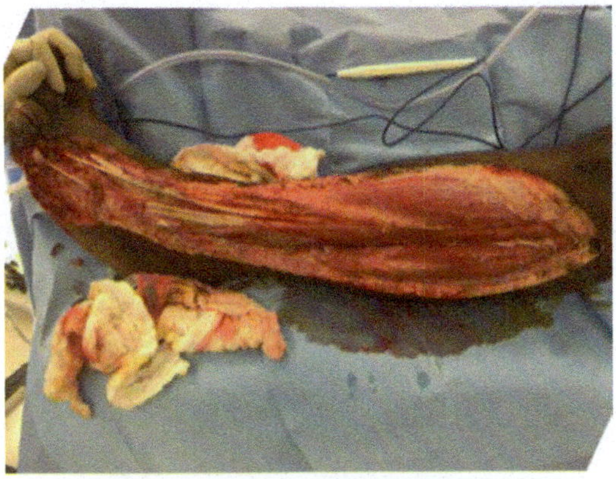

Fig. 23 Case Study Deep Third-Degree Burn from prolonged exposure to hot pavement in Las Vegas. Dual mechanism of integumentary insult; both deep tissue injury (from prolonged pressure) and thermal injury from hot pavement. First debridement in the operating room to remove all of the necrotic tissue exposing common extensor tendons and anterior tibialis tendon. At this time Hyalomatrix was placed in the OR under negative pressure wound therapy (NPWT)

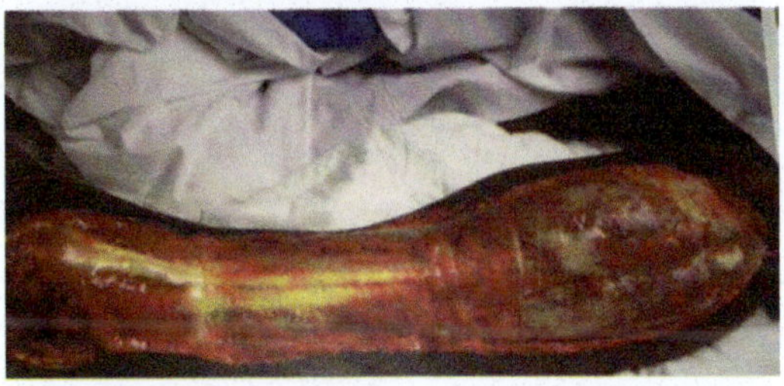

Fig. 24 Case Study Deep Burn. Granulation over extensor tendon sheaths and anterior tibialis muscle belly proximally at the first NPWT change. Note the decreased depth and the shiny healthy appearance of the tendon sheaths

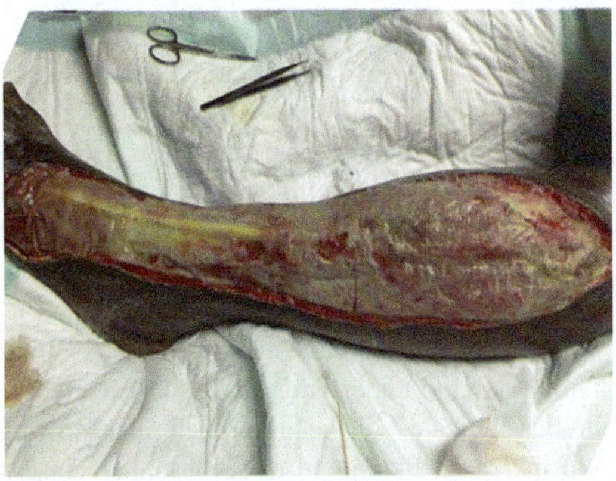

Fig. 25 Case Study Deep Burn. The extensor tendons are completely granulated over, and the wound depth is minimal in comparison to the initial debridement

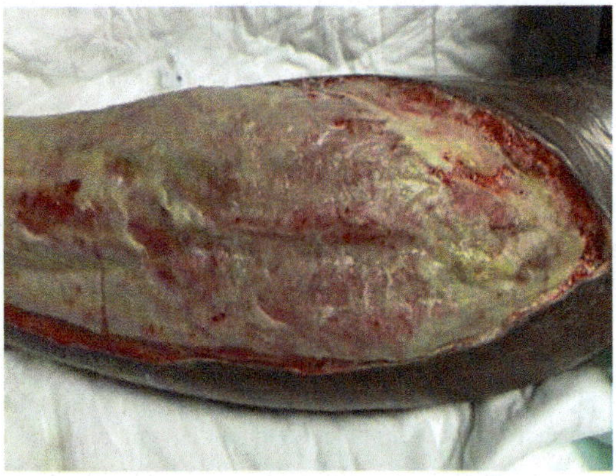

Fig. 26 Case Study Deep Burn: The extensor tendons are completely granulated over, and the wound depth is minimal in comparison to the initial debridement

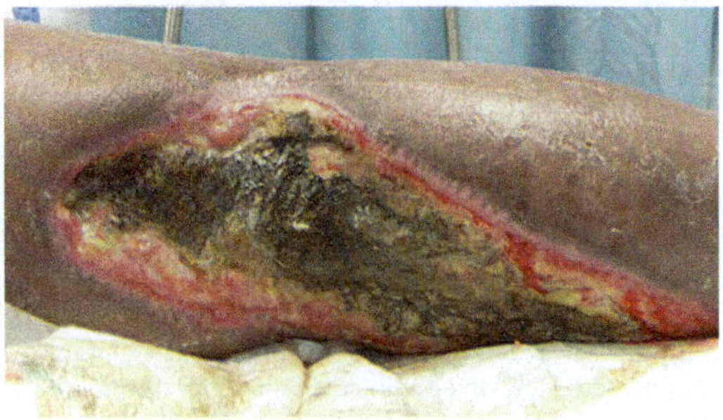

Fig. 27 Case Study Failed Femoral Popliteal Graft initial presentation

appearance of the wound after 10 days under NPWT with HA. The extensor tendons are completely granulated over, and the wound depth is minimal in comparison with the initial debridement. The wound was then terminally closed with a STSG with good coverage and preservation of the function of the extremity.

9.2 Case 2: Failed Femoral Popliteal Graft (Figs. 27, 28, 29, and 30)

Elderly female who had a femoral bypass which subsequently failed and developed a severe knee flexion contracture. In a relatively brief period of time, the patient underwent serial debridements and placement of HA.

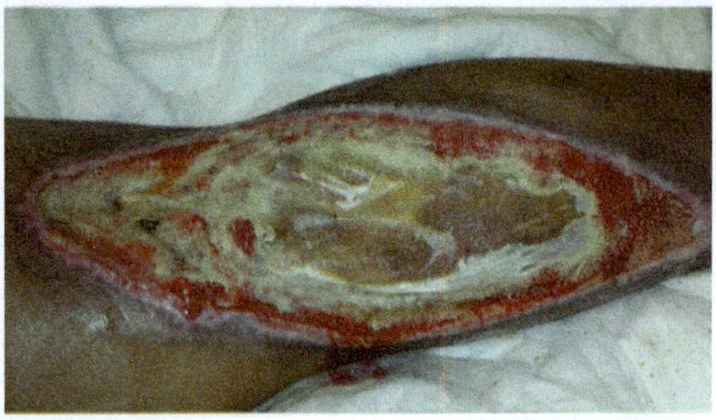

Fig. 28 Case Study Failed Femoral Popliteal Graft after the first application of fenestrated HA placed under NPWT for 5 days

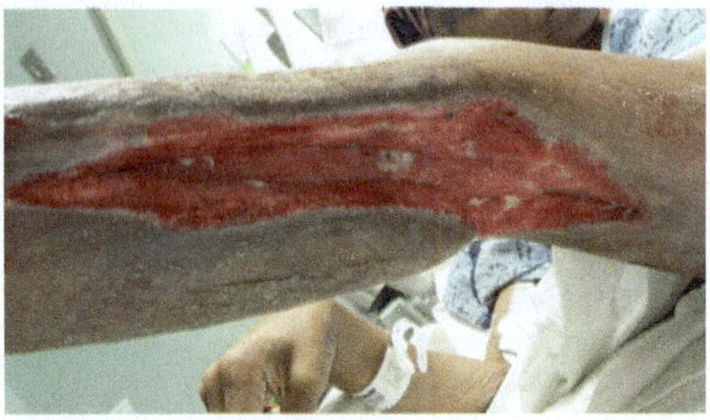

Fig. 29 Case Study Failed Femoral Popliteal Graft—wound bed after two additional applications of fenestrated HA under NPWT changed approximately every 5 days

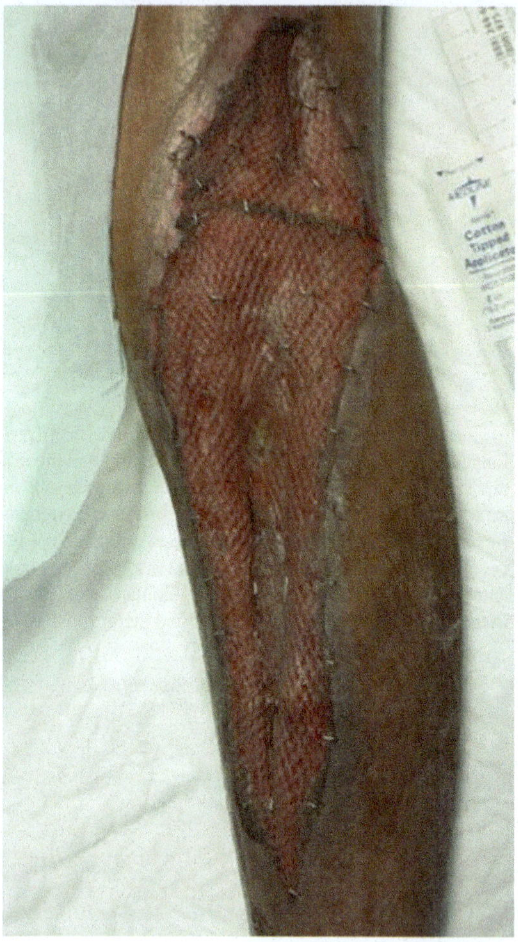

Fig. 30 Case Study Failed Femoral Popliteal Graft—split-thickness skin graft (STSG) placed with NPWT. STSG after 5 days under NPWT

9.3 Case 3: Necrotizing Fasciitis (Figs. 31, 32, 33, 34, and 35)

This case is of a 72-year-old female with known hypertension, elevated BMI, and diabetes who presented to the ER with a leg wound that had been present for some time. The wound became infected and she developed rapidly expanding necrotizing fasciitis. She subsequently went into acute respiratory failure and developed metabolic acidosis.

9.4 Case 4: Open Abdomen (Figs. 36, 37, 38, and 39)

The open abdomen is a relatively new and increasingly common strategy for the management of abdominal emergencies in both trauma and general surgery. The open abdomen can reduce mortality associated with conditions such as abdominal compartment syndrome, bowel perforation, and internal organ laceration. However, the resulting open abdomen is a complex clinical problem [110–114]. Advanced techniques and improved technologies are now readily available, allowing management of the open abdomen as well as the progressive reduction of the resulting abdominal and underlying fascial defect. Recent studies indicate both an improved survival rate and increased likelihood to successfully close a large proportion of patients, treated with open abdomen technique (OAT). Moreover, these

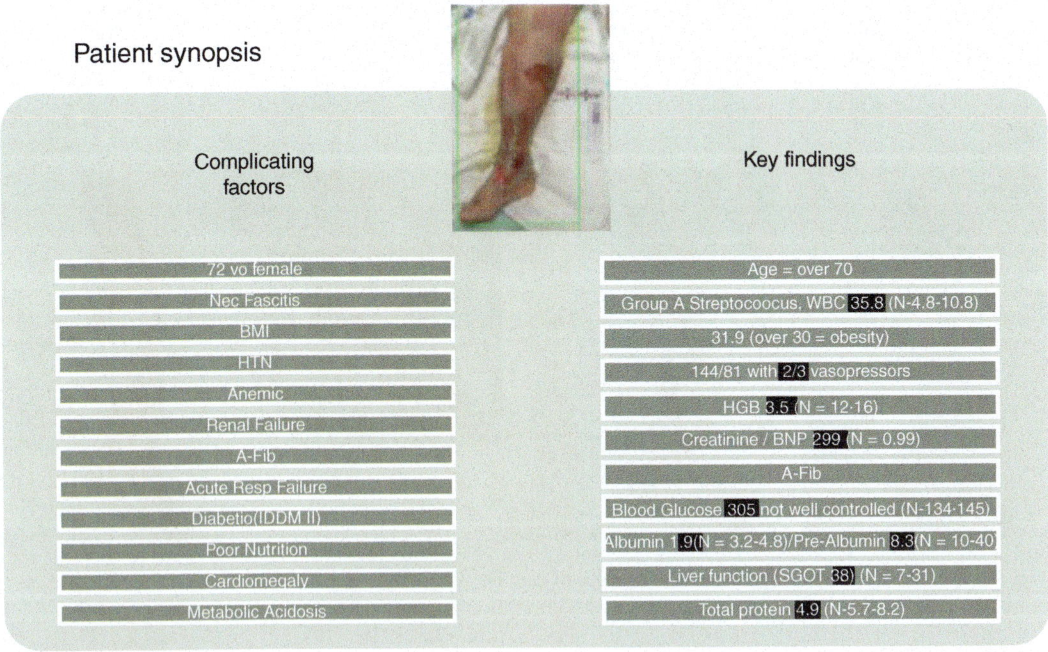

Fig. 31 Case Study Necrotizing Fasciitis. Overall case synopsis with significant number of abnormal lab values complicating care

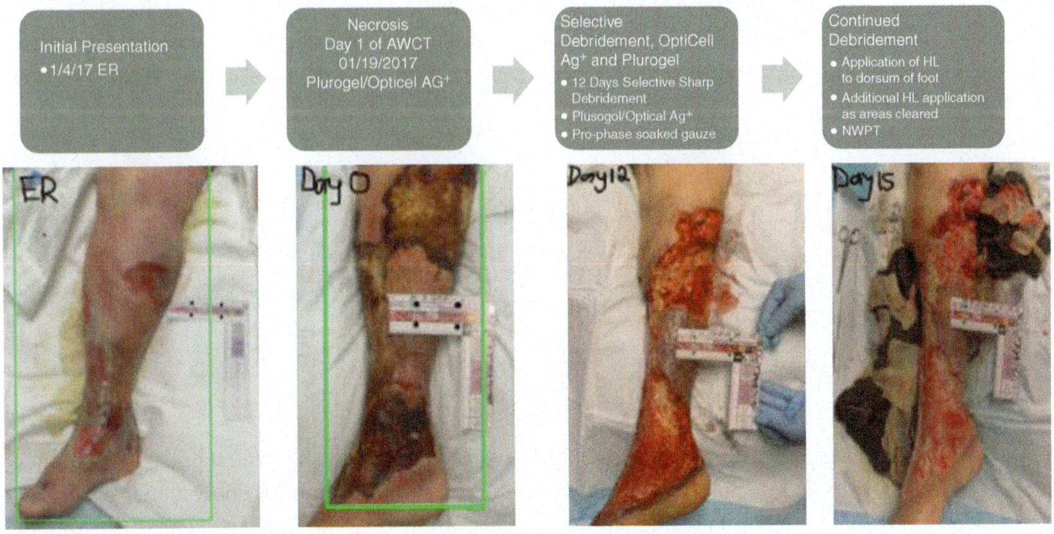

Fig. 32 Case Study Necrotizing Fasciitis—sequence of care Days 0–15

patients can now be closed within the initial hospitalization. These techniques and technologies include the appropriate use of negative pressure wound therapy (NPWT) [5] and synthetic or biologic repair materials [6]. It is essential that general and trauma surgeons understand the core principles underlying the need for and management of the open abdomen.

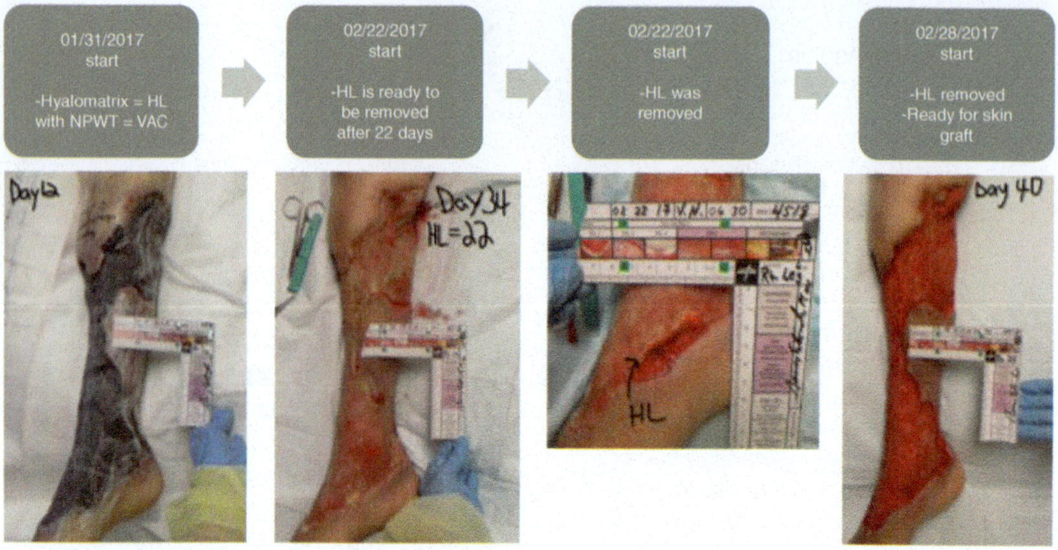

Fig. 33 Case Study Necrotizing Fasciitis—sequence of care Days 12–40

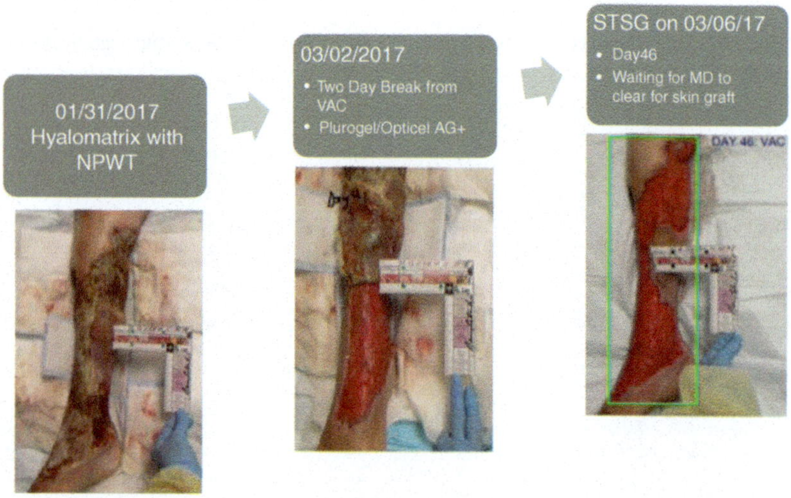

Fig. 34 Case Study Necrotizing Fasciitis—summary to Day 46

As described by the Open Abdomen Advisory Panel [115], the open abdomen technique (OAT) is widely utilized in life-threatening trauma, intra-abdominal sepsis, and abdominal compartment syndrome. The OAT poses a variety of critical care challenges, inclusive of surgical, metabolic, and nutritional complications, as well as infections both local and systemic. Negative pressure wound therapy (NPWT) [11] has become increasingly common for the management of the open abdomen. NPWT does not completely overcome the challenges posed by mesh degradation, inevitable epiboly at the peri-wound, or complex wound gutters. This case demonstrates a novel approach to complex open abdomen wound management utilizing NPWT in combination with two unique dressings, chitosan and hyaluronic acid. Chitosan fiber dressing, impregnated with silver (Ag+1), has antimicrobial properties, promotes hemostasis, decreases inflammation via cellular pathways, and is compatible with NPWT because of the fiber vertical

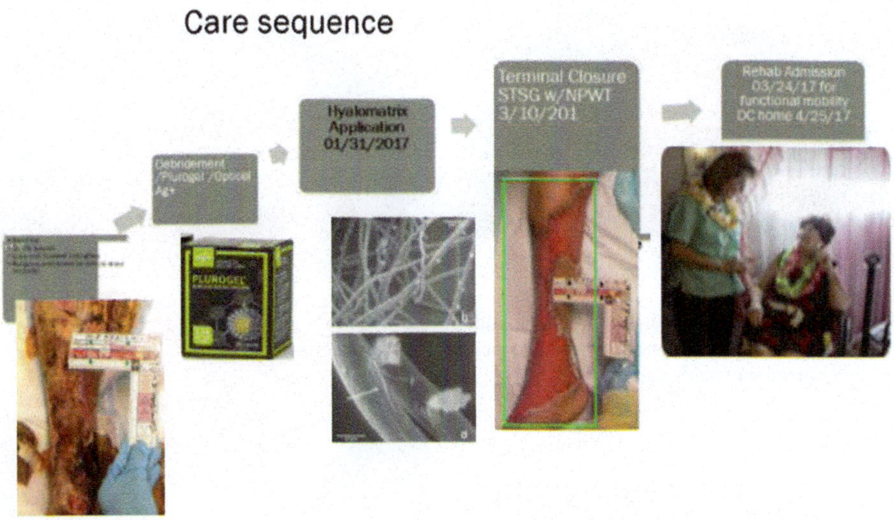

Fig. 35 Case Study Necrotizing Fasciitis—patient discharged home on April 25, 2017 (initial admission on January 4, 2017), with durable integumentary coverage and a functional lower extremity for standing, transfers, and ambulation with front wheeled walker

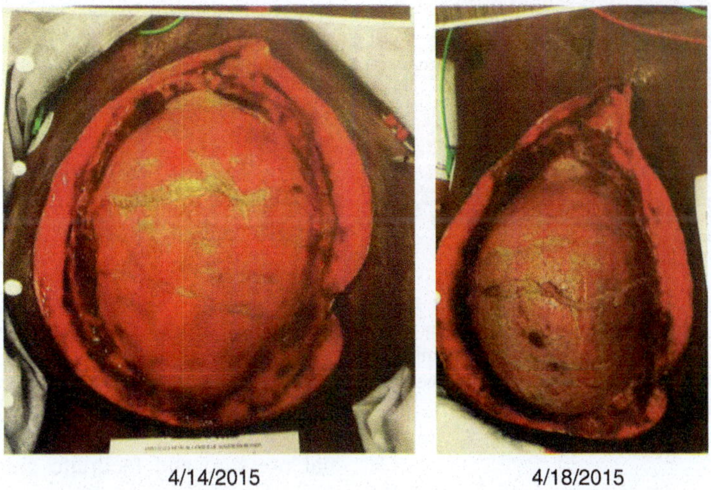

Fig. 36 Case Study Open Abdomen. Trauma patient admitted secondary to machete wound with intestinal complication, open abdomen. MM is a 45-year-old man who sustained multiple knife stab wounds to his abdomen. He was immediately transferred to a Level I Trauma Center. After initial assessment, the patient underwent emergent exploratory laparotomy and was found to have multiple penetrating organ injuries. Damage control surgery was performed. The patient was left in discontinuity, open abdomen with NPWT to manage exudate and provide barrier mechanism. Patient was transferred in critical condition to the trauma intensive critical care unit (TICU). MM underwent aggressive resuscitation with multiple abdominal washouts and ultimately placement of a polyglactin 910 mesh to approximate the fascia; NPWT was placed in the OR theater to manage drainage and abdominal pressure and facilitate granulation. NPWT set at continuous pressure at 100 mmHg. Unfortunately, within 7 days, the inevitable occurred: necrosis of the overlying mesh with combined areas of tissue necrosis and mesh degradation. Large wound gutters began forming at the peri-wound interface, particularly in the inferior quadrants. Biofilm/bioburden formation consistent with multibacterial colonization was confirmed with laboratory analysis. NPWT was discontinued and wet-to-dry gauze dressings instituted. Further degradation and thickening of the peri-wound margins continued with the formation of yellow-green biofilm over the polyglactin 910 mesh. The top right is at initiation of NPWT, Hyalomatrix® and Opticell Ag®. The lower left is after 4 days of NPWT with Opticell Ag® and Hyalomatrix® circumferentially in gutters with attention to promote granulation over Vicryl mesh

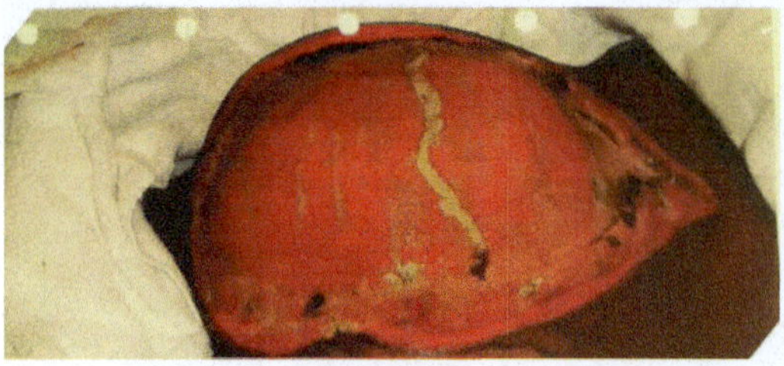

04/25/2015

Fig. 37 Case Study Open Abdomen—improved granulation, stabilization of Vicryl mesh, and continued decrease in depth of peri-wound gutters at margins

05/07/2015

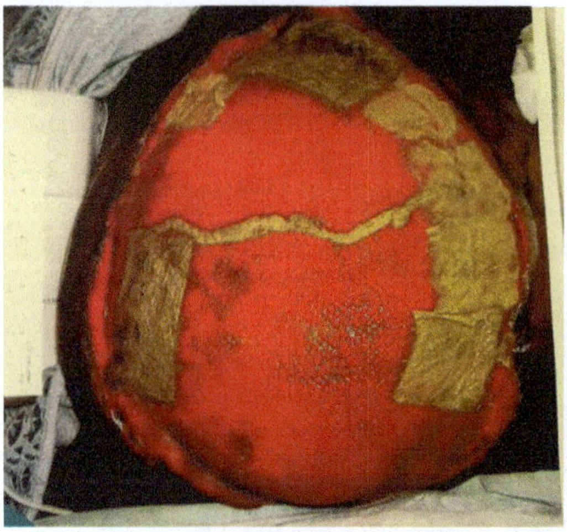

Fig. 38 Case Study Open Abdomen—Opticell Ag at wound margins; HA is visible at the top left upper quadrant. Here what is visible is the clear silicone membrane. The actual HA has incorporated into the wound bed and instilled a proliferative bias

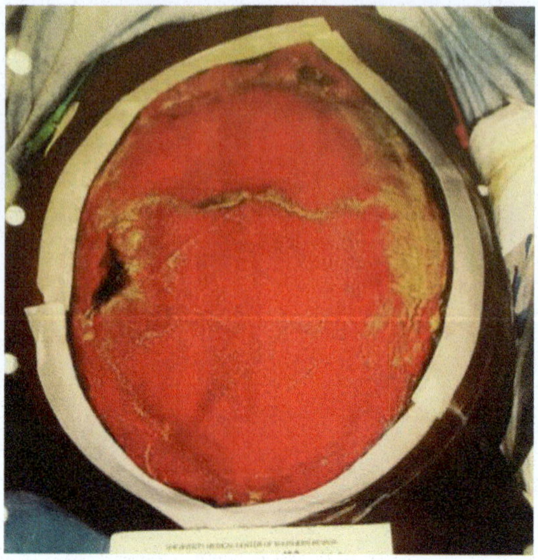

5/19/15 Terminal STSG 5/21/15

Fig. 39 Case Study Open Abdomen—improved healing evidenced by decreased depth of gutters, improved granulation, and increased abdominal stabilization. Terminal closure was achieved with a STSG on May 21, 2015

wicking (as opposed to horizontal) [116–118]. The unique combination of chitosan and HA resulted in cellular proliferation, neovascularization, and reduction of infection, providing the basis for terminal reepithelialization sufficient to support terminal closure by split-thickness skin graft (STSG).

The 45-year-old man sustained multiple knife stab wounds to his abdomen. He was immediately transferred to a Level I Trauma Center. After initial assessment, the patient underwent emergent exploratory laparotomy and was found to have multiple penetrating organ injuries. Damage control surgery was performed. The patient was left in discontinuity, open abdomen with NPWT to manage exudate and provide barrier mechanism. Patient was transferred in critical condition to the trauma intensive critical care unit (TICU). MM underwent aggressive resuscitation with multiple abdominal washouts and ultimately placement of a polyglactin 910 mesh to approximate the fascia; NPWT was placed in the OR theater to manage drainage and abdominal pressure and facilitate granulation. NPWT set at continuous pressure at 100 mmHg. Unfortunately, within 7 days, the inevitable occurred: necrosis of the overlying mesh with combined areas of tissue necrosis and mesh degradation. Large wound gutters began forming at the peri-wound interface, particularly in the inferior quadrants. Biofilm/bioburden formation consistent with multibacterial colonization was confirmed with laboratory analysis. NPWT was discontinued and wet-to-dry gauze dressings instituted. Further degradation and thickening of the peri-wound margins continued with the formation of yellow-green biofilm over the polyglactin 910 mesh.

The patient's open abdominal wound with bacterial colonization and mesh degradation posed a difficult dilemma for the medical team. He was not acutely septic from his wounds, providing an opportunity to avert utilization of traditional surgical pathway, i.e., repeated abdominal washout in the OR theater with explantation of mesh. This treatment approach could have been potentially catastrophic for this patient. Instead, a decision was made to opt for a broad-spectrum antimicrobial treatment (chitosan Ag+1) in combination with a molecular biologic substrate (HA) that would facilitate angiogenesis, fibroblast migration, and deposition of ECM components. The utilization of chitosan Ag+1 to mitigate bioburden and the use of HA in combination with NPWT (at a lower setting 50–75 mmHg) was selected to manage wound exudate, abdominal pressures, and exudate. Prior to the application of the chitosan/HA/NPWT combination, the wound surface area was 750 cm^2 (Figs. 36, 37, 38, and 39). Figure 37 shows the appearance of the chitosan dressing (yellowish) and the hyaluronic acid dressing (clear and shiny). Note that different dressings under the NPWT are used in areas appropriate for the properties of that specific dressing—chitosan, antibacterial effect, versus hyaluronic acid, neoangiogenic effect. MM was closed after 17 days using a split-thickness skin graft over a good granulation base with no additional complications and no readmission.

9.5 Case 5: Bilateral LE Burn (Figs. 40, 41, 42, 43, and 44)

This case illustrates the use of HA over a deep third-degree burn requiring surgical debridement to the level of cortical bone and excision of a substantial portion of the anterior tibialis muscle belly. The 54-year-old female patient had multiple comorbidities including nutrition, renal, and liver failure.

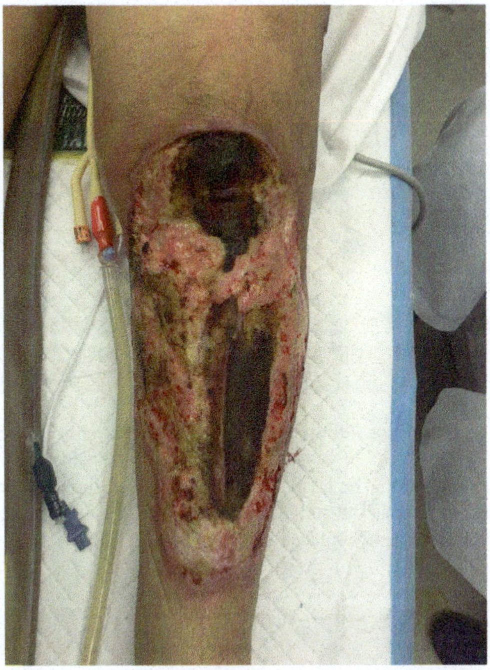

Fig. 40 Case Study Bilateral Lower Extremity Deep Third-Degree Burns. Initial presentation

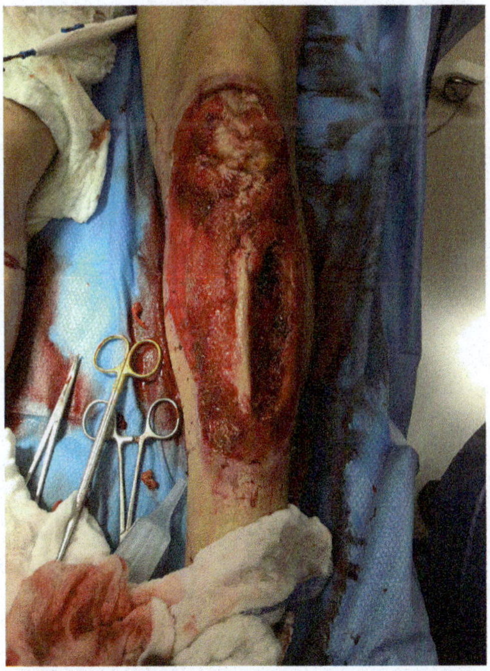

Fig. 41 Case Study Bilateral Lower Extremity Deep Third-Degree Burns—debridement intraoperatively. Note the exposed tibial crest, lateral anterior tibialis muscle defect secondary to necrosis that required extensive excision

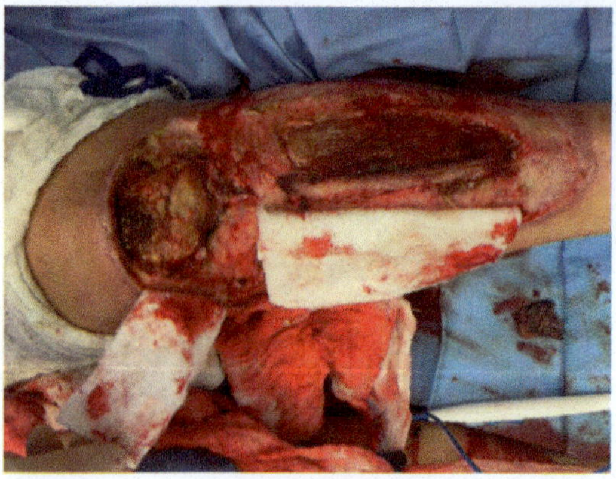

Fig. 42 Case Study Bilateral Lower Extremity Deep Third-Degree Burns—intraoperative placement of Hyalomatrix. The Hyalomatrix is the white fibrous material visible at the lower margin of the leg. It has been fenestrated and is placed under NPWT

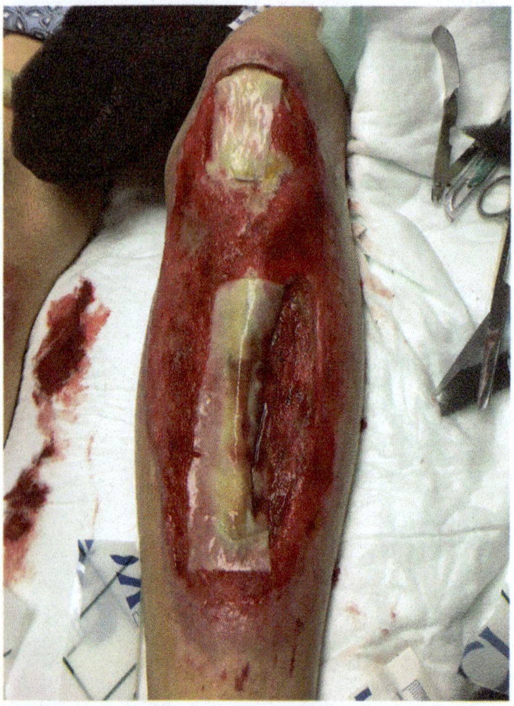

Fig. 43 Case Study Bilateral Lower Extremity Deep Third-Degree Burns—intraoperative takedown of NPWT exposing intact Hyalomatrix. A substantial portion of the Hyalomatrix has incorporated into the wound. Note the varied areas of clear Hyalomatrix (HMWHA) and areas of increased inflammatory response (LMWHA) seen as opaque fluid collection. The patient did not have an elevated white blood count

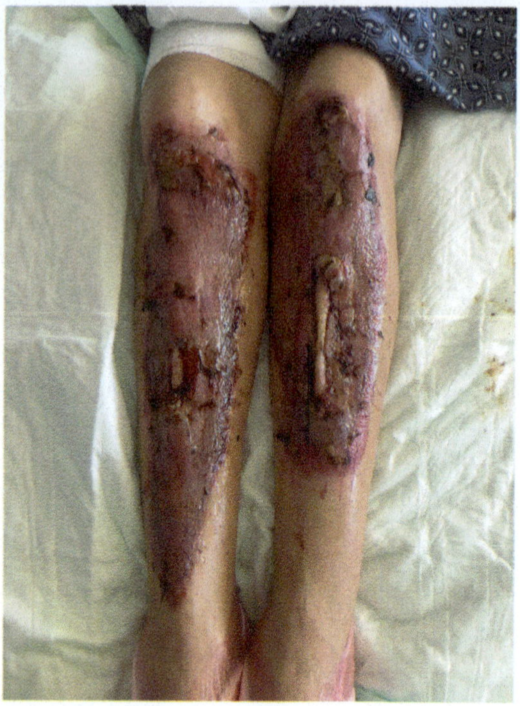

Fig. 44 Case Study Bilateral Lower Extremity Deep Third-Degree Burns—bilateral LE after STSG placement under NPWT with a complicated course of aftercare secondary to a urinary tract infection, sepsis, and inappropriate wound care. Despite adversity, the wounds did continue to closure. Of significant importance was the preservation of functional dorsiflexion

Conclusions

Mediators and mechanisms of inflammation and inflammatory resolution and repair do not exist in isolation, as an "either or" on or off state. Tissue injury either surgical, traumatic, or pathological that creates a full-thickness defect in the skin poses very unique obstacles for healing and restoration of function. Typically, tissue injury causes an immediate onset of inflammation mediated by chemoattractants derived from plasma proteins, resident and recruited hematopoietic cells, extracellular matrix, and bacteria. Progression to complete wound healing is accompanied by resolution of the inflammatory mediators and the reconstitution of normal microvascular

Table 1 Resolution of inflammation is directed by downregulation of the pro-inflammatory mediators and restoration of microvascular permeability

Dynamic components of inflammation	Processes in inflammatory resolution
Plasma protein-derived chemoattractant (C5, fibrinopeptides, 2-thrombin)	Reconstruction and reconstitution of vascular permeability
Chemokines (MCP, MIP, RANTES)	Anti-inflammatory cytokines (IL-10, TGF-β, IL-1 ra)
Growth factors (TNF-α, OL-1, I-6, PDGF TGF-β)	Mediators of apoptosis (CD44, caspases)
Eicosanoids (prostaglandins, leukotrienes)	Transcription factors (NRf-2, NF-Kβ)
ECM fragments (fibronectin, elastin, collagen)	Receptor downregulation with proteolysis of chemokines
ROS	Lymphatic drainage
Nitric oxide	
Bacterial-derived chemoattractants	

permeability, which will in turn contribute to the cessation of local pro-inflammatory response. Resolution of inflammation is directed by downregulation of the pro-inflammatory mediators and restoration of microvascular permeability. Together these things contribute to the cessation of local chemoattractants, synthesis of anti-inflammatory mediators, apoptosis, and lymphatic drainage. These are presented in summary in Table 1. An excessive or prolonged inflammatory response results in increased tissue injury and, therefore, poor healing. Successful wound repair requires the coordinated expression of both inflammation and the resolution of inflammation and the restoration of stable tissue.

In one wound there are simultaneous areas of granulation/proliferative bias and an inflammation bias. The inflammation bias occurs first and is collocated with necrotic tissue, debris, nonviable tissue, or areas where, despite best efforts, bacteria may exist. As the areas of inflammation resolve, proliferation follows restoring tissue stability.

The HA polymer Hyalomatrix® is a commercially available 3D scaffold that responds to the varied environments of the wound milieu. HA is a biologically active molecule that differentially responds based on the chemokines, cytokines, cells, and molecules in the ECM. Often areas of inflammation are predominately in areas of wounds that are deeper and in and around significant structures, tendons, and neurovascular bundles. Alternatively, proliferative areas tend to predominate along the edges of wounds or in juxtaposition to hair follicles that remain. Areas of granulation can also migrate out from hair follicles circumferentially, 360°.

Rain drops into a puddle of water are an elegant way to visualize the many microenvironments and the continuum between areas of inflammation or proliferation. Each drop represents an area that is either in a predominate state of inflammation or proliferation (Fig. 45). The ripples moving out from the center of inflammation or proliferation (droplets) gradually decrease in intensity and influence on the surrounding ECM. The ECM is a fluid and dynamic environment that responds to change and interacts with both intrinsic and extrinsic stimuli. Figure 46 represents the puddle analogy of the ECM being both varied and dynamic, a cumulation of all of the various cellular and matrix signals that are either dampened or amplified based on the microwound milieu.

HA is a recognized, biologically active molecule that naturally regulates all phases of tissue repair on multiple levels and should be considered as a safe and effective option to be used in skin repair [119–124]. HA in the form of Hyalomatrix® is presented here in five case studies where significant soft tissue defect occurred either from wounding, NF, or the subsequent debridement.

In deep burns there is a significant loss of the ECM and the required growth factors due to debridement and the associated zone of injury [125]. In necrotizing fasciitis (NF),

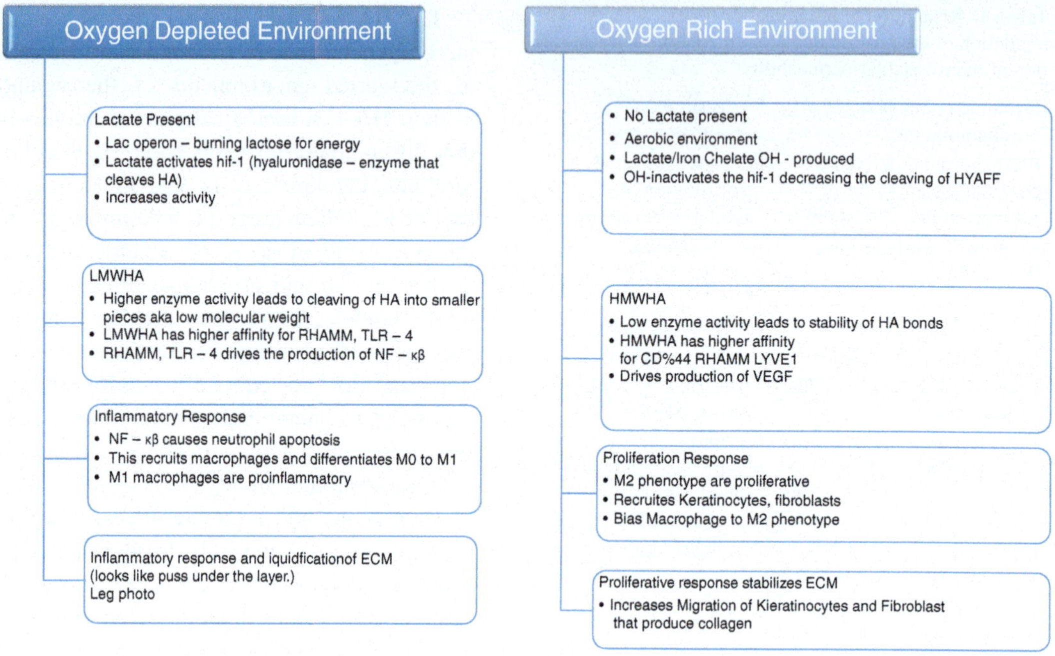

Fig. 45 Summary chart of the continuum for inflammation and resolution of inflammation

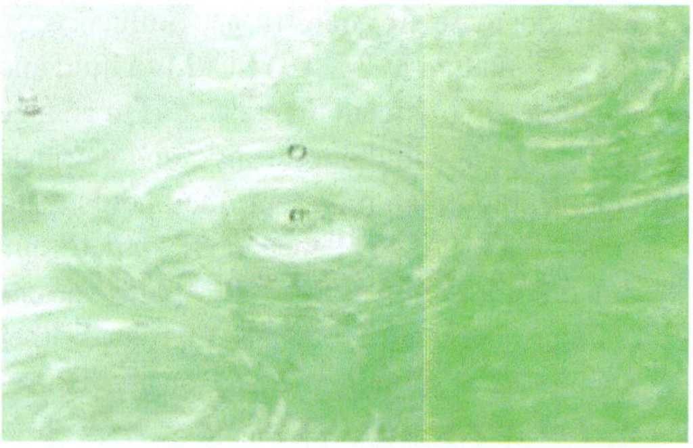

Fig. 46 Imagery of a puddle—abstract representation of the effects of wounding (rain drops) and the diminishing amplitude of the waves of inflammation dispersing and interacting with areas of extracellular matrix that are stable. The ECM is dynamic and ever changing in response to wounding

there is a substantial loss of tissue due to repeated selective sharp debridements and the associated physical destruction during the removal of the epidermis and dermal components. Degloving injuries and necrotizing fasciitis (NF) pose unique challenge as the delamination of the skin and immediate integument decrease blood supply and viable remaining tissue including the ECM and component growth factors, cytokines and chemokines.

Four varied case studies are presented where HYAFF was incorporated into the treatment process to both expedite closure and improve the result.

References

1. Jiang D, Liang J, Noble PW (2011) Hyaluronan as an immune regulator in human diseases. Physiol Rev 91(1):221–264
2. Weissmann B, Meyer K, Sampson P, Linker A (1954) Isolation of oligosaccharides enzymatically produced from hyaluronic acid. J Biol Chem 208(1):417–429
3. Coleman PJ, Scott D, Mason RM, Levick JR (1999) Characterization of the effect of high molecular weight hyaluronan on trans-synovial flow in rabbit knees. J Physiol 514(Pt 1):265–282
4. Scott JE, Heatley F (1999) Hyaluronan forms specific stable tertiary structures in aqueous solution: a 13C NMR study. Proc Natl Acad Sci U S A 96(9):4850–4855
5. Bates EJ, Harper GS, Lowther DA, Preston BN (1984) Effect of oxygen-derived reactive species

on cartilage proteoglycan-hyaluronate aggregates. Biochem Int 8(5):629–637
6. Bates EJ, Lowther DA, Handley CJ (1984) Oxygen free-radicals mediate an inhibition of proteoglycan synthesis in cultured articular cartilage. Ann Rheum Dis 43(3):462–469
7. Weigel PH, Fuller GM, LeBoeuf RD (1986) A model for the role of hyaluronic acid and fibrin in the early events during the inflammatory response and wound healing. J Theor Biol 119(2):219–234
8. McKee CM, Penno MB, Cowman M, Burdick MD, Strieter RM, Bao C, Noble PW (1996) Hyaluronan (HA) fragments induce chemokine gene expression in alveolar macrophages. The role of HA size and CD44. J Clin Invest 98(10):2403–2413
9. Papakonstantinou E, Roth M, Karakiulakis G (2012) Hyaluronic acid: a key molecule in skin aging. Dermatoendocrinol 4(3):253–258
10. McKee CM, Lowenstein CJ, Horton MR, Wu J, Bao C, Chin BY, Choi AM, Noble PW (1997) Hyaluronan fragments induce nitric-oxide synthase in murine macrophages through a nuclear factor kappaB-dependent mechanism. J Biol Chem 272(12):8013–8018
11. Prehm P (1984) Hyaluronate is synthesized at plasma membranes. Biochem J 220(2):597–600
12. Jiang M, Osterlund P, Sarin LP, Poranen MM, Bamford DH, Guo D, Julkunen I (2011) Innate immune responses in human monocyte-derived dendritic cells are highly dependent on the size and the 5′ phosphorylation of RNA molecules. J Immunol 187(4):1713–1721
13. Toole BP (1990) Hyaluronan and its binding proteins, the hyaladherins. Curr Opin Cell Biol 2(5):839–844
14. Herishanu Y, Gibellini F, Njuguna N, Hazan-Halevy I, Farooqui M, Bern S, Keyvanfar K, Lee E, Wilson W, Wiestner A (2011) Activation of CD44, a receptor for extracellular matrix components, protects chronic lymphocytic leukemia cells from spontaneous and drug induced apoptosis through MCL-1. Leuk Lymphoma 52(9):1758–1769
15. Ioachim E, Goussia A, Agnantis NJ (1999) Glycoprotein CD44 expression in colorectal neoplasms. An immuno-histochemical study including correlation with cathepsin D, extracellular matrix components, p53, Rb, bcl-2, c-erbB-2, EGFR and proliferation indices. Virchows Arch 434(1): 45–50
16. Radotra B, McCormick D, Crockard A (1994) CD44 plays a role in adhesive interactions between glioma cells and extracellular matrix components. Neuropathol Appl Neurobiol 20(4):399–405
17. Hardwick C, Hoare K, Owens R, Hohn HP, Hook M, Moore D, Cripps V, Austen L, Nance DM, Turley EA (1992) Molecular cloning of a novel hyaluronan receptor that mediates tumor cell motility. J Cell Biol 117(6):1343–1350
18. Turley EA (1992) Hyaluronan and cell locomotion. Cancer Metastasis Rev 11(1):21–30
19. Mohapatra S, Yang X, Wright JA, Turley EA, Greenberg AH (1996) Soluble hyaluronan receptor RHAMM induces mitotic arrest by suppressing Cdc2 and cyclin B1 expression. J Exp Med 183(4):1663–1668
20. Al-Mulla F, Leibovich SJ, Francis IM, Bitar MS (2011) Impaired TGF-beta signaling and a defect in resolution of inflammation contribute to delayed wound healing in a female rat model of type 2 diabetes. Mol Biosystems 7(11):3006–3020
21. Ekholm EC, Ravanti L, Kahari V, Paavolainen P, Penttinen RP (2000) Expression of extracellular matrix genes: transforming growth factor (TGF)-beta1 and ras in tibial fracture healing of lathyritic rats. Bone 27(4):551–557
22. Gong D, Shi W, Yi SJ, Chen H, Groffen J, Heisterkamp N (2012) TGFbeta signaling plays a critical role in promoting alternative macrophage activation. BMC Immunol 13:31
23. Heinemeier K, Langberg H, Olesen JL, Kjaer M (2003) Role of TGF-beta1 in relation to exercise-induced type I collagen synthesis in human tendinous tissue. J Appl Physiol (1985) 95(6):2390–2397
24. Kihara Y, Tashiro M, Nakamura H, Yamaguchi T, Yoshikawa H, Otsuki M (2001) Role of TGF-beta1, extracellular matrix, and matrix metalloproteinase in the healing process of the pancreas after induction of acute necrotizing pancreatitis using arginine in rats. Pancreas 23(3):288–295
25. Leask A (2006) Scar wars: is TGFbeta the phantom menace in scleroderma? Arthritis Res Ther 8(4):213
26. Leask A, Abraham DJ (2004) TGF-beta signaling and the fibrotic response. FASEB J 18(7):816–827
27. Meyer-ter-Vehn T, Han H, Grehn F, Schlunck G (2011) Extracellular matrix elasticity modulates TGF-beta-induced p38 activation and myofibroblast transdifferentiation in human tenon fibroblasts. Invest Ophthalmol Vis Sci 52(12):9149–9155
28. Ripellino JA, Bailo M, Margolis RU, Margolis RK (1988) Light and electron microscopic studies on the localization of hyaluronic acid in developing rat cerebellum. J Cell Biol 106(3):845–855
29. Tammi R, Ripellino JA, Margolis RU, Tammi M (1988) Localization of epidermal hyaluronic acid using the hyaluronate binding region of cartilage proteoglycan as a specific probe. J Invest Dermatol 90(3):412–414
30. Batzios SP, Zafeiriou DI, Papakonstantinou E (2013) Extracellular matrix components: an intricate network of possible biomarkers for lysosomal storage disorders? FEBS Lett 587(8):1258–1267
31. Hamm R (2015) Text and atlas of wound diagnosis and treatment. McGraw Hill, New York, NY
32. Kazlauskas A (2005) The priming/completion paradigm to explain growth factor-dependent cell cycle progression. Growth Factors 23(3):203–210
33. Grotendorst GR, Okochi H (1996) Hayashi N. A novel transforming growth factor beta response element controls the expression of the connective tissue growth factor gene. Cell Growth Differ 7(4):469–480

34. Igarashi A, Okochi H, Bradham DM, Grotendorst GR (1993) Regulation of connective tissue growth factor gene expression in human skin fibroblasts and during wound repair. Mol Biol Cell 4(6):637–645
35. Desmouliere A, Geinoz A, Gabbiani F, Gabbiani G (1993) Transforming growth factor-beta 1 induces alpha-smooth muscle actin expression in granulation tissue myofibroblasts and in quiescent and growing cultured fibroblasts. J Cell Biol 122(1):103–111
36. Figg W, Folkman J (2008) Angiogenesis. Springer Science and Business Media, LLC, New York, NY
37. Schaber JA, Triffo WJ, Suh SJ, Oliver JW, Hastert MC, Griswold JA (2007) Pseudomonas aeruginosa forms biofilms in acute infection independent of cell-to-cell signaling. Infect Immun 75:3715–3721
38. Stout RD, Suttles J (1997) T cell signaling of macrophage function in inflammatory disease. Front Biosci 2:d197–d206
39. Bhowmick S, Rother S, Zimmermann H, Lee PS, Moeller S, Schnabelrauch M, Koul V, Jordan R, Hintze V, Scharnweber D (2017) Biomimetic electrospun scaffolds from main extracellular matrix components for skin tissue engineering application—the role of chondroitin sulfate and sulfated hyaluronan. Mater Sci Eng C Mater Biol Appl 79:15–22
40. Campo GM, Avenoso A, Campo S, D'Ascola A, Traina P, Samà D, Calatroni A (2008) NF-kB and caspases are involved in the hyaluronan and chondroitin-4-sulphate-exerted antioxidant effect in fibroblast cultures exposed to oxidative stress. J Appl Toxicol 28(4):509–517
41. Morioka Y, Yamasaki K, Leung D, Gallo RL (2008) Cathelicidin antimicrobial peptides inhibit hyaluronan-induced cytokine release and modulate chronic allergic dermatitis. J Immunol 181(6):3915–3922
42. Ng CK, Handley CJ, Preston BN, Robinson HC (1992) The extracellular processing and catabolism of hyaluronan in cultured adult articular cartilage explants. Arch Biochem Biophys 298(1):70–79
43. Ng CK, Handley CJ, Preston BN, Robinson HC, Bolis S, Parker G (1995) Effect of exogenous hyaluronan and hyaluronan oligosaccharides on hyaluronan and aggrecan synthesis and catabolism in adult articular cartilage explants. Arch Biochem Biophys 316(1):596–606
44. Rock K, Grandoch M, Majora M, Krutmann J, Fischer JW (2011) Collagen fragments inhibit hyaluronan synthesis in skin fibroblasts in response to ultraviolet B (UVB): new insights into mechanisms of matrix remodeling. J Biol Chem 286(20):18268–18276
45. Sadeghi N, Camby I, Goldman S, Gabius HJ, Balériaux D, Salmon I, Decaesteckere C, Kiss R, Metens T (2003) Effect of hydrophilic components of the extracellular matrix on quantifiable diffusion-weighted imaging of human gliomas: preliminary results of correlating apparent diffusion coefficient values and hyaluronan expression level. AJR Am J Roentgenol 181(1):235–241
46. Suwiwat S, Ricciardelli C, Tammi R, Tammi M, Auvinen P, Kosma VM, LeBaron RG, Raymond WA, Tilley WD, Horsfall DJ (2004) Expression of extracellular matrix components versican, chondroitin sulfate, tenascin, and hyaluronan, and their association with disease outcome in node-negative breast cancer. Clin Cancer Res 10(7):2491–2498
47. Travis JA, Hughes MG, Wong JM, Wagner WD, Geary RL (2001) Hyaluronan enhances contraction of collagen by smooth muscle cells and adventitial fibroblasts: role of CD44 and implications for constrictive remodeling. Circ Res 88(1):77–83
48. Yagi M, Sato N, Mitsui Y, Gotoh M, Hamada T, Nagata K (2010) Hyaluronan modulates proliferation and migration of rabbit fibroblasts derived from flexor tendon epitenon and endotenon. J Hand Surg Am 35(5):791–796
49. Gough MJ, Killeen N, Weinberg AD (2012) Targeting macrophages in the tumour environment to enhance the efficacy of alphaOX40 therapy. Immunology 136(4):437–447
50. Herwig R, Pelzer A, Horninger W, Rehder P, Klocker H, Ramoner R, Pinggera GM, Gozzi C, Konwalinka G, Bartsch G (2004) Measurement of intracellular versus extracellular prostate-specific antigen levels in peripheral macrophages: a new approach to noninvasive diagnosis of prostate cancer. Clin Prostate Cancer 3(3):1848
51. Joshi AD, Oak SR, Hartigan AJ, Finn WG, Kunkel SL, Duffy KE, Das A, Hogaboam CM (2010) Interleukin-33 contributes to both M1 and M2 chemokine marker expression in human macrophages. BMC Immunol 11:52
52. Katschke KJ, Rottman JB, Ruth JH, Qin S, Wu L, LaRosa G, Ponath P, Park CC, Pope RM, Koch AE (2001) Differential expression of chemokine receptors on peripheral blood, synovial fluid, and synovial tissue monocytes/macrophages in rheumatoid arthritis. Arthritis Rheum 44:1022–1032
53. Kawamura H, Kawamura T, Kanda Y, Kobayashi T, Abo T (2012) Extracellular ATP-stimulated macrophages produce macrophage inflammatory protein-2 which is important for neutrophil migration. Immunology 136(4):448–458
54. Kessler L, Tritschler S, Bohbot A, Sigrist S, Karsten V, Boivin S, Dufour P, Belcourt A, Pinget M (2001) Macrophage activation in type 1 diabetic patients with catheter obstruction during peritoneal insulin delivery with an implantable pump. Diabetes Care 24(2):302–307
55. Lawrence T, Natoli G (2011) Transcriptional regulation of macrophage polarization: enabling diversity with identity. Nat Rev Immunol 11(11):750–761
56. Leibovich SJ, Ross R (1975) The role of the macrophage in wound repair. A study with hydrocortisone and antimacrophage serum. Am J Pathol 78(1):71–100
57. Martinez FO, Helming L, Gordon S (2009) Alternative activation of macrophages: an

immunologic functional perspective. Annu Rev Immunol 27:451–483
58. Marzotto M, Bonafini C, Olioso D, Baruzzi A, Bettinetti L, Di Leva F, Galbiati E, Bellavite P (2016) Arnica montana stimulates extracellular matrix gene expression in a macrophage cell line differentiated to wound-healing phenotype. PLoS One 11(11):e0166340
59. Minton K (2011) Macrophages: a transcription factor to call their own. Nat Rev Immunol 11(2):74
60. Papatriantafyllou M (2011) Macrophages: support from the locals. Nat Rev Immunol 11(7):442
61. Patterson AM, Schmutz C, Davis S, Gardner L, Ashton BA, Middleton J (2002) Differential binding of chemokines to macrophages and neutrophils in the human inflamed synovium. Arthritis Res 4:209–214
62. Reece P, Baatjes AJ, Cyr MM, Sehmi R, Denburg JA (2013) Toll-like receptor-mediated eosinophil-basophil differentiation: autocrine signalling by granulocyte-macrophage colony-stimulating factor in cord blood haematopoietic progenitors. Immunology 139(2):256–264
63. Rodero MP, Khosrotehrani K (2010) Skin wound healing modulation by macrophages. Int J Clin Exp Pathol 3(7):643–653
64. Ruth JH, Shahrara S, Park CC, Morel JC, Kumar P, Qin S, Koch AE (2003) Role of macrophage inflammatory protein-3alpha and its ligand CCR6 in rheumatoid arthritis. Lab Investig 83:579–588
65. St Pierre BA, Tidball JG (1994) Macrophage activation and muscle remodeling at myotendinous junctions after modifications in muscle loading. Am J Pathol 145(6):1463–1471
66. Stout RD (2010) Editorial: macrophage functional phenotypes: no alternatives in dermal wound healing? J Leukoc Biol 87(1):19–21
67. Stout RD, Bottomly K (1989) Antigen-specific activation of effector macrophages by IFN-gamma producing (TH1) T cell clones. Failure of IL-4-producing (TH2) T cell clones to activate effector function in macrophages. J Immunol 142(3):760–765
68. Stout RD, Suttles J (1987) Functional characteristics of in vitro generated macrophages: a transient refractory state precedes reinducibility of a spatially restricted, possibly contact-dependent, cytostatic mechanism. Cell Immunol 105(1):33–44
69. Stout RD, Watkins SK, Suttles J (2009) Functional plasticity of macrophages: in situ reprogramming of tumor-associated macrophages. J Leukoc Biol 86(5):1105–1109
70. Scott A, Lian O, Roberts CR, Cook JL, Handley CJ, Bahr R, Samiric T, Ilic MZ, Parkinson J, Hart DA, Duronio V, Khan KM (2008) Increased versican content is associated with tendinosis pathology in the patellar tendon of athletes with jumper's knee. Scand J Med Sci Sports 18(4):427–435
71. Chang MY, Tanino Y, Vidova V, Kinsella MG, Chan CK, Johnson PY, Wight TN, Frevert CW (2014) A rapid increase in macrophage-derived versican and hyaluronan in infectious lung disease. Matrix Biol 34:1–12
72. Kramer RH, Rosen SD, McDonald KA (1988) Basement-membrane components associated with the extracellular matrix of the lymph node. Cell Tissue Res 252(2):367–375
73. Miyata K, Takaya K (1981) Elastic fibers associated with collagenous fibrils surrounded by reticular cells in lymph nodes of the rat as revealed by electron microscopy after orcein staining. Cell Tissue Res 220:445–448
74. Xu H, Guan H, Zu G, Bullard D, Hanson J (2001) The role of ICAM-1 molecule in the migration of Langerhans cells in the skin and regional lymph node. Eur J Immunol 31:3085–3093
75. Erdelyi I, van Asten AJ, van Dijk JE, Nederbragt H (2005) Expression of versican in relation to chondrogenesis-related extracellular matrix components in canine mammary tumors. Histochem Cell Biol 124(2):139–149
76. Nara Y, Kato Y, Torii Y, Tsuji Y, Nakagaki S, Goto S, Isobe H, Nakashima N, Takeuchi J (1997) Immunohistochemical localization of extracellular matrix components in human breast tumours with special reference to PG-M/versican. Histochem J 29(1):21–30
77. Merrilees MJ, Falk BA, Zuo N, Dickinson ME, May BC, Wight TN (2017) Use of versican variant V3 and versican antisense expression to engineer cultured human skin containing increased content of insoluble elastin. J Tissue Eng Regen Med 11(1):295–305
78. Wight TN, Kang I, Merrilees MJ (2014) Versican and the control of inflammation. Matrix Biol 35:152–161
79. Wight TN, Kinsella MG, Evanko SP, Potter-Perigo S, Merrilees MJ (2014) Versican and the regulation of cell phenotype in disease. Biochim Biophys Acta 1840(8):2441–2451
80. Andersson-Sjoland A, Hallgren O, Rolandsson S, Weitoft M, Tykesson E, Larsson-Callerfelt AK, Rydell-Törmänen K, Bjermer L, Malmström A, Karlsson JC, Westergren-Thorsson G (2015) Versican in inflammation and tissue remodeling: the impact on lung disorders. Glycobiology 25(3):243–251
81. Chang MY, Tanino Y, Vidova V, Kinsella MG, Chan CK, Johnson PY, Wight TN, Frevert CW (2014) Reprint of: a rapid increase in macrophage-derived versican and hyaluronan in infectious lung disease. Matrix Biol 35:162–173
82. Akhtar S, Meek KM, James V (1999) Immunolocalization of elastin, collagen type I and type III, fibronectin, and vitronectin in extracellular matrix components of normal and myxomatous mitral heart valve chordae tendineae. Cardiovasc Pathol 8(4):203–211
83. Brasselet C, Durand E, Addad F, Al Haj Zen A, Smeets MB, Laurent-Maquin D, Bouthors S, Bellon G, de Kleijn D, Godeau G, Garnotel R, Gogly B, Lafont A (2005) Collagen and elastin cross-linking:

a mechanism of constrictive remodeling after arterial injury. Am J Physiol Heart Circ Physiol 289(5):H2228–H2233
84. Finlay GA, O'Donnell MD, O'Connor CM, Hayes JP, FitzGerald MX (1996) Elastin and collagen remodeling in emphysema. A scanning electron microscopy study. Am J Pathol 149(4): 1405–1415
85. Lamme EN, de Vries HJ, van Veen H, Gabbiani G, Westerhof W, Middelkoop E (1996) Extracellular matrix characterization during healing of full-thickness wounds treated with a collagen/elastin dermal substitute shows improved skin regeneration in pigs. J Histochem Cytochem 44(11):1311–1322
86. Steed MM, Tyagi N, Sen U, Schuschke DA, Joshua IG, Tyagi SC (2010) Functional consequences of the collagen/elastin switch in vascular remodeling in hyperhomocysteinemic wild-type, eNOS-/-, and iNOS-/- mice. Am J Physiol Lung Cell Mol Physiol 299(3):L301–L311
87. Schultz GS, Wysocki A (2009) Interactions between extracellular matrix and growth factors in wound healing. Wound Repair Regen 17(2):153–162
88. Schultz GS, Barillo DJ, Mozingo DW, Chin GA, Wound Bed Advisory Board Members (2004) Wound bed preparation and a brief history of TIME. Int Wound J 1(1):19–32
89. Schultz GS, Sibbald RG, Falanga V, Ayello EA, Dowsett C, Harding K, Romanelli M, Stacey MC, Teot L, Vanscheidt W (2003) Wound bed preparation: a systematic approach to wound management. Wound Repair Regen 11(Suppl 1):S1–S28
90. Pacilli A, Pasquinelli G (2009) Vascular wall resident progenitor cells: a review. Exp Cell Res 315(6):901–914
91. Pasquinelli G, Vinci MC, Gamberini C, Orrico C, Foroni L, Guarnieri C, Parenti A, Gargiulo M, Ledda F, Caldarera CM, Muscari C (2009) Architectural organization and functional features of early endothelial progenitor cells cultured in a hyaluronan-based polymer scaffold. Tissue Eng Part A 15(9):2751–2762
92. Cheshire PA, Herson MR, Cleland H, Akbarzadeh S (2016) Artificial dermal templates: a comparative study of NovoSorb biodegradable temporising matrix (BTM) and Integra((R)) dermal regeneration template (DRT). Burns 42(5):1088–1096
93. Fourman MS, Phillips BT, Fritz JR, Conkling N, McClain SA, Simon M, Dagum AB (2014) Laser-assisted indocyanine green dye angiography accurately predicts the split-thickness graft timing of integra artificial dermis. Ann Plast Surg 73(2):150–155
94. Guldberg RE, Oest M, Lin AS, Ito H, Chao X, Gromov K, Goater JJ, Koefoed M, Schwarz EM, O'Keefe RJ, Zhang X (2004) Functional integration of tissue-engineered bone constructs. J Musculoskelet Neuronal Interact 4(4):399–400
95. Kim PJ, Attinger CE, Steinberg JS, Evans KK (2014) Integra(R) bilayer wound matrix application for complex lower extremity soft tissue reconstruction. Surg Technol Int 24:65–73
96. Lee SM, Stewart CL, Miller CJ, Chu EY (2015) The histopathologic features of Integra(R) dermal regeneration template. J Cutan Pathol 42(5):368–369
97. Vithlani G, Santos Jorge P, Brizman E, Mitsimponas K (2017) Integra((R)) as a single-stage dermal regeneration template in reconstruction of large defects of the scalp. Br J Oral Maxillofac Surg 55(8):844–846
98. Wosgrau AC, Jeremias Tda S, Leonardi DF, Pereima MJ, Di Giunta G, Trentin AG (2015) Comparative experimental study of wound healing in mice: Pelnac versus Integra. PLoS One 10(3):e0120322
99. Harding K, Sumner M, Cardinal M (2013) A prospective, multicentre, randomised controlled study of human fibroblast-derived dermal substitute (Dermagraft) in patients with venous leg ulcers. Int Wound J 10(2):132–137
100. Hart CE, Loewen-Rodriguez A, Lessem J (2012) Dermagraft: use in the treatment of chronic wounds. Adv Wound Care 1(3):138–141
101. Marston WA (2004) Dermagraft, a bioengineered human dermal equivalent for the treatment of chronic nonhealing diabetic foot ulcer. Expert Rev Med Devices 1(1):21–31
102. Browne AC, Vearncombe M, Sibbald RG (2001) High bacterial load in asymptomatic diabetic patients with neurotrophic ulcers retards wound healing after application of Dermagraft. Ostomy Wound Manage 47(10):44–49
103. Edmonds ME, Foster AV, McColgan M (1997) 'Dermagraft': a new treatment for diabetic foot ulcers. Diabet Med 14(12):1010–1011
104. Spielvogel RL (1997) A histological study of Dermagraft-TC in patients' burn wounds. J Burn Care Rehabil 18(1 Pt 2):S16–S18
105. Purdue GF (1997) Dermagraft-TC pivotal efficacy and safety study. J Burn Care Rehabil 18(1 Pt 2):S13–S14
106. Purdue GF, Hunt JL, Still JM Jr, Law EJ, Herndon DN, Goldfarb IW, Schiller WR, Hansbrough JF, Hickerson WL, Himel HN, Kealey GP et al (1997) A multicenter clinical trial of a biosynthetic skin replacement, Dermagraft-TC, compared with cryopreserved human cadaver skin for temporary coverage of excised burn wounds. J Burn Care Rehabil 18(1 Pt 1):52–57
107. Hansbrough JF, Mozingo DW, Kealey GP, Davis M, Gidner A, Gentzkow GD (1997) Clinical trials of a biosynthetic temporary skin replacement, Dermagraft-transitional covering, compared with cryopreserved human cadaver skin for temporary coverage of excised burn wounds. J Burn Care Rehabil 18(1 Pt 1):43–51
108. Gentzkow GD, Iwasaki SD, Hershon KS, Mengel M, Prendergast JJ, Ricotta JJ, Steed DP, Lipkin S (1996) Use of dermagraft, a cultured human dermis, to treat diabetic foot ulcers. Diabetes Care 19(4):350–354
109. Economou TP, Rosenquist MD, Lewis RW 2nd, Kealey GP (1995) An experimental study to

determine the effects of Dermagraft on skin graft viability in the presence of bacterial wound contamination. J Burn Care Rehabil 16(1):27–30
110. Burlew CC, Moore EE, Cuschieri J, Jurkovich GJ, Codner P, Crowell K, Nirula R, Haan J, Rowell SE, Kato CM, MacNew H, Ochsner MG et al (2011) Sew it up! A western trauma association multi-institutional study of enteric injury management in the postinjury open abdomen. J Trauma 70(2):273–277
111. Diaz JJ Jr, Cullinane DC, Dutton WD, Jerome R, Bagdonas R, Bilaniuk JW, Collier BR, Como JJ, Cumming J, Griffen M, Gunter OL, Kirby J, Lottenburg L et al (2010) The management of the open abdomen in trauma and emergency general surgery: part 1-damage control. J Trauma 68(6):1425–1438
112. Diaz JJ Jr, Cullinane DC, Khwaja KA, Tyson GH, Ott M, Jerome R, Kerwin AJ, Collier BR, Pappas PA, Sangosanya AT et al (2013) Eastern association for the surgery of trauma: management of the open abdomen, part III-review of abdominal wall reconstruction. J Trauma Acute Care Surg 75(3):376–386
113. Diaz JJ Jr, Dutton WD, Ott MM, Cullinane DC, Alouidor R, Armen SB, Bilanuik JW, Collier BR, Gunter OL et al (2011) Eastern Association for the Surgery of trauma: a review of the management of the open abdomen – part 2 “Management of the open abdomen”. J Trauma 71(2):502–512
114. Johnston M, Safcsak K, Cheatham ML, Smith CP (2015) Management of the open abdomen in obese trauma patients. Am Surg 81(11):1134–1137
115. Abstracts of the Annual Congress of the British Society for Immunology. December 5-8, 2011, Liverpool, United Kingdom (2011). Immunology, 135(Suppl 1):1–228
116. Anas A, Paul S, Jayaprakash NS, Philip R, Bright Singh IS (2005) Antimicrobial activity of chitosan against vibrios from freshwater prawn Macrobrachium rosenbergii larval rearing systems. Dis Aquatic Organ 67(1–2):177–179
117. Kumar MN, Muzzarelli RA, Muzzarelli C, Sashiwa H, Domb AJ (2004) Chitosan chemistry and pharmaceutical perspectives. Chem Rev 104(12):6017–6084
118. Kurita K (2006) Chitin and chitosan: functional biopolymers from marine crustaceans. Mar Biotechnol 8(3):203–226
119. Larraneta E, Henry M, Irwin NJ, Trotter J, Perminova AA, Donnelly RF (2018) Synthesis and characterization of hyaluronic acid hydrogels crosslinked using a solvent-free process for potential biomedical applications. Carbohydr Polym 181:1194–1205
120. Law N, Doney B, Glover H, Qin Y, Aman ZM, Sercombe TB, Liew LJ, Dilley RJ, Doyle BJ (2018) Characterisation of hyaluronic acid methylcellulose hydrogels for 3D bioprinting. J Mech Behav Biomed Mater 77:389–399
121. Lou J, Stowers R, Nam S, Xia Y, Chaudhuri O (2018) Stress relaxing hyaluronic acid-collagen hydrogels promote cell spreading, fiber remodeling, and focal adhesion formation in 3D cell culture. Biomaterials 154:213–222
122. Ma X, Xu T, Chen W, Qin H, Chi B, Ye Z (2018) Injectable hydrogels based on the hyaluronic acid and poly (gamma-glutamic acid) for controlled protein delivery. Carbohydr Polym 179:100–109
123. Payne WM, Svechkarev D, Kyrychenko A, Mohs AM (2018) The role of hydrophobic modification on hyaluronic acid dynamics and self-assembly. Carbohydr Polym 182:132–141
124. Westbrook AW, Ren X, Moo-Young M, Chou CP (2018) Engineering of cell membrane to enhance heterologous production of hyaluronic acid in Bacillus subtilis. Biotechnol Bioeng 115(1):216–231
125. Loos MS, Freeman BG, Lorenzetti A (2010) Zone of injury: a critical review of the literature. Ann Plast Surg 65(6):573–577

Part III

Wound Management

Negative-Pressure Wound Therapy for Large Burn Wounds

David E. Varon, Jessica D. Smith, Riyam Mistry, Neel A. Kantak, and Eric G. Halvorson

1 Introduction

Over the last 20 years, negative-pressure wound therapy (NPWT) has become a widely used and well-described treatment for acute and chronic wounds. NPWT works by removing exudate, creating a sterile and moist environment, increasing diffusion of blood and nutrients to the wound, and promoting re-epithelialization of the damaged tissue [1–3]. NPWT has been used to treat a wide variety of wounds including diabetic foot ulcers, pressure ulcers, sternal wounds, open abdominal wounds following peritonitis and abdominal aneurysm rupture, severe open fractures of the lower extremities, and burns. Additionally, it is frequently used to prepare a wound bed for skin grafting and then as a bolster dressing to enhance skin graft take [1]. Until recently, however, NPWT has been most commonly used on smaller burns. Extra-large (XL) NPWT, used to treat burn wounds ≥15% TBSA, is relatively new and has been described sporadically in existing literature [4].

Steinstraesser et al. [5] first described XL-NPWT in a 2009 case report. In this report, NPWT was used to secure split-thickness skin grafts (STSGs) covering 18% of the patient's body following multiple debridements to eradicate fulminant necrotizing fasciitis. After 7 days, the authors reported a 90% graft take and determined that NPWT is a treatment option for large skin-grafted areas. In 2010, Chong et al. [6] were the first to report that XL-NPWT is an ideal option for treating burn patients with wounds ≥15% TBSA. Since then, several studies have further discussed the use of XL-NPWT for large burns [4, 7–9]. Randomized studies regarding the effectiveness of XL-NPWT have yet to be conducted. However, the reported benefits of XL-NPWT are so encouraging that it should be considered as a treatment option for large wounds [4]. This chapter will discuss when and how to utilize XL-NPWT, as well as the benefits of this technique in managing large burn wounds.

D. E. Varon (✉)
University of Michigan Medical School, Ann Arbor, MI, USA
e-mail: dvaron@umich.edu

J. D. Smith
University of Utah School of Medicine, Salt Lake City, UT, USA

R. Mistry
Department of Plastic Surgery, Royal Devon and Exeter Hospital, NHS Foundation Trust, Exeter, UK

N. A. Kantak
Department of Plastic Surgery, Mid-Atlantic Permanente Medical Group, Upper Malboro, MD, USA

E. G. Halvorson
Plastic Surgery Center of Asheville, Asheville, NC, USA

Recent Clinical Techniques, Results, and Research in Wounds (2018)
https://doi.org/10.1007/15695_2018_112, © Springer International Publishing AG
Published Online: 05 July 2018

2 Advantages of XL-NPWT for Large Burns

Although NPWT has been utilized to treat a plethora of acute and chronic wounds, XL-NPWT has only recently been described as a treatment for large burn wounds and as a bolster dressing for extensive STSGs. As the most common cause of wounds ≥15% TBSA are burns, the current literature focuses primarily on the indications for XL-NPWT in the management of burn wounds [4, 6–9]. Large burns damage the skin, suppress the body's immune response, and cause extreme fluid shifts. XL-NPWT aims to address these effects and should be utilized to prevent infection, promote re-epithelialization, and aid in estimating fluid loss so that fluid resuscitation can be more precise and effective. There are numerous secondary benefits of using NPWT for large burns that will also be discussed.

3 Infection Prevention

When a thermal or chemical burn occurs, the skin, which serves as the body's primary barrier and first line of defense to pathogens, is compromised. Microorganisms from the patient's skin, gastrointestinal system, respiratory system, and external environment immediately enter the burned area. These microbes utilize the protein exudate that the wound produces to colonize the area within the first 48 h following injury. Microbial colonization does not always lead to infection, but the microorganisms can certainly cause serious and life-threatening infections [10–12]. Severe burns damage the subdermal plexus of vessels, impairing the body's ability to deliver erythrocytes and immune cells to the wound [4, 13–16]. Furthermore, the body decreases its production of granulocytes and monocytes [10, 17] and simultaneously releases inflammatory mediators, which induce immunosuppression, increase vascular permeability, and shift fluid to extravascular spaces [4, 18–20]. As a result, the body's ability to prevent and fight infection is greatly impaired following a large burn, and burn patients are susceptible to infection-related mortality. Sepsis due to burn wound infections or infectious complications cause approximately 75% of deaths in patients who suffer >40% TBSA burns [10].

To effectively treat a burn, it is therefore paramount that the risk of infection be reduced. Traditional burn dressings are changed in a nonsterile environment. Despite antimicrobial additives, there is often significant colonization evident at each dressing change. Such dressings do not maintain a sterile wound environment. As bacteria colonizing burn wounds cause the majority of infections in burn patients, it is possible that maintaining a more sterile wound-healing environment would reduce the risk of such infections. XL-NPWT dressings are placed in a sterile environment (the operating room), with the occlusive dressing and negative pressure effectively sealing off the wound [4]. These dressings are not changed on a daily basis, thus preventing continued colonization of the wounds. It is our belief that maintaining a more sterile wound environment may lead to improved wound healing and a lower risk of infection.

4 Promoting Re-epithelialization

Re-epithelialization is integral to wound healing. However, after a burn has occurred and dermal vessels have been damaged, the body's ability to create new epithelial tissue is impaired [4]. Re-epithelialization requires wound neovascularization and increased blood flow, so damage of the dermal vessels is particularly detrimental. Treatment of burns, therefore, needs to promote angiogenesis in order to enhance re-epithelialization and burn wound healing [21]. This is particularly important because studies have shown that epithelialization of deep wounds is frequently inhibited and, as a result, a patient's risk of infectious morbidity and mortality is increased [4, 22]. Additionally, burn wounds tend to require autologous skin grafting procedures, which create donor sites. STSG donor sites can be painful and debilitating and should be treated in a manner that promotes healing and reduces pain [9]. All too often, donor sites are neglected and treated in ways we would never treat a burn wound (e.g., leaving them open to air).

A patient's survival is undeniably linked to the take and success of the skin grafts, so wound dressings need to promote graft survival and take. NPWT has been shown to promote angiogenesis and, in turn, wound healing [22]. Improved angiogenesis allows for blood, nutrients, growth factors, and cytokines to be delivered more efficiently and in greater quantities to the wound, and multiple studies have reported that wound healing is enhanced as a result [21, 23–26]. Given the dangerous nature of large burns and the fact that they frequently require skin grafting procedures, optimizing re-epithelialization is an important goal.

XL-NPWT has shown to enhance graft take with reports of 95% [7] and 97% [4] graft take. A prospective randomized controlled trial by Petkar et al. [27] comparing the use of NPWT to standard dressings in 30 burn patients found that mean graft take was higher in the NPWT group than in the control group (96.7% vs. 87.5%, $p < 0.001$) on STSGS. Normally larger burns, especially those involving areas that experience shear forces (e.g., mobile joints, posterior trunk, the perineum, etc.), have higher rates of graft loss. XL-NPWT, in particular the traditional technique described by Fischer et al. [4], addresses the issue of shear force by protecting these vulnerable areas with two layers of occlusive dressing and securing it with sutures or staples. It is postulated that XL-NPWT also improves graft take by preventing shifting or "floating" of skin grafts. The constant removal of exudate precludes fluid from accumulating under the graft and, therefore, allows for contact between the skin graft and wound bed to be maintained [7]. The removal of exudate allows for the dressing to stay fixed in one location, reducing external shear and patient pain [9]. Additionally, removing the exudate may accelerate re-epithelialization because it eliminates an extrinsic impediment of microcirculation and improves the area's blood supply [7, 28, 29]. NPWT creates mechanical tension, which may encourage cell proliferation and the formation of granulation tissue. However, Fischer et al. suggest that increased graft take may not be seen when the "total body wrap" concept is utilized because sponges are not placed to cover all grafted areas; use of the traditional method of application is, therefore, encouraged [4, 28, 30].

Rapid healing of autograft donor sites is also important to consider in terms of pain, given the associated pain levels that patients frequently report and the potential need to use the same donor sites for further skin grafts [9]. Genecov et al. [31] investigated re-epithelialization of donor sites in both a porcine and human model, and found that NPWT significantly increased the rate of re-epithelialization compared to an adhesive film dressing (OpSite, Smith and Nephew, UK) dressing. Similar to the reasons for improved graft take, they report that the enhanced healing rate may be due to the mechanical forces provided by the vacuum, which improve angiogenesis, and/or the removal of third-space fluid and wound exudate, which allows for restored local blood flow. Although Genecov et al. [31] did not investigate XL-NPWT and its effects on larger wounds; it is likely that the benefits seen with the smaller donor sites are similar to those for larger donor sites. Further investigation of donor and recipient site re-epithelialization due to XL-NPWT is necessary, as is the effect of healing and patients' length of stay.

5 Fluid Management

Large burns disturb the body's ability to maintain fluid homeostasis. Fluid loss, especially burn shock, must be treated effectively to reduce morbidity and mortality. Fluid resuscitation plays an integral role in this treatment [22]. However, there are a wide variety of resuscitation protocols, and it can be difficult to determine the amount of fluid resuscitation necessary to treat individual patients [22, 32]. Currently fluid loss and resuscitation are estimated with a variety of parameters including body weight, heart rate, blood pressure, urine output, and laboratory values [4]. Though useful, these parameters are imprecise and can lead to over- or under-resuscitation, which can cause pulmonary edema, acute kidney injury, renal failure, and death [4, 33–36]. To further complicate fluid management, the amount of fluids that a patient needs tend to fluctuate. Fluid resuscitation is most crucial immediately following a burn, after surgical debridement, and following autologous skin grafting because the affected body surface area is increased by the addition of donor sites [4, 37]. Given the complicated nature of fluid management following a burn, a more accurate method for estimating fluid loss would be beneficial.

XL-NPWT, addresses these problems by consistently removing exudate and maintaining a beneficial healing environment with minimal dressing changes. Fischer et al. state that burn patients with ≥15% TBSA burns required a maximum of two dressing changes, while Low et al. [8], Chong et al. [6], and Kamolz et al. [7] report dressing changes once every 4 days [4, 6–8]. A reduction in dressing changes decreases the amount of tedious work that nurses have to perform and, most importantly, has been associated with a decrease in patients' anxiety and pain according to nurses involved in their care [9]. Kantak et al. [9] also suggest that patient-reported pain levels may be lower overall with XL-NPWT because NPWT may modify the inflammatory response, which modulates pain perception, and decreases the amount of shear on affected areas. Lastly, Fischer et al. [4] and Kamolz et al. [7] reported no infections when XL-NPWT was utilized.

When using standard dressings on patients with large burns, insensible fluid loss through the wounds is both significant and difficult to estimate. The classic calculation for insensible losses is inherently inaccurate, as it does not take into account differences in fluid losses for different size burns and the change in rate of fluid loss over time. Although studies have not been conducted to specifically evaluate the use of XL-NPWT as a method for estimating and treating fluid loss, the studies conducted by Fischer et al. [4] and Chong et al. [6] have noted that XL-NPWT may aid in determining the proper amount of fluid resuscitation. Low et al. [8] also suggest that utilizing XL-NPWT is beneficial because fewer VAC machines are needed, which makes charting fluid output more convenient and accurate. Fischer et al. [4] utilized the VAC output measurements to assess fluid management and found that average fluid loss was highest on day 1 after grafting and declined with time. They also found that donor sites produced more than twice as much output as recipient sites. Similarly, Lamke and Liljedahl [38] reported that fluid loss was three times higher from donor sites compared to recipient sites. This information may be useful to other burn centers as they try to determine the amount of required fluid resuscitation. It should be noted, however, that Fischer et al. [4] had two patients develop acute kidney injuries, which they report may be due to a lack of experience estimating fluid needs based on XL-NPWT outputs [4, 38]. Ultimately, with proper technique, XL-NPWT has the potential to improve fluid management by providing ICU teams with a more accurate determination of insensible losses that can be incorporated into clinical decision-making.

6 Techniques

There are two previously described methods of application for XL-NPWT in existing literature. Chong et al. [6] describe the "total body wrap" or "sandwich" technique, in which affected areas are sandwiched between large polyurethane dressings. Small slits are made in the dressing away from the grafted areas, and small sponges are placed to act as wicks for the exudative fluid. The sponges are placed away from the grafts so as to avoid disrupting the grafts and to allow for easy visualization of the wounds through the dressing. The polyurethane dressings adhere to one another around the periphery and create a seal when suction is applied. They recommend initially applying negative pressure at 250 mmHg and then decreasing the pressure to 125 mmHg after the seal is created. Low et al. [8] (from the same burn center) further describe this technique and suggest placing long, thin strips of NPWT sponges to span the entire length of an affected limb. They also recommend placing the suction tubing in a dependent position and intraoperatively connecting it to wall suction to improve the vacuum seal and enhance wound exudate clearance. Postoperatively, the suction can be transferred to a NPWT vacuum machine unit and set on 125 mmHg.

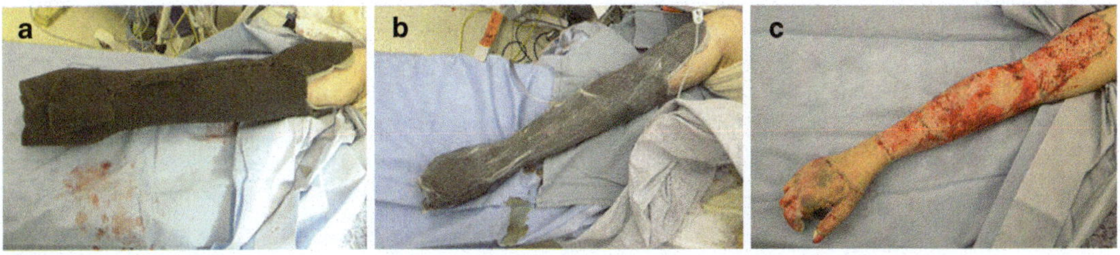

Fig. 1 (**a**) Modified technique of NPWT applied to an STSG recipient site on the right arm. (**b**) Covered with occlusive dressing to obtain a seal. (**c**) Showing skin graft take after NPWT is removed

7 The Brigham and Women's Hospital Experience

At our institution we employed a different, more traditional technique with the intent of improving graft fixation [4]. Initially, nonadherent fine mesh gauze (N-TERFACE, Winfield Laboratories, Richardson, Texas, USA, and/or Xeroform Covidien, Mansfield, MA, USA) was contoured to match the affected area and used to cover graft recipient sites, while silver-impregnated nonadherent foam (Mepilex Ag, Molnlycke Health Care, Gothenburg, Sweden) was similarly contoured and used to cover donor sites [4]. Recently we simplified this technique. Silver-impregnated nonadherent foam (Mepilex Ag, Molnlycke Health Care, Gothenburg, Sweden) is applied to both recipient and donor sites, as well as over any intervening intact skin or burn wound. This allows for an entire body area to be covered safely with the two-layered dressing [9], without the need for contouring, greatly simplifying the dressing application process. Extremities can simply be wrapped circumferentially. NPWT sponges (V.A.C. GranuFoam, KCI, San Antonio, TX, and/or Ioban, 3M, St. Paul, MN) are then applied to cover the area completely, transparent self-adhesive drapes (V.A.C. Drape, KCI, San Antonio, TX, and/or Ioban, 3M, St. Paul, MN) are placed, and a suction pad (Sensa T.R.A.C. Pad, KCI, San Antonio, TX) is attached (Fig. 1) [4, 9].

On the extremities and in areas of shear or moisture (e.g., perineum, non-excised burn, open tissue), however, additional strategies are necessary to maintain the seal. For the limb, tincture of benzoin is applied to dry, healthy skin, and then the limb NPWT sponges are then sandwiched between large sheets of occlusive dressing. Wall suction is utilized to create the initial seal and more difficult areas are sealed last to ensure complete seal. For areas of shear or moisture, two layers of occlusive dressing are applied and secured to the tissues with staples or sutures (Fig. 2). Suction pads are placed strategically in the most dependent areas, and one suction pump (V.A.C. Therapy Unit, KCI, San Antonio, TX) is utilized for every 9% TBSA involved, as seen in Figs. 3 and 4 [4]. Similar to Chong et al. and Low et al., the machine is set to apply negative pressure at 125 mmHg [4, 6, 8]. If the machine cannot maintain the seal and standard troubleshooting does not identify any problems, the suction pad can be switched to wall suction [4].

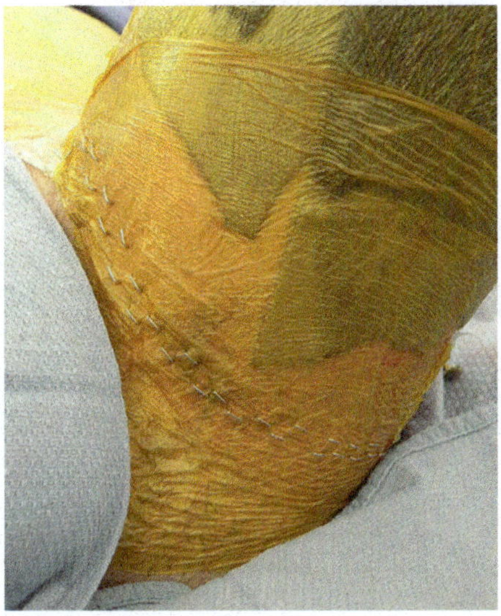

Fig. 2 Application of modified technique of NPWT to the groin area: in this case two layers of occlusive dressing and two rows of staples facilitate the maintenance of a seal to overcome shear forces and moisture

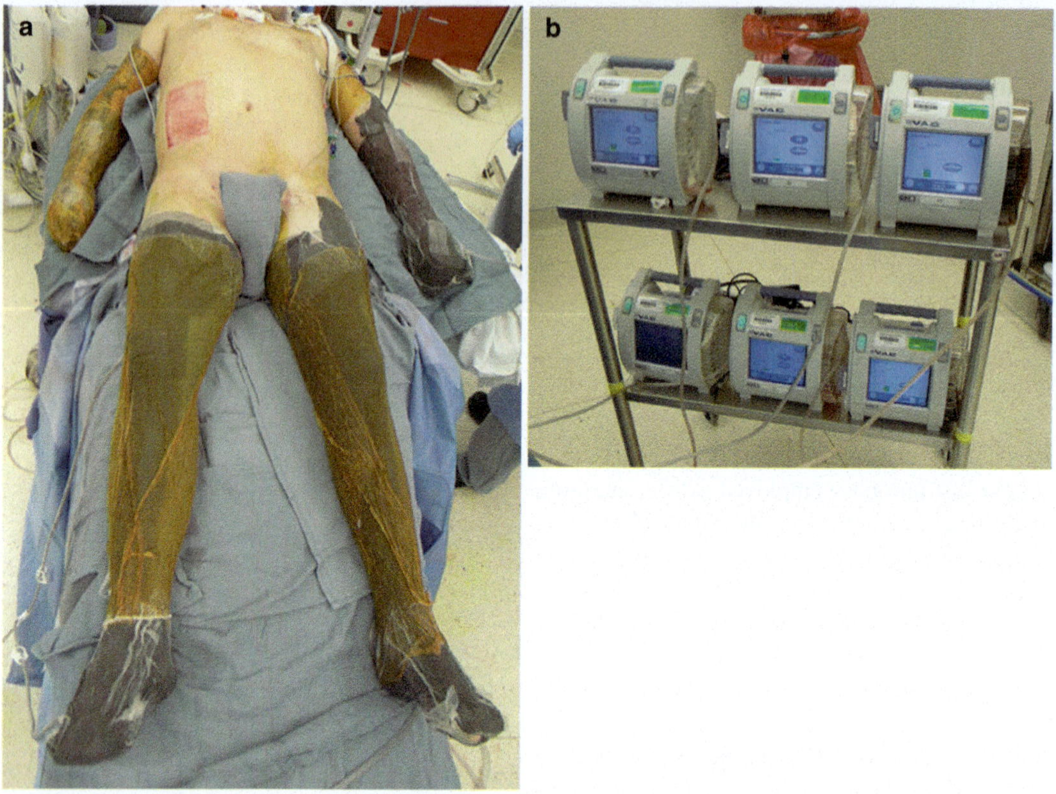

Fig. 3 (**a**) Application of extra-large NPWT dressing: in this case a seal was obtained by sandwiching extremities between large sheets of occlusive dressing. (**b**) Applying suction pads to the most dependent areas, with one pump used per arm and two pumps per leg

The use of NPWT to treat various burn and donor site wounds has become a loved technique in the burn unit at the Brigham and Women's Hospital (BWH). In our preliminary study of XL-NPWT for large burn wounds, 12 patients had a graft take average of 97% with the STSG donor sites re-epithelializing in an average of 11.25 days, which corroborates the study by Genecov et al., which showed that NPWT enhanced donor site re-epithelialization [4, 30]. Our graft take results were similar to those achieved by Petkar et al. [27], although our burn wounds were much greater than the 10% TBSA burns in their study.

The length of stay (LOS) for our patients averaged 37.9 days (median 32.5, range 19–66), and all patients survived without any wound infections. Although our sample size is too small to make reliable conclusions on the effect of LOS, the two patients who had burns of TBSA>35%, their LOS was found to be shorter than the American Burn Association's burn respiratory national averages (39 vs. 62 days and 50 vs. 68 days, respectively).

Surgeons and nurses in the burn unit noted a considerable decrease in pain and anxiety experienced by patients when compared to the standard of care. Although most patients experience very little to no pain following surgery, pain is intrinsically related to dressing changes. Most patients experience increased pain after the dressing is removed at 5–7 days. Decreased pain exhibited by patients who received NPWT as a burn dressing suggests that NPWT modifies the inflammatory response that modulates pain perception or that the lack of motion and sheer minimizes pain [4].

As reported by Fischer et al. [4] and Lamke and Liljedahl [38], the results from our study followed a similar trend [38]. Fluid outputs from the wounds during the first 5 days of grafting aver-

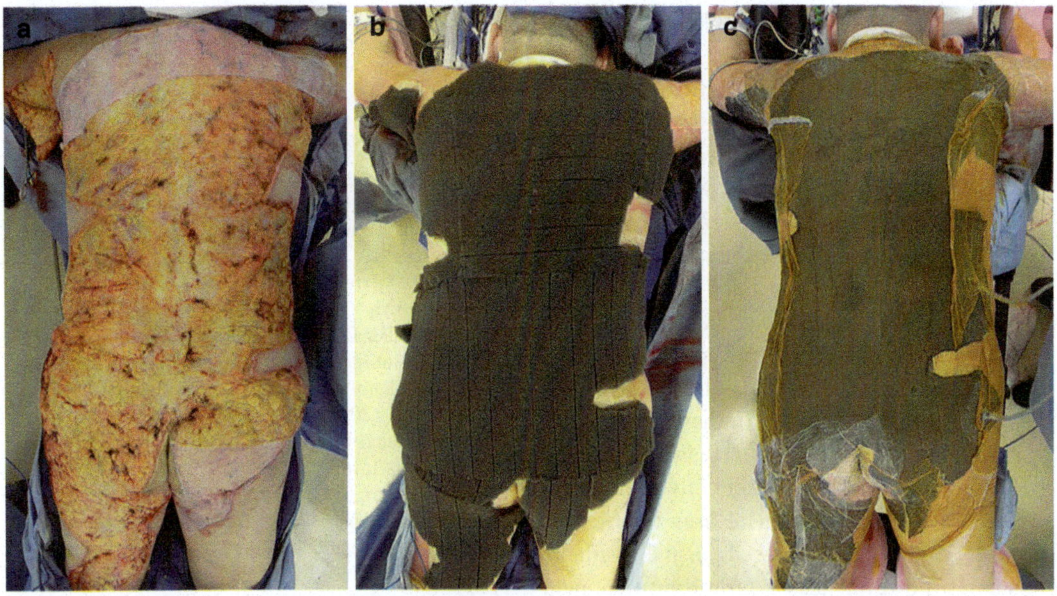

Fig. 4 (**a**) Application of extra-large NPWT dressing: large campfire burn of the posterior trunk and buttocks. (**b**) Covered with xeno- and autografts followed by a microporous nonadherent foam with a silicone contact layer followed by conventional NPWT sponge. (**c**) Proximal thighs were then circumferentially wrapped and sealed using an occlusive dressing sandwich technique, and staples/sutures were used in the perineum. This seal held for 6 days

aged 101 ± 66 mL/%TBSA covered per day. Average output for the donor sites was double that of the recipient site at 132 ± 83 mL/%TBSA vs. 61 ± 37 mL/%TBSA, respectively. These numbers can be used to predict fluid loss from burn wounds covered with NPWT dressings, although measuring actual output is obviously more accurate.

Two of our patients developed acute kidney (AKI) injury that was resolved, and one patient developed a hematoma within 12 h of surgery that was quickly evacuated without further complications. The development of AKI may have been due to a lack of experience in using XL-NPWT and an underestimation of fluid loss. On the other end of the fluid resuscitation spectrum, however, none of our patients developed lung edema from over-resuscitation, and they were able to discontinue manual ventilation earlier than burn patients in other studies, although our study is too small to perform meaningful statistical analysis.

We ultimately found that our modified NPWT dressing is a safe and effective dressing for treating large burn wounds, and a technology-based improvement for patients, nurses, and surgeons alike.

Conclusions

Though relatively new, XL-NPWT has proven to be safe and effective in treating burns ≥15% TBSA. To date, there are no randomized studies that have proven the benefits of XL-NPWT; however, early results suggest that XL-NPWT may have multiple benefits including decreasing a patient's risk of infection, improving healing of donor and recipient sites, decreasing the number of necessary dressing changes, and aiding in more accurate fluid resuscitation. Numerous secondary benefits have also been observed. Most importantly, we have noted that patients have greatly reduced pain following debridement and grafting procedures, particularly at the donor sites. Because of this, and because dressings are not changed daily, patients require much less narcotic and potentially less ventilator time. This has the potential to decrease morbidity related to prolonged ICU/ventilator time and large quantity narcotic use.

Although there is a lack of literature regarding the use XL-NPWT, the initial literature suggests that it is safe, effective, and with benefits when treating patients who have burns ≥15% TBSA. XL-NPWT seems to reduce the risk of infection, improve the rate of re-epithelialization of both donor and recipient sites, reduce the number of necessary dressing changes and associated pain and anxiety, and allow for more effective fluid resuscitation. Further investigation into these benefits is warranted, as is further research regarding length of stay, the cost-effective nature of XL-NPWT, and its clinical uses for treating other large wounds. Based on the available studies, however, it is a promising treatment option for wounds ≥15% TBSA.

References

1. Orgill DP, Bayer LR (2011) Update on negative-pressure wound therapy. Plast Reconstr Surg 127(Suppl 1):105S–115S
2. Wang X, Zhang Y, Han C (2014) Topical negative pressure improves autograft take by altering nutrient diffusion: a hypothesis. Med Sci Monit 20:61–63
3. Xia CY, Yu AX, Qi B, Zhou M, Li ZH, Wang WY (2014) Analysis of blood flow and local expression of angiogenesis associated growth factors in infected wounds treated with negative pressure wound therapy. Mol Med Rep 9:1759–1754
4. Fischer S, Wall J, Pomahac B, Riviello R, Halvorson EG (2016) Extra-large negative pressure wound therapy dressings for burns – initial experience with technique, fluid management, and outcomes. Burns 42(2):457–465
5. Steinstraesser L, Sand M, Steinau HU (2009) Giant VAC in a patient with extensive necrotizing fasciitis. Int J Low Extrem Wounds 8(1):28–30
6. Chong SJ, Liang WH, Tan BK (2010) Use of multiple VAC devices in the management of extensive burns: the total body wrap concept. Burns 36(7):e127–e129
7. Kamolz LP, Lumenta DB, Parvizi D, Wiedner M, Justich I, Keck M, Pfurtscheller K, Schintler M (2014) Skin graft fixation in severe burns: use of topical negative pressure. Ann Burns Fire Disasters 27(3):141–145
8. Low OW, Chong SJ, Tan BK (2013) The enhanced total body wrap – the new frontier in dressing care for burns. Burns 39(7):1420–1422
9. Kantak NA, Mistry R, Halvorson EG (2016) A review of negative-pressure wound therapy in the management of burn wounds. Burns 42(8):1623–1633
10. Church D, Elsayed S, Reid O, Winston B, Lindsay R (2006) Burn wound infections. Clin Microbiol Rev 19(2):403–434
11. Erol S, Altoparlak U, Akcay MN, Celebi F, Parlak M (2004) Changes of microbial flora and wound colonization in burned patients. Burns 30(4):357–361
12. Sheridan RL (2000) Evaluating and managing burn wounds. Dermatol Nurs 12(1):17–18 21–28
13. Watts AM, Tyler MP, Perry ME, Roberts AH, McGrouther DA (2001) Burn depth and its histological measurement. Burns 27(2):154–160
14. Papp A, Kiraly K, Harma M, Lahtinen T, Uusaro A, Alhava E (2004) The progression of burn depth in experimental burns: a histological and methodological study. Burns 30(7):684–690
15. Kloppenberg FW, Beerthuizen GI, ten Duis HJ (2001) Perfusion of burns wounds assessed by laser Doppler imaging is related to burn depth and healing time. Burns 27(4):359–363
16. Monstrey S, Hoeksema H, Verbelen J, Pirayesh A, Blondeel P (2008) Assessment of burn depth and burn wound healing potential. Burns 34(6):761–769
17. Gamelli RL, He LK, Liu H (1994) Marrow granulocyte-macrophage progenitor cell response to burn injury as modified by endotoxin and indomethacin. J Trauma 37(3):339–346
18. Kim GH, Oh KH, Yoon JW, Koo JW, Kim HJ, Chae DW, Noh JW, Kim JH, Park YK (2003) Impact of burn size and initial serum albumin level on acute renal failure occurring in major burn. Am J Nephrol 23(1):55–60
19. Demling RH, Kramer G, Harms B (1984) Role of thermal injury-induced hypoproteinemia on fluid flux and permeability in burned and nonburned tissue. Surgery 95(2):136–144
20. Lehnhardt M, Jafari HJ, Druecke D, Steinstraesser L, Steinau HU, Klatte W, Schwake R, Homann HH (2005) A qualitative and quantitative analysis of protein loss in human burn wounds. Burns 31(2):159–167
21. Ma Z, Shou K, Li Z, Jian C, Qi B, Yu A (2016) Negative pressure wound therapy promotes vessel destabilization and maturation at various stages of wound healing and thus influences wound prognosis. Exp Ther Med 11(4):1307–1317
22. Rex S (2012) Burn injuries. Curr Opin Crit Care 18(6):671–676
23. Greene AK, Puder M, Roy R, Arsenault D, Kwei S, Moses MA, Orgill DP (2006) Microdeformational wound therapy: effects on angiogenesis and matrix metalloproteinases in chronic wounds of 3 debilitated patients. Ann Plast Surg 56(4):418–422
24. Chen SZ, Li J, Li XY, Xu LS (2005) Effects of vacuum-assisted closure on wound microcirculation: an experimental study. Asian J Surg 28(3):211–217

25. Grimm A, Dimmler A, Stange S, Labanaris A, Sauer R, Grabenbauer G, Horch RE (2007) Expression of HIF-1 alpha in irradiated tissue is altered by topical negative-pressure therapy. Strahlenther Onkol 183(3):144–149
26. Labler L, Rancan M, Mica L, Harter L, Mihic-Probst D, Keel M (2009) Vacuum-assisted closure therapy increases local interleukin-8 and vascular endothelial growth factor levels in traumatic wounds. J Trauma 66(3):749–757
27. Petkar KS, Dhanraj P, Kingsly PM, Sreekar H, Lakshmanarao A, Lamba S, Shetty R, Zachariah JR (2011) A prospective randomized controlled trial comparing negative pressure dressing and conventional dressing methods on split-thickness skin grafts in burned patients. Burns 37(6):925–929
28. Moisidis E, Heath T, Boorer C, Ho K, Deva AK (2004) A prospective, blinded, randomized, controlled clinical trial of topical negative pressure use in skin grafting. Plast Reconstr Surg 114(4):917–922
29. Banwell PE, Musgrave M (2004) Topical negative pressure therapy: mechanisms and indications. Int Wound J 1(2):95–106
30. Kamolz LP, Andel H, Haslik W, Winter W, Meissl G, Frey M (2004) Use of subatmospheric pressure therapy to prevent burn wound progression in human: first experiences. Burns 30(3):253–258
31. Genecov DG, Schneider AM, Morykwas MJ, Parker D, White WL, Argenta LC (1998) A controlled subatmospheric pressure dressing increases the rate of skin graft donor site reepithelialization. Ann Plast Surg 40(3):219–225
32. Greenhalgh DG (2010) Burn resuscitation: the results of the ISBI/ABA survey. Burns 36:176–182
33. Fahlstrom K, Boyle C, Makic MB (2013) Implementation of a nurse-driven burn resuscitation protocol: a quality improvement project. Crit Care Nurse 33(1):25–35
34. Walker TL, Rodriguez DU, Coy K, Hollen LI, Greenwood R, Young AE (2014) Impact of reduced resuscitation fluid on outcomes of children with 10-20% body surface area scalds. Burns 40(8):1581–1586
35. Imm A, Carlson RW (1993) Fluid resuscitation in circulatory shock. Crit Care Clin 9(2):313–333
36. Aboelatta Y, Abdelsalam A (2013) Volume overload of fluid resuscitation in acutely burned patients using transpulmonary thermodilution technique. Burn Care Res 34(3):349–354
37. Boswick JA, Thompson JD, Kershner CJ (1977) Critical care of the burned patient. Anesthesiology 47(2):164–170
38. Lamke LO, Liljedahl SO (1971) Evaporative water loss from burns, grafts and donor sites. Scand J Plast Reconstr Surg 5:17–22

Negative Pressure Wound Therapy for the Treatment of Complex Spinal Wounds

Joseph S. Cheng, Rani Nasser, Brittany Staarmann, George Yang, Juan C. Mejia-Munne, and Justin Gibson

1 Introduction

The treatment of postoperative spinal infections and wound dehiscence, especially if instrumentation is involved, is a costly endeavor not only in financial terms but also in health-related quality of life for patients. Prolonged immobilization due to open wounds places patients at risk for pressure sores, deep vein thrombosis, and pulmonary complications.

Techniques for avoidance of spinal infections include the use of perioperative antibiotics, gentle handling of tissue intraoperatively, as well as the quantity and type of spinal instrumentation used. Titanium bears properties of resistance to glycocalyx (biofilm) formation and decreased inflammation/corrosion as compared to stainless steel [1–3]. Some authors have described good results in treating spinal infections with microbial-guided pharmacotherapy and debridement without removal of titanium instrumentation in conjunction with NPWT [4].

Negative pressure wound therapy (NPWT) has been used for several decades to assist in closure of large or necrotic wounds in general and orthopedic surgery and has recently been demonstrated to be a useful technique for complex spinal wounds. Unfortunately, randomized clinical trials of NPWT in spinal surgery are lacking to guide surgeons in the use of this treatment modality. This chapter is intended to summarize current uses and controversies of NPWT in spine surgery.

2 Mechanisms of NPWT Affecting Wound Healing

The ability of negative pressure wound therapy (NPWT) to improve healing in complex surgical wounds is multifactorial and continues to be elucidated by basic science research and clinical trials. Below are discussed several factors through which NPWT contributes to wound healing.

A negative pressure wound therapy system acts as a sterile barrier and additionally helps debride necrotic tissue from the wound bed [5]. Negative pressure closure improves arteriolar dilation to facilitate microcirculation and decreases excess edema and fluid surrounding wound site helping to decrease bacterial colonization. NPWT also increases granulation tissue formation and accelerates wound healing [6].

NPWT may also help increase antibiotic concentration to the wound bed according to a randomized controlled trial to evaluate antibiotic concentration in wounds in patients undergoing vacuum-assisted closure versus traditional dressing changes. Patients in the study had ulcers

J. S. Cheng (✉) · R. Nasser · B. Staarmann
G. Yang · J. C. Mejia-Munne · J. Gibson
Department of Neurosurgery, University of Cincinnati College of Medicine, Cincinnati, OH, USA
e-mail: chengj6@uc.edu

Recent Clinical Techniques, Results, and Research in Wounds (2018)
https://doi.org/10.1007/15695_2018_115, © Springer International Publishing AG
Published Online: 30 June 2018

infected with daptomycin-sensitive bacteria; biopsies of the lesions were taken to determine concentration of drug at time zero and after wound therapy regimens. Preliminary analysis demonstrated an increase in antibiotic concentration in tissues following VAC therapy compared to traditional therapy [7].

The negative pressure contracts wound edges in large wounds and deceases edema, both mechanisms leading to a decrease in wound size. In a prospective randomized clinical trial of 30 patients with open musculoskeletal injuries at a tertiary care hospital by Sinha et al. [8], patients were randomized to either vacuum-assisted closure (necrotic tissues debrided prior to VAC placement with dressing changes every 3–4 days) versus standard wound therapy (debridement followed by dressing changes daily). The study showed that the size of the soft tissue defects was reduced 5–25 mm (mean decrease of 26.6%) in the vacuum-assisted closure group versus less than 5 mm in patients in the standard therapy group.

3 Indications for Negative Pressure Wound Therapy

Ousey et al. [9] performed a systematic review in 2013 evaluating NPWT for spinal wounds; no randomized controlled trials were available, ten retrospective reviews and four case studies of patients with spinal wound complications. Further research into the indications for NPWT in spinal wounds is indicated.

Studies of NPWT for spinal patients have been primarily focused on those patients who have had postoperative infection. In 2014, Adogwa et al. [6] published a retrospective study comparing the use of NPWT to traditional closure in patients with long-segment (defined as four or more vertebral levels) deformity correction with posterior instrumentation of the thoracolumbar spine. In the treatment arm of the study, a negative pressure device was placed over the incisional area and a continuous −80 mmHg negative pressure wound therapy device was left in place for 3 days postoperatively. Subfascial drains were used in both the control and the treatment arms and were continued until postoperative day #2 or until drain output was less than 80 mL per 24 h. The authors reported that use of negative pressure wound therapy resulted in 50% decrease in incidence of wound dehiscence and approximately 30% reduction in surgical site infections. These findings indicate that use of negative pressure wound therapy as a prophylactic measure in patients undergoing long-segment posterior thoracolumbar fusion may reduce wound dehiscence and surgical site infections. Importantly, there was no significant difference in length of hospital stay or 30-day readmission rates between the two groups.

The use of NPW therapy in high-risk surgical closures in patients with multiple comorbidities was evaluated in a prospective randomized controlled study by Masden et al. [10]. Eighty-one patients were randomized to receive NPW versus traditional closure utilizing silver-impregnated dressing, and there was no statistically significant difference in incidence of infection or dehiscence between the two groups. Of note in this study, 74 of the 81 patients underwent lower extremity closures and results may or may not be generalized to spinal wound closure.

Horn et al. [11] noted that use of NPWT closure in pediatric spinal wounds is good alternative to leaving wound packed between surgical procedures as it acted as continuous barrier in patients with incontinence. This paper also points to importance of monitoring patients with neuromuscular scoliosis (such as those with myelomeningocele) for urinary tract infection prior to operative treatments in order to start appropriate antibiotic regimen prior to surgery to decrease risk of postoperative wound contamination.

The use of negative pressure wound therapy has been demonstrated to be a cost-effective modality in the management of postoperative spinal wound complications by reducing the complexity of surgery needed (decreased instrumentation removal, decreased usage of flap for wound coverage) and by expediting patients' care transition to the outpatient setting [12].

4 Procedure Notes for Negative Pressure Wound Vacuum Placement

The use of NPWV occurs following aggressive debridement and washout of surgical bed. The importance of adequate debridement of necrotic and purulent tissue cannot be overemphasized. An open-pore polyurethane sponge is then prepared to size, and placed into the surgical bed. It is important to remove all infected or devitalized tissue prior to wound vacuum sponge placement. The sponge is ideally placed such that it is adjacent to bone and hardware deep within wound so no cavity is left that could become loculated or re-inhabited by infection. The sponge should not be placed against skin as suction over skin may lead to blistering. A sealant drape is sealed over the sponge and should span at least 5 cm beyond margins of wound to ensure airtight suction. The vacuum pump and collection canister are then connected. The vacuum pump is typically set at 125 mmHg [9]. For patients with exposed dura, the use of a lower negative pressure (50 mmHg) should be considered given risks of cerebrospinal fluid leakage if there is an occult leak [13]. As device is turned on sponge is inspected as it contracts and margins are pulled in toward center from all sides. Ideally, the sponge will cover all tissue where granulation is desired but will avoid contact with the skin.

Dressing changes are performed every 2–3 days. Care must be taken that all components of sponge are removed during dressing changes [14]. The dressing changes may occur at bedside or in operating room depending on patient's ability to tolerate procedure and physician discretion. If dressing changes are to occur at bedside, it is prudent to ensure adequate pain medication and sedation have been given prior to initiating dressing changes. Frequent dressing changes not only allow assessment of the wound but also prevent granulation tissue from growing into the sponge and potentially being traumatized at subsequent dressing changes, thereby compromising the wound. Pediatric patients may have accelerated healing which necessitates more frequent dressing changes than adults to prevent granulation tissue adherence to sponge [15].

Animal studies have demonstrated that optimal healing occurs at 125 mmHg of subatmospheric pressure at interval of 3 min on time followed by 5 min off time. Due to patient discomfort associated with alternating settings (intermittent suction), NPW therapy vacuums are typically set to continuous negative pressure [16].

Duration of NPWT will vary by patient's wound size and response to therapy. Table 1 shows the average durations of VAC therapy and number of dressing changes reported by previous studies [16–19].

Ultimately, the decision for final closure of the wound depends on the patient being medically ready to return to the operating room and on the wound bed having healthy granulation tissue visualized throughout which is amenable to closure [16]. Patients with MRSA or multibacterial infections typically are more likely to need repeat debridement and longer NPWT duration before definitive wound closure [19].

More recently, negative pressure wound therapy with instillation and dwell time (NPWTi-d) has been developed wherein a topical solution is delivered directly over the wound and then is allowed to dwell in the wound bed for programmed amount of time before the negative pressure phase is begun and the solution is removed. There is debate regarding the most appropriate solution to use; however normal saline, Dakin's solution, and polyhexanide solutions have been tried. Further prospective

Table 1 The average durations of VAC therapy and number of dressing changes

Study	Avg. dressing changes	VAC duration
Karaaslan et al., 2015 ($n = 6$)	5.1 (range 3–8)	15.5 days (range 9–24 days)
Mehbod et al., 2005 ($n = 20$)	2.2 (2–3)	7 days (range 5–14 days)
Ploumis et al., 2008 ($n = 73$)	1.4	7 days (range 5–14 days)
Zehnder and Place, 2007 ($n = 11$)	Unreported (approx. q 2–3 days)	26 (range 11–47 days)

randomized clinical trials are warranted to evaluate this technique further; however early studies indicate that this may be a useful option [20].

Systemic antibiotics are frequent utilized in conjunction with wound vacuum closure [9]. Selection of antibiotic regimen should obtain broad-spectrum antimicrobial coverage initially and may be narrowed as cultures demonstrate sensitivities. Should instrumentation be maintained, intravenous antibiotics should be followed by long-term oral suppressive therapy [21].

5 Risks Associated with Negative Pressure Wound Therapy

Skin irritation from adhesive or sponge contact is one of the most commonly reported adverse reactions with NPW therapy. It is estimated that skin irritation occurs in 2.2% of the population treated with vacuum therapy and typically resolves within 48 h [15].

NPWT should not be used in active CSF leak, patients with bleeding diathesis, patients with allergies to NPW dressing, and neoplastic disease in wound [9]. Care and attention is needed to remove all portions of the sponge, given reports of persistent infections due to sponge pieces left in wound [22].

While NPWT should not be used in patients with active CSF leakage, a study by Lee et al. [13] provides evidence that VAC therapy is safe and effective in postoperative spine infections with exposed dura in a retrospective review of prospectively collected data of 40 patients with postoperative wound infections. Thirty-one patients had exposed dura noted at time of washout and 28 had VAC sponge applied directly to dura (wound vac pressure of 50 mmHg, interface of Mepitel, and white foam) with minimum of 1 week of NWP therapy and dressing changes 2–3 days prior to final closure. Nine patients who did not have exposed dura underwent washout and NPW therapy with wound VAC pressure of 125 mmHg. From the 31 patients with dura exposed, two patients died prior to final closure due to unrelated complications and three patients required a muscle flap. All other patients (in both dura exposed and non-exposed groups) achieved wound closure in delayed manner. Of note, study does not mention if there was any concern for CSF leak in patients prior to VAC placement and a decreased suction pressure was used in patients with exposed dura.

Highlighting the importance of not using NPWT in the presence of an active CSF leak is a case report of a 23-year-old patient with open pelvic fracture requiring VAC therapy for wound closure [23]. After initiation of VAC therapy, the patient was noted to have deterioration of neurological status with subsequent imaging showing tear in the dural sac at L5-S1 and CT head demonstrating crowding of basal cisterns and sagging of cerebellar tonsils. Patient required dural patch repair for cerebrospinal fluid leak exacerbated by VAC and had improvement of neurological status following resolution of intracranial hypotension.

6 Care of Patients Undergoing NPWT

Certain aspects of patient care merit specific mention for patients undergoing NPWT. It is important that patients continue to have mobilization regimens unless instability caused by hardware removal precludes activity [14]. Portable NPWT systems are now available which may allow patients to return to home or work.

It is important that patients undergoing VAC therapy have optimization of nutritional parameters. Healing of wounds requires a large amount of energy and protein; additionally vitamin C and iron are needed for proper collagen formation [24]. Additionally, ingrowth of granulation tissue into the foam sponge can lead to wound breakdown and bleeding during dressing change. This complication can be avoided by maintaining regularly scheduled dressing changes [25].

Adequate analgesia is important when wound vacuum dressings are changed. If the patient is unable to tolerate bedside changing of dressings, it may be prudent to return to the operating room for dressing changes. Some papers have even reported returning to the operating room for the first dressing change. It is not uncommon for patients to experience discomfort when the wound vacuum suction is initiated after a dressing change, and patients should be prepared for such.

It is important that caregivers and providers be aware of potential hardware problems which may cause malfunction of the NPWT system. Blockages or leakage of tubes or seals can prevent proper functioning of the system. Overfilling of the collection canister will also lead to poor function of the vacuum system, with unpleasant fluid spillage an added concern. Many NPWT systems have sensing devices to prevent this.

Conclusions

Negative pressure wound therapy (NPWT) is a technique used commonly in plastic and general surgery but should also be considered in the neurosurgeon's armamentarium for treating postoperative spinal infections and wound complications. More research is needed to clearly understand the mechanism by which NPWT assists in wound healing and to help delineate the applications of NPWT in spinal surgery. In appropriately selected patients, NPWT is a potential strategy to assist in closure of complex spinal wounds.

References

1. Arens S, Schlegel U, Printzen G, Ziegler WJ, Perren SM, Hansis M (1996) Influence of materials for fixation implants on local infection. An experimental study of steel versus titanium DCP in rabbits. J Bone Joint Surg Br 78:647–651
2. Emery BE, Dixit R, Formby CC, Biedlingmaier JF (2003) The resistance of maxillofacial reconstruction plates to biofilm formation in vitro. Laryngoscope 113:1977–1982
3. Soultanis KC, Pyrovolou N, Zahos KA, Karaliotas GI, Lenti A, Liveris I, Babis GC, Soucacos PN (2008) Late postoperative infection following spinal instrumentation: stainless steel versus titanium implants. J Surg Orthop Adv 17:193–199
4. Ahmed R, Greenlee JD, Traynelis VC (2012) Preservation of spinal instrumentation after development of postoperative bacterial infections in patients undergoing spinal arthrodesis. J Spinal Disord Tech 25:299–302
5. Kale M, Padalkar P, Mehta V (2017) Vacuum-assisted closure in patients with post-operative infections after instrumented spine surgery: a series of 12 cases. J Orthop Case Rep 7:95–100
6. Adogwa O, Fatemi P, Perez E, Moreno J, Gazcon GC, Gokaslan ZL, Cheng J, Gottfried O, Bagley CA (2014) Negative pressure wound therapy reduces incidence of postoperative wound infection and dehiscence after long-segment thoracolumbar spinal fusion: a single institutional experience. Spine J 14:2911–2917
7. Lo Torto F, Ruggiero M, Parisi P, Borab Z, Sergi M, Carlesimo B (2017) The effectiveness of negative pressure therapy on infected wounds: preliminary results. Int Wound J 14(6):909–914
8. Sinha K, Chauhan VD, Maheshwari R, Chauhan N, Rajan M, Agrawal A (2013) Vacuum assisted closure therapy versus standard wound therapy for open musculoskeletal injuries. Adv Orthop 2013:245940
9. Ousey KJ, Atkinson RA, Williamson JB, Lui S (2013) Negative pressure wound therapy (NPWT) for spinal wounds: a systematic review. Spine J 13:1393–1405
10. Masden D, Goldstein J, Endara M, Xu K, Steinberg J, Attinger C (2012) Negative pressure wound therapy for at-risk surgical closures in patients with multiple comorbidities: a prospective randomized controlled study. Ann Surg 255:1043–1047
11. Horn PL, Ruth B, Kean JR (2007) Use of wound V.A.C. therapy in pediatric patients with infected spinal wounds: a retrospective review. Orthop Nurs 26:317–322
12. Kim JJ, Franczyk M, Gottlieb LJ, Song DH (2017) Cost-effective alternative for negative-pressure wound therapy. Plast Reconstr Surg Glob Open 5:e1211
13. Lee R, Street J, Boyd M, Fisher C, Dvorak M, Paquette S, Kwon B (2016) Management of post-operative spine wound infections using vacuum assisted closure (VAC) therapy. Spine J 16:S68–S69
14. Jones GA, Butler J, Lieberman I, Schlenk R (2007) Negative-pressure wound therapy in the treatment of complex postoperative spinal wound infections: complications and lessons learned using vacuum-assisted closure. J Neurosurg Spine 6:407–411
15. Husted D, Grauer JN, Hilibrand AS (2004) The use of wound vacuums in the management of postoperative wound infections. Semin Spine Surg 16:182–187
16. Zehnder SW, Place HM (2007) Vacuum-assisted wound closure in postoperative spinal wound infection. Orthopedics 30:267–272
17. Karaaslan F, Erdem S, Mermerkaya MU (2015) Wound management with vacuum-assisted closure in postoperative infections after surgery for spinal stenosis. Int Med Case Rep J 8:7–11
18. Mehbod AA, Ogilvie JW, Pinto MR, Schwender JD, Transfeldt EE, Wood KB, Le Huec JC, Dressel T (2005) Postoperative deep wound infections in adults after spinal fusion: management with vacuum-assisted wound closure. J Spinal Disord Tech 18:14–17
19. Ploumis A, Mehbod AA, Dressel TD, Dykes DC, Transfeldt EE, Lonstein JE (2008) Therapy of spinal wound infections using vacuum-assisted wound

closure: risk factors leading to resistance to treatment. J Spinal Disord Tech 21:320–323
20. Anghel EL, Kim PJ, Attinger CE (2016) A solution for complex wounds: the evidence for negative pressure wound therapy with instillation. Int Wound J 13(Suppl 3):19–24
21. Lall RR, Wong AP, Lall RR, Lawton CD, Smith ZA, Dahdaleh NS (2015) Evidence-based management of deep wound infection after spinal instrumentation. J Clin Neurosci 22:238–242
22. Topkoru BC, Kaner T (2015) Negative pressure wound therapy (VAC) for the treatment of spinal surgical site infections. World Spinal Column J 1:46–49
23. Sporns PB, Zimmer S, Hanning U, Zoubi T, Wölfer J, Herbort M, Schwindt W, Niederstadt T (2015) Acute tonsillar cerebellar herniation in a patient with traumatic dural tear and VAC therapy after complex trauma. Spine J 15:e13–e16
24. Wild T, Rahbarnia A, Kellner M, Sobotka L, Eberlein T (2010) Basics in nutrition and wound healing. Nutrition 26:862–866
25. Canavese F, Krajbich JI (2010) Use of vacuum assisted closure in instrumented spinal deformities for children with postoperative deep infections. Indian J Orthop 44:177–183

Potential Mechanisms and Application of Honeybee Products in Wound Management: Wound Healing by Apitherapy

Ahmad Oryan and Esmat Alemzadeh

1 Introduction

Traditional medicine refers to a wide range of the indigenous drugs from plants and animals. Practices of traditional medicines include Iranian, Herbal, Ayurveda, Chinese, Acupuncture, Siddha, Unani, Islamic, Vietnamese, Muti, Ifá, and African may be based on historical or cultural traditions [1–3]. Currently, many plants and remedies have been investigated for potential therapeutic effects and have shown evidence of healing activities [4–10]. Based upon the recent studies conducted by the World Health Organization (WHO), about 80% of the total population in the developing countries uses traditional medicine for healthcare [11].

Since natural sources are inexpensive, available, and affordable, they are widely used for wound healing purposes and other skin diseases. However, the use of traditional medicine is a subject of controversy around the world, and the safety of such treatment modalities needs to be evaluated through scientific standardization. One natural medicine is apitherapy which is the medicinal use of bee products. These products are honey, propolis, royal jelly, bee pollen, and bee venom. Today, apitherapy is recognized among contemporary and conventional treatment methods, and an increasing amount of literature is available in this therapeutic modality. Perhaps the most significant advantage of apitherapy is its low cost and the fact that honey is an effective antimicrobial agent against resistant hospital pathogens [12, 13].

This chapter throws a light on the use of honey and more briefly the other bee products in healthcare and illustrates the action mechanisms of honey in wound healing processes. Honey accelerates healing by decreasing inflammation and stimulating immune response, autolytic debridement, and antioxidant activities. These therapeutic properties make honey a rational and accepted natural agent for healing. Therefore, honey being simply and easily available is a valuable and popular material in developing countries and is considered as a promising treatment in regenerative medicine.

2 Healing History

Throughout history, honey has been considered both as a medicine and as a food. The exact origin of apitherapy has not been traced; however, Muslims, ancient Greeks, ancient Egyptians, Chinese, and people from other countries and nations have used honey as a treatment for several diseases. The Egyptians were the first people to use honey as a treatment strategy in wound healing.

A. Oryan, D.V.M., Ph.D. (✉) • E. Alemzadeh
Department of Biotechnology, School of Veterinary Medicine, Shiraz University, Shiraz, Iran
e-mail: oryan@shirazu.ac.ir; esmat.alemzadeh@gmail.com

Recent Clinical Techniques, Results, and Research in Wounds (2017)
DOI 10.1007/15695_2017_38, © Springer International Publishing AG
Published Online: 24 October 2017

In the oldest human scriptures from Sumer dated back to about 2000 BC, honey was used for treating wounds [14], and based on the Smith papyrus (1700 BC), honey was used as an effective therapeutic regimen in wound healing and regenerative medicine. The Quran mentions honey as a protective agent for humankind and says "thy Lord taught the bee to build its cells in hills, on trees and in men's habitations… there issues from within their bodies a drink of varying colors, wherein is healing for mankind" (Quran 16:68–69).

Until the early twentieth century, the use of honey as a wound dressing was a common practice in wound care, but with the advent of antibiotics in the early 1900s, honey was neglected and consigned to items of historical interest. Today, with the emergence of resistant bacteria, honey has again caught the attention of medical researchers because it is a nontoxic antimicrobial agent which can be used for therapeutic purposes [15, 16].

3 Biochemical and Physicochemical Properties of Honey

Honey as a natural sweet substance is composed of sugars and other constituents such as enzymes, amino acids, organic acids, carotenoids, vitamins, minerals, and aromatic substances [17]. The composition, color, aroma, and flavor of honey are rather variable and depend on its floral source, geographical regions, and seasonal and environmental factors [18, 19]. In general, honey contains approximately 75–80% carbohydrates, 17–20% water, and 1–2% mineral and organic matters. The physical properties of honey have a determining role in its price and acceptability by consumers. On the other hand, the chemical composition determines the physicochemical characteristics of honey including color, pH, water activity, and so on.

Honey contains numerous types of sugars including 75% monosaccharides, 10–15% disaccharides, and small amounts of other sugars which are responsible for properties such as energy value, viscosity, and hygroscopicity which result in enhanced angiogenesis, mesenchymal cell proliferation, collagen deposition, and tissue maturation [20]. Honey is a supersaturated solution, and sugar as the main constituent accounts for 95–99% of its dry matter. Fructose and glucose are the major sugars almost in all honey types, and their amounts depend largely on the source of the nectar, regions, and climate conditions [21]. The concentration of fructose and glucose and their ratio are effective indicators for evaluation of crystallization and floral sources of honey [22]. In addition, the sucrose content in honey is a useful parameter in identifying any improper manipulation, and high level of sucrose may indicate a variety of adulterations [23]. Honey also contains organic acids, minerals, and proteins. Organic acids are derived from sugars by enzymes secreted by honeybees and are responsible for acidity, color, pH, and electrical conductivity [24]. During ripening, honeybees provide glucose oxidase which is responsible in gluconic acid production which is the predominant acid in honey [25]. Gluconic acid and citric acid can be used as reagents to differentiate two types of honey, floral and honeydew, and to measure purity and authenticity [24].

Honey contains about 0.2% protein, which varies according to the species of the honeybees [26]. The most popular amino acids in honey are glutamic acid, phenylalanine, tyrosine, leucine, alanine, and isoleucine [27]. The amount of proline is a useful index in determining both purity and maturation of honey, and a maximum value of 180 mg/kg^{-1} of proline may be indicative of impure honey [28]. Various groups of macro- and microelement minerals such as potassium, magnesium, calcium, iron, phosphorus, sodium, manganese, iodine, zinc, lithium, cobalt, nickel, cadmium, copper, barium, chromium, selenium, arsenic, and silver are found in different honeys. Many factors such as soil type, floral sources, climatic conditions, and fertilization impact mineral composition of honey [29]. The mineral elements, in contrast to vitamins and amino acids, do not degrade by exposure to heat, light, oxidizing agents, and extreme pH [18].

The US Department of Agriculture has classified honey into seven color categories including water white, extra white, white, extra light white, light amber, amber, and dark amber. The honey coloring components are plant pigments and are related to floral origin, the content of pollen, mineral composition, total phenolics, and hydroxymethyl furfural. It has been shown that dark-colored honeys have higher phenolic content and antioxidant capacities [30]. A variety of environmental conditions such as crystallization, storage time, and temperature may change the color. It has been proved that a dark color develops as a result of temperature and storage time, whereas crystallization deduces a light color in honey. Lower water content and higher glucose concentration lead to faster crystallization. Since the glucose crystals are white once crystallized, the crystalized honey turns lighter in color [18, 31].

Water is the second largest constituent, and its content depends on the botanical origin of honey, the storage condition, and the level of maturity achieved in the hive. The free water is defined as the water activity (a_w) [29] and is the amount of water available to microorganisms. Most microorganisms need an a_w higher than 0.91 to grow, and the mean value a_w for honey is between 0.5 and 0.65. Many studies have noted the importance of a_w, because the osmophilic yeasts present in honey result in fermentation of honey, forming ethyl alcohol and carbon dioxide, thereby changing the quality of honey [15, 21, 32]. Moreover, the moisture content of honey influences the viscosity and crystallization, as well as other parameters such as color, flavor, taste, specific gravity, solubility, and conservation. Higher glucose concentration and lower water content result in faster crystallization [22, 32].

4 Application of Honey in Wound Healing and Regenerative Medicine

Several studies have described the effectiveness of honey in the healing processes [5, 33, 34]. Honey enhances wound contraction, promotes epithelialization, elevates granulation tissue formation, improves wound healing, and stimulates tissue growth, synthesis of collagen, and development of new blood vessels in the bed of wounds. Furthermore, honey is able to reduce the postoperative adhesion; subside inflammation, pain, and edema; and facilitate debridement (Fig. 1) [5, 35–37].

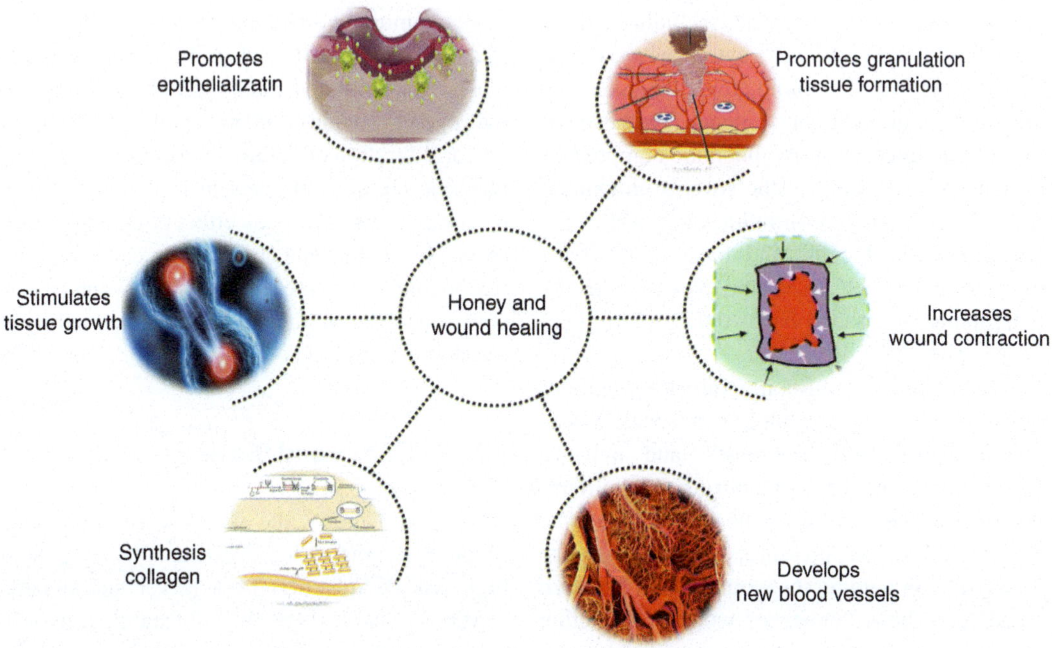

Fig. 1 Therapeutic effects of honey on wound healing

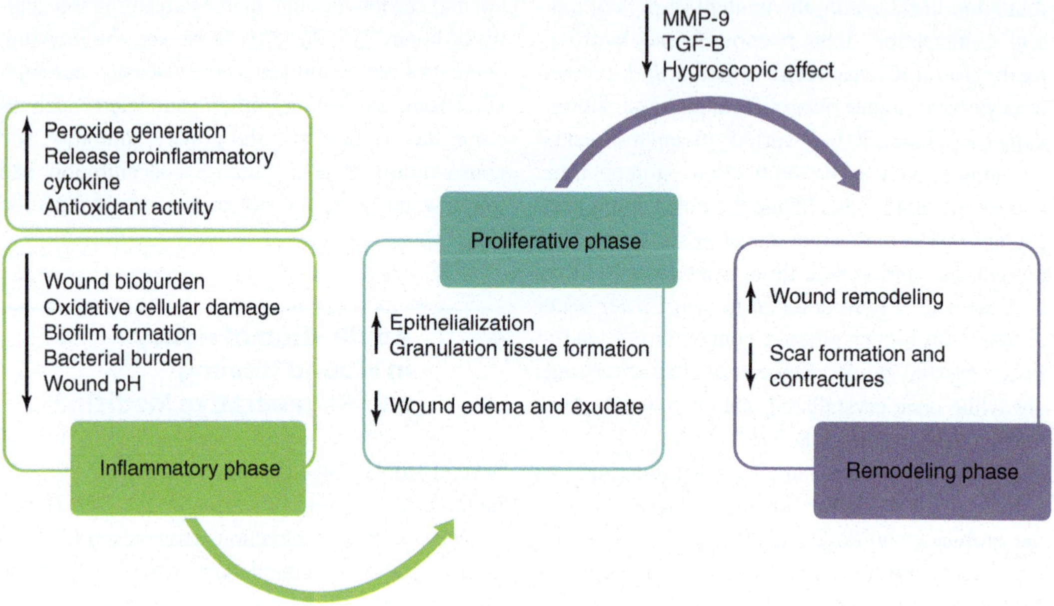

Fig. 2 The regulatory effects of honey on normal phases of wound healing

Wound healing is arranged in three interrelated dynamic phases including inflammation, proliferation, and remodeling, and honey has an effective role in these stages (Fig. 2) [38]. Honey stimulates monocytes in inflammatory phase, to release inflammatory cytokines including TNF-a, IL-6, IL-1b, and NO. These cytokines are essential in initiation of inflammatory processes and are capable of inducing collagen synthesis by fibroblasts. In contrast, the phenolic components present in honey control the severity inflammation. Moreover, honey stimulates removal of tissue debris, dead cells, and bacteria from the wound site by cell lyses and phagocytosis by neutrophils and macrophages during the inflammatory phase [39, 40].

The acidic nature of honey initiates release of oxygen from the hemoglobin to stimulate angiogenesis, proliferate fibroblasts, and enhance granulation tissue formation during the proliferative or fibroplasia phase in the wound area [41]. The high osmotic pressure of honey is also responsible in holding the wound edges together. In addition, honey enhances wound contraction by stimulating fibroblasts and myofibroblasts to deposit more collagen. Honey also significantly promotes reepithelialization in wounds [42]. Glucose present in honey provides required energy for the epithelial cells and facilitates their migration across the wound surface [43]. Production of hydrogen peroxide at low levels in honey stimulates development of new capillaries [42, 43] and growth and proliferation of fibroblasts and epithelial cells [41, 44]. Presence of hydrogen peroxide in honey enables it to stimulate proliferation of cultured fibroblasts. Also, the phenolic components present in honey can protect cells against the toxic effect of hydrogen peroxide [45]. In the final phase, honey can accelerate remodeling of the cutaneous wounds by contracting the wound environment and reducing the scar tissue [46].

4.1 Honey and Burns

During burn injury, the skin loses its protective function against microorganisms, leading to a high risk of infection [47]. Silver sulfadiazine (SSD) is considered as the gold standard in burn wounds, and when topically applied, it is able to release silver and absorb the burn exudates.

However, application of silver sulfadiazine has severe adverse effects and delays wound healing processes [48, 49]. Recently, topical application of honey has reemerged, as a treatment option, in burn wound management [50]. Many studies have demonstrated the role of honey in burn wound healing [44, 51, 52]. Aziz and Hassan (2017) [53] included nine studies in conducting a systematic review and meta-analysis of the impact of honey compared to silver sulfadiazine in treatment of burn wounds. Three options including healing time, number of wounds healed, and number of infected wounds rendered sterile were investigated quantitatively in this review. The data showed a statistically significant difference between the two groups in the time of healing, the proportion of patients with healed wounds, and proportion of infected wounds rendered sterile favoring the honey group. It was concluded that honey has statistically significant beneficial effects compared to SSD in superficial or partial-thickness burns.

4.2 Honey and Skin Ulcers

Leg ulcers are defects in the epidermis and typically are chronic. Venous disease, in most instances, is the main reason for leg ulcers. Compression therapy (phlebological compression bandages, medical compression stockings) is the standard treatment for venous ulcers, and honey therapy currently has gained popularity in leg ulcer treatment [54, 55]. Sloughy venous ulcer is an appropriate environment for infection, prolongs inflammation, and delays wound healing. Migration of neutrophils and release of proteolytic enzymes and oxygen-free radicals lead to tissue hypoxia and promote further bacterial proliferation and tissue destruction. Application of honey can be an effective treatment regime to control the infection. Honey removes necrotic tissues by the autolytic action of tissue proteases and cleans the wound bed [56]. In comparing between honey and phenytoin, it has been shown that there is no significant difference between these two treatment regimes in treatment of chronic ulcers [57]. Honey is able to mitigate pain, reduce scar tissue formation, contract the wound size, and decrease the healing time [58].

Ulceration of the foot is the most common complication among diabetic patients, and it may lead to amputation of the lower leg [59]. Topical application of honey has been considered as a treatment option in treatment of diabetic foot ulcer (DFU), and several clinical studies have reported the beneficial effects of honey in treating these ulcers [60–62]. Insani and coworkers (2016) planned a systematic review and meta-analysis to investigate the efficacy of honey in management of diabetic foot ulcers. Five clinical trials with 517 patients were included. They reported that dressing the wounds with honey showed beneficial effects in decreasing mean duration of wound healing, eradication of infection, formation of granulation tissue, and experience of pain in comparison to the control groups (normal saline, alginate, and povidone iodine). Honey maintains moisture and prevents adhesion of dressing to wound surface, and these result in attenuation of pain level. In addition, it has been reported that honey can decrease edema and malodorous discharge of the wound area [63].

5 Mechanism of Action of Honey on Wound Healing

Many investigations have proved that honey is a reputable and effective therapeutic agent in wound healing. Its useful actions have been endorsed to its antimicrobial, anti-inflammatory, antioxidant activities, boosting effect on the immune system and debridement action.

5.1 Antimicrobial Activity of Honey and Its Mechanisms of Action

The antimicrobial therapy is an important matter when the body's immune response is insufficient to clear the infection. Many studies have noted the ability of honey against pathogenic and nonpathogenic microorganisms including bacteria, fungi, and viruses [64–66]. Honey can act as both bacteriostatic and bactericidal depending on the concentration used; however, it should be kept in mind that the botanical origin of honey is one of the most important criteria which can impact its medicinal value, for example, Brudzynski et al. (2012) [67] showed that the bactericidal effect of manuka honey was higher than blueberry honey.

Despite the improvement of surgical techniques and using antibiotics, wound infections remain a health problem. Antibiotics are always necessary in bacterial infection, but the indiscriminate use of antibiotics has led to the emergence of antibiotic-resistant strains [38]. Since the new series of antibiotics need huge investments and this will not occur soon, the researchers have promoted their efforts to find alternatives to antibiotic-resistant bacteria in the recent years. Recent evidences have suggested that honey can be an efficient remedy in the treatment of infected wounds. One unanticipated finding was that honey has high in vitro activity against both gram-positive and gram-negative bacteria. Surprisingly, it has also been found that resistance to honey has never been observed to date, and a possible explanation for this might be due to the multifactorial nature of the antimicrobial properties of honey that affects more than one target site [68, 69].

Biofilms are a collection of microorganisms containing bacteria and fungi that impair epithelialization and granulation tissue formation [70]. Biofilms protect bacteria from antimicrobial agents and have complementary metabolic strategies in obtaining nutrients from the host and degrading its immune modulatory molecules [3]. Many studies have confirmed the antibiofilm properties of honey [66, 71, 72]. Honey significantly inhibits bacterial attachment to a vinyl substrate and reduces further early biofilm development. According to the classification of Al-Waili et al. (2011), the antimicrobial mechanisms of honey are direct and indirect. In direct action the bacteria are directly eliminated by honey, and factors such as hydrogen peroxide factors, high osmolality, acidity, non-peroxide factors, and phenols are involved in this mechanism. Indirect action is the antibacterial response of the whole organism toward bacteria and includes recruitment of lymphocytes and antibody production and release of nitric oxide, cytokines, and immunomodulation [73].

5.1.1 Hydrogen Peroxide and Non-peroxide Activity

Hydrogen peroxide (H_2O_2) is an important antiseptic which kills microorganisms by oxidizing them [74]. During the honey-making process, honeybees add glucose oxidase to the collected nectar. Glucose oxidase converts the glucose into hydrogen peroxide and gluconic acid which is inactive during honey ripening but regains its efficiency when the honey is diluted [15]. When interacted with wound exudates, the honey becomes diluted and produces low level of H_2O_2 which is nontoxic to host but harbors a long-lasting antiseptic effect against the wound contaminants [74]. The concentration of hydrogen peroxide produced in honey is much lower than those typically applied to a contaminated wound. Wounds indicate a biphasic response to topical application of H_2O_2. It has been shown that low concentrations of H_2O_2 promote wound healing, while at high levels, it delays healing [75].

Although the antibacterial activity depends on the presence of hydrogen peroxide, in most honeys, exceptionally, some honeys including manuka honey maintains its antibacterial activity even after H_2O_2 removal. In this regard, Kwakman et al. [68] suggested that non-peroxide factors are responsible for the antimicrobial activity of manuka honey. The content of non-peroxide compounds can be influenced by the floral sources, harvest season, and geographical location. Several compounds such as methyl syringate, defensin 1, and methylglyoxal (MGO) contribute to the non-peroxide activity of honey [76]. MGO is an active ingredient of manuka and is derived from the nonenzymatic conversion of dihydroxyacetone which is found in high levels in the nectar of manuka flowers [77]. Antibacterial activity of MGO has also been attributed to disruption of collagen that promotes fibrosis in chronic tissue infections [78]. MGO also can also negatively affect glucose oxidase and H_2O_2 generation. Reaction of MGO with the glucose oxidase results in formation of high molecular weight adducts which reduce enzymatic activity of glucose oxidase, and this may be a possible explanation for suppressing H_2O_2 generation in manuka honey [79]. What we know about MGO is largely based upon its electrophilic properties that can bind to DNA and proteins and alter proteins' structure, function, and synthesis. MGO effectively inhibits growth and multiplication of gram-positive and gram-negative bacteria. By binding the MGO to fimbriae and flagella proteins, it results in reduced structural integrity and subsequently impaired function [80].

In the honeybee, defensins exist in the form of two different peptides – defensins 1 and 2. Defensins have cytotoxic activity against gram-positive bacteria, some species of gram-negative bacteria, mycelia fungi, yeasts, protozoa, mites, and viruses. It has been indicated that defensin 2 is responsible for antibacterial activity in bees and contributes in antimicrobial activity of honey. Bee defensin 1 is present in the bee salivary gland and is linked to the honey royal jelly which is associated with the insect's immune response and provides the social immunity of the colony, while defensin 2 plays an important role in the honeybee individual immunity [81].

5.1.2 Osmolarity and Acidity

Honey is a saturated solution of sugars. Sugars present in honey interact with water molecules and leave very few of the available water molecules for microorganisms. Due to the osmolarity activity, honey draws out edematous fluid through the wound tissue and contributes in removal of debris, necrotic and devitalized tissue [82]. The flow of the lymph creates a moist healing environment and provides oxygenation and nutrification for the traumatized tissue. Although osmolarity of honey decreases during its dilution, it generates hydrogen peroxide which is an antimicrobial product. It has been shown that honey is more effective than sugar in reducing bacterial contamination and promoting wound healing [83].

The range of acidic pH of honey is between 3.2 and 4.5, during the dilution stage of honey, which is due to formation of gluconic acid. It has been indicated that neutral or slightly alkaline environment is suitable for growth of wound pathogenic bacteria. Besides, the optimum pH for protease activity is about 7.3. Acidification of honey is able to assist in the antibacterial action of macrophages and prevents ammonia produced by the bacterial metabolism to harm body tissues [84–86].

5.2 Anti-inflammatory Activity

One of the therapeutic benefits of honey is its anti-inflammatory activity. The ability of honey to decrease the damage caused by the free radicals may contribute in reducing damage and breakdown of lipids, proteins, and nucleic acids and thus prevent further tissue necrosis [87, 88]. In the inflammatory phase, the reactive oxygen species induce the activity of the fibroblasts and further production of the collagen fibers of scar tissue. Hence, prolongation of the inflammatory phase may result in hyper-granulation and fibrosis. The transcription factor nuclear factor-kappa beta (NF-KB) as an important marker of inflammation enhances proinflammatory activity and activates genes encoding for proinflammatory cytokines – interleukin (IL)-6, IL-8, and tumor necrosis factor-α (TNF-α) [43, 89]. Honey prevents a prolonged inflammatory response by inhibition of nitric oxide (NO) production and NF-KB activation [90].

A large and growing body of literature has showed that several mechanisms including inhibition of the classical complement pathway, inhibition of reactive oxygen species (ROS) formation, inhibition of leukocyte infiltration, inhibition of matrix metallopeptidase 9 (MMP-9), and inhibition of cyclooxygenase-2 (COX-2) and inducible NO synthase expression can describe the anti-inflammatory properties of honey. It has been demonstrated that honey is able to affect NF-κB signaling pathway and decreases inflammation. Since NF-κB controls many genes involved in inflammation, the major focus has been on inhibiting NF-kB activation and its translocation into the nucleus. It has been shown that honey can suppress the gene expressions of NF-κB (p65 and p50) and IκBα. In addition, honey decreases degradation of the IkB proteins

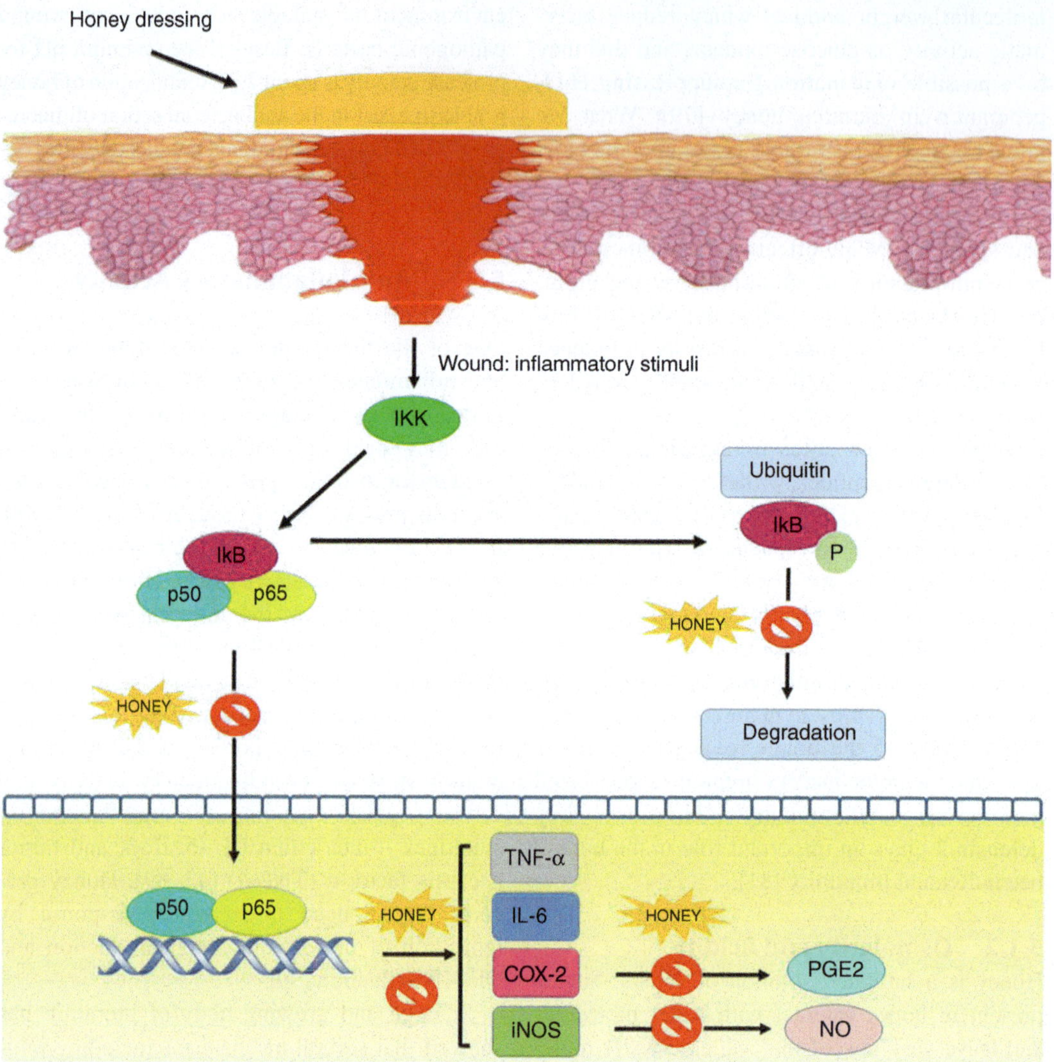

Fig. 3 Mechanisms of action of honey as an anti-inflammatory agent

and prevents the translocation of NF-κB subunits (p65 and p50) into the nucleus and finally leads to reduction of inducible nitric oxide synthase (iNOS), COX-2, TNF-α, and IL-6 expressions as well as prostaglandin E2 (PGE2) and NO production (Fig. 3) [91].

Prostaglandins are mediators of inflammation and pain which can decrease B- and T-lymphocyte functions. Honey decreases the concentrations of plasma prostaglandin to reduce edema and inflammation and activates lymphocytes to produce antibodies against wound pathogens. In addition, the phenolic compounds of honey are responsible in inhibiting of PGE2 release from monocytes in inflamed tissues. It has also been shown that other phenolic compounds such as quercetin, chrysin, and luteolin have inhibitory effects on interleukin-1b and COX-2 expression, PGE2 synthesis, and NF-κB stimulation [92].

5.3 Antioxidant Activity

Free radicals disrupt the structure of other molecules and result in cellular damage. Antioxidants neutralize the free radicals and protect cell from damage [93]. The presence of phenolic compounds such as ellagic, caffeic, p-coumaric, and ferulic acids and flavonoids including apigenin, pinocembrin, kaempferol, quercetin, galangin, chrysin, and hesperetin makes honey a rich source of natural antioxidants. Different honeys have a considerable variation of antioxidant activities due to different floral and geographical origins. In addition, darker honeys have more antioxidant activities [94, 95].

Neutrophils and macrophages release high level of ROS against invading bacteria, in the chronic wounds. ROSs mediate the TNF-α-induced cytotoxicity, and honey is a treatment strategy that can inhibit the TNF-α-induced cytotoxicity with its antioxidant activity [96]. In addition, honey is capable to inhibit NO production by macrophages in a dose-dependent manner [97]. Honey is considerably potent in protecting DNA against damages and has a great role in free radical scavenging, lipid peroxidation inhibition, and antioxidant activity [98].

5.4 Role of Honey in Debridement of Wounds

Debridement is the process of removing any necrotic tissue from a wound to induce granulation tissue formation and tissue maturation. As necrotic tissues can lead to growth of infecting bacteria and induce wound to become chronic, it is imperative to remove any dead tissue [99]. It has been reported that honey has debridement action, but the mechanisms of its action are almost unknown. However, honey facilitates autolytic debridement by its high osmotic pressure and activation of protease to remove the attached slough and necrotic tissue (Fig. 4) [100]. Interestingly, honey has been shown to increase the activity of the enzyme plasmin in the culture medium. Plasmin degrades the fibrin which is attached to the debris in wound bed, while it is not able to digest the collagen matrix needed for tissue repair. It has been shown that inflammation enhances production of the plasminogen activator inhibitor (PAI) and honey is capable to inhibit this pathway. Therefore, reduction in production of PAI by honey is a good reason for its anti-inflammatory activity [101].

5.5 Immunostimulatory Action

Honey can act as an immunomodulator during wound healing [102]. It stimulates cells of the immune system to be infiltrated in the wound site [103]. In addition, honey is capable to stimulate

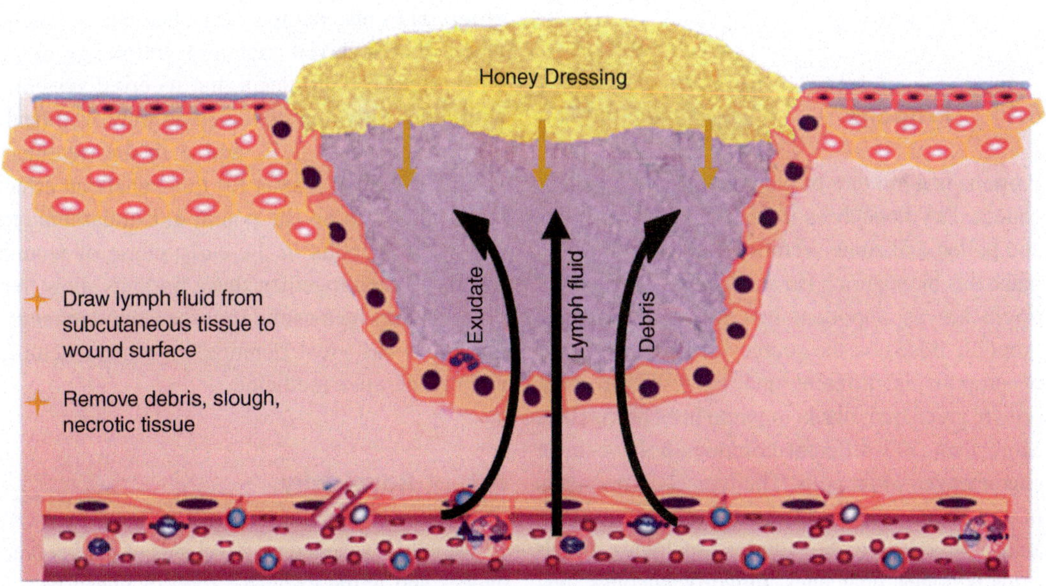

Fig. 4 The debridement action of honey in wound healing processes

the release of TNF-α from monocytes/macrophages. Gannabathula et al. [104] indicated that the arabinogalactan proteins (AGPs) and apisimin present in honey are, at least partly, responsible for stimulating the release of TNF-α. The major glycoproteins in honey, namely, apalbumin 1 (Apa1, 56 kDa), apalbumin 2 (Apa2, 49 kDa), and apalbumin 3 (Apa3, 70 kDa), also stimulate macrophages to release TNF-α [102]. Based on the type of honey, there is variation in immunostimulatory activity. By decreasing the concentration of prostaglandins and increasing NO, honey may induce antibody production and enhance humoral immunity. On the other hand, presence of prebiotic oligosaccharides in honey enables it to support and amplify the immune responses [73, 105].

6 Bee Products and Their Potential Value in Wound Healing

Besides, honeybees produce various derivatives including beeswax, venom, propolis, pollen, and royal jelly that have beneficial roles in human health. Among these products, beeswax, venom, and royal jelly are chemically synthesized by the bees themselves, and the others are derived from plants and are modified and engineered by the bees for their own use.

6.1 Propolis

Propolis is a mixture of plant resins and exudates collected by honeybees in combination with wax and pollen and some secretions added by bees to make this biomaterial. Botanical and geographical origin has an important role in composition of propolis. Based on the sources of resin, the color of propolis is different and ranges from dark brown, green, red, black, to white hues [106, 107]. More than 300 different compounds have been characterized in propolis. The typical components of propolis are the aliphatic acids, esters, aromatic acids, fatty acids, carbohydrates, aldehydes, amino acids, ketones, chalcones, dihydrochalcones, terpenoids, vitamins, and inorganic substances [108]. In particular, propolis has antioxidant, anti-inflammatory, and antimicrobial effects, and these make it a useful product to be applied in wound healing [109]. In addition, topical application of propolis decreases the number of mast cells, and this effect speeds up the regeneration process and has high potential in wound healing [110]. Several in vivo studies have indicated the role of propolis in treating the burn, diabetic, excisional, and incisional wounds [111–113].

Based on in vivo evidences, propolis shortens the inflammatory phase of wound healing by debriding activity and reducing the number of mast cells and neutrophils. Wound contraction is an essential process of repair and is associated with collagen synthesis. Propolis stimulates expression of collagen type I during the initial stage of wound healing and facilitates wound closure [112, 114–116]. Propolis also is responsible for restoring TGF-β expression and signaling, mediating HoxD3 (a homeobox transcription factor) and Smad, to accelerate collagen expression [111]. Combination of propolis and honey has a synergistic effect and can hasten tissue repair [116, 117]. In a pilot study, Henshaw et al. [118] evaluated the role of propolis in the healing of human diabetic foot ulcers (DFU). At weeks 1 and 3, the healing rate was significantly faster in the propolis-treated patients than the control group. They also compared the healing rate in the ulcers that received systemic antibiotics along with propolis with ulcers that received systemic antibiotics only and indicated an improved healing rate at weeks 1, 3, and 4 in the treatment group. The main reason for this beneficial effect was claimed to be the potent anti-inflammatory effects of propolis in the early phase of wound healing. Taken together, these findings show that propolis may be a useful tool for wound management and has great potential in wound healing and regenerative medicine.

6.2 Royal Jelly

Royal jelly is secreted by the glands of worker honeybees and is the exclusive food of queen bee. It consists of water, proteins, carbohydrates, lipids, mineral salts, vitamins, and a series of bioactive substances such as 10-hydroxyl-2-decenoic acid and several insulin-like peptides. In addition, RJ contains phenolic compounds, a potent antibacterial protein (royalisin), and 10-hydroxy decenoic acid [119–123]. It has been demonstrated that topical application of RJ is effective on wound healing, and such beneficial effect has been correspondent to its anti-inflammatory activity. RJ efficiently inhibits the production of proinflammatory cytokines including TNF-α, IL-6, and IL-1 by lipopolysaccharide/interferon-gamma (LPS/IFN-γ)-activated macrophages [124]. Kim et al. (2010) demonstrated that 5 ug/mL of decocted RJ enhances migration of fibroblasts in humans and increases the level of sphingolipids in an in vitro wound healing model [125]. Several studies have confirmed the potential of RJ against different bacteria especially the gram-positive bacteria [126, 127].

It has been stated the RJ reduced the duration of wound recovery and compared with nitrofurazone ointment (positive control) had a better effect on wound healing [128]. It has been shown that daily oral administration of RJ at doses of 10, 100, and 1000 mg/kg body weight possesses no insulin-like activity. However, RJ can shorten the duration of wound recovery by decreasing exudation and accelerating collagen formation in the wound bed [129]. RJ creates an alkaline environment in the wound area, and its antimicrobial, immunomodulating, and nutritional properties can eliminate infection and promote wound healing [130]. It can be concluded that royal jelly is effective on wound restoration; however, further studies with more focus on humans are suggested.

6.3 Beeswax

Beeswax is a natural wax which is secreted by wax glands of honeybees. Chemically, beeswax mainly contains esters of fatty acids and various long-chain alcohols. Its main components are palmitate, palmitoleate, and oleate esters of long-chain (30–32 carbons) aliphatic alcohol [131]. Mendoza et al. [132, 133] indicated that D-002 (a mixture of beeswax alcohols) has potential anti-inflammatory action on osteoarthritis. Moustafa et al. [134] compared the healing of deep second-degree burns treated with silver sulfadiazine (SSD) and a mixture of honey, beeswax, and olive oil (MHBO) and revealed that wound contraction was significantly higher in the MHBO group than both SSD and the control groups. In addition, inflammatory reaction and exudation were less in MHBO group than the SSD and control groups. Beeswax is significantly able to shorten the wound area and healing time. It also obviously improves the number of fibroblasts and new blood capillaries. It is believed that the beeswax ointment has remarkable therapeutic effects on wound healing in diabetic rabbits [135].

6.4 Bee Pollen

Bee pollen is the pollen ball that is collected by bees and is packed in honeycomb cells. Bees collect pollen from different plants and mix it with a small dose of their salivary glands' secretion or nectar. It has been stated that the bee pollen is antifungal, antimicrobial, antiviral, anti-inflammatory, immunostimulating, and local analgesic and also facilitates proliferation of endothelial cells and mesenchymal cells and deposition of collagen matrix in granulation tissue of the burn wounds in humans [136, 137]. Based on the plant sources and geographical origins, the composition of the bee pollen is variable. The typical compounds in bee pollen are proteins, amino acids, carbohydrates, lipids, fatty acids, phenolic compounds, enzymes, and coenzymes as well as vitamins and bioelements [138, 139]. Flavonoids and phenolic acids are important components in the bee pollen and play key roles in anti-inflammatory and antibacterial activity [140, 141]. It has been shown that bee pollen has a strong antibiotic activity against fungi and gram-negative and gram-positive bacteria [141, 142]. The mechanism of anti-inflammatory effect of bee pollen is relative to inhibiting the cyclooxygenase and lipoxygenase activities which flavonoids and phenolic acids as well as fatty acids and phytosterols are responsible for this activity [140]. Several studies have shown the important role of bee pollen in healing and showed that bee pollen is a strong anti-inflammatory agent and is able to decrease the healing time and the discomfort of both the duration period and the intensity of ailments [140, 143]. Kaempferol is a natural flavonol founded in bee pollen and is responsible to inhibit the activity of hyaluronidase and elastase. In fact, kaempferol prevents depolymerization of hyaluronic acid, strengthens the connective tissue, and seals blood vessels [144, 145]. Infection is one of the factors interrupting the healing process, and the necrotic tissues are good environments for microorganisms [146]. It has been shown that bee pollen ointment has an effective antimicrobial activity in postburn wounds [147].

6.5 Bee Venom

Bee venom is a natural toxin produced by the honeybee and had been used as a traditional medicine to treat chronic inflammatory and skin diseases [149, 150]. Bee venom possesses various components including peptides, enzymes, and biologically active and non-peptide components [151]. The bee venom has long been known to have therapeutic properties including antimicrobial, anti-inflammatory, antioxidant, and antitumor properties [152–155]. It has been suggested as an effective treatment for healing. The application of the bee venom is a successful treatment in diabetic wound healing, and it significantly increases wound closure by increasing collagen production and restores the levels of inflammatory cytokines, free radical, TGF-β, and VEGF [152].

Conclusions

Although honey is an ancient wound dressing, it has been considered as a modern type of wound dressing nowadays because of its bioactive material. Honey has all beneficial criteria to be used in treating infected wounds and is a good alternative option to antibiotics due to its antibacterial activity. It is believed that honey and other bee products could be used in wound healing because it has many advantageous effects to enhance wound healing. Such beneficial influences are results of the antibacterial, anti-inflammatory, and antioxidant properties and debridement action of honey. In addition, honey boosts the immune system and stimulates fibroplasia and angiogenesis in the wound bed. However, further studies are recommended to compare the effectiveness of composition, characteristics, and biological properties of different kinds of honeys on wound healing in order to illustrate a guideline for medical application.

References

1. Dorai AA (2012) Wound care with traditional, complementary and alternative medicine. Indian J Plast Surg 45(2):418–424
2. Kigen GK, Ronoh HK, Kipkore WK, Rotich JK (2013) Current trends of traditional herbal medicine practice in Kenya: a review. Afr J Pharmacol Therapeut 2(1):32–37
3. Rickard AH, Gilbert P, High NJ, Kolenbrander PE, Handley PS (2003) Bacterial coaggregation: an integral process in the development of multi-species biofilms. Trends Microbiol 11(2):94–100
4. Oryan A, Mohammadalipour A, Moshiri A, Tabandeh MR (2016) Topical application of aloe vera accelerated wound healing, modeling, and remodeling: an experimental study. Ann Plast Surg 77(1):37–46
5. Oryan A, Zaker S (1998) Effects of topical application of honey on cutaneous wound healing in rabbits. Zentralbl Veterinärmed A 45(3):181–188
6. Oryan A, Mohammadalipour A, Moshiri A, Tabandeh MR (2015) Avocado/soybean unsaponifiables: a novel regulator of cutaneous wound healing, modelling and remodelling. Int Wound J 12(6):674–685
7. Padhi S, Panda SK (2017) Evaluation of wound healing potential of crude leave extracts of Bixa Orellana Linn. in wistar rat. World J Pharm Phamaceut Sci 5(8):1388–1395
8. Tabandeh MR, Oryan A, Mohhammad-Alipour A, Tabatabaei-Naieni A (2013) Silibinin regulates matrix metalloproteinase 3 (stromelysine1) gene expression, hexoseamines and collagen production during rat skin wound healing. Phytother Res 27(8):1149–1153
9. Oryan A, Naeini AT, Nikahval B, Gorjian E (2010) Effect of aqueous extract of Aloe vera on experimental cutaneous wound healing in rat. Veterinarski Arhiv 80(4):509–522
10. Tabandeh MR, Oryan A, Mohammadalipour A (2014) Polysaccharides of Aloe vera induce MMP-3 and TIMP-2 gene expression during the skin wound repair of rat. Int J Biol Macromol 65:424–430
11. Lim M, Sadarangani P, Chan H, Heng J (2005) Complementary and alternative medicine use in

multiracial Singapore. Complement Ther Med 13(1):16–24
12. Fratellone PM, Tsimis F, Fratellone G (2016) Apitherapy products for medicinal use. J Altern Complement Med 22(12):1020–1022
13. Majtán J (2009) Apitherapy--the role of honey in the chronic wound healing process. Epidemiol Mikrobiol Imunol 58(3):137–140
14. Lusby P, Coombes A, Wilkinson J (2002) Honey: a potent agent for wound healing? J Wound Ostomy Continence Nurs 29(6):295–300
15. McLoone P, Warnock M, Fyfe L (2016) Honey: a realistic antimicrobial for disorders of the skin. J Microbiol Immunol Infect 49(2):161–167
16. Murray J (2005) Honey--a modern wound management product. Nurs Standard 19(51):36–37
17. Alqarni AS, Owayss AA, Mahmoud AA (2016) Physicochemical characteristics, total phenols and pigments of national and international honeys in Saudi Arabia. Arab J Chem 9(1):114–120
18. da Silva PM, Gauche C, Gonzaga LV, Costa ACO, Fett R (2016) Honey: chemical composition, stability and authenticity. Food Chem 196:309–323
19. Alvarez-Suarez JM, Gasparrini M, Forbes-Hernández TY, Mazzoni L, Giampieri F (2014) The composition and biological activity of honey: a focus on Manuka honey. Foods 3(3):420–432
20. Kamal MA, Klein P (2011) Determination of sugars in honey by liquid chromatography. Saudi J Biol Sci 18(1):17–21
21. Tornuk F, Karaman S, Ozturk I, Toker OS, Tastemur B, Sagdic O, Dogan M, Kayacier A (2013) Quality characterization of artisanal and retail Turkish blossom honeys: determination of physicochemical, microbiological, bioactive properties and aroma profile. Industrial Crops Prod 46:124–131
22. Escuredo O, Dobre I, Fernández-González M, Seijo MC (2014) Contribution of botanical origin and sugar composition of honeys on the crystallization phenomenon. Food Chem 149:84–90
23. Puscas A, Hosu A, Cimpoiu C (2013) Application of a newly developed and validated high-performance thin-layer chromatographic method to control honey adulteration. J Chromatogr A 1272:132–135
24. Mato I, Huidobro JF, Simal-Lozano J, Sancho MT (2006) Rapid determination of nonaromatic organic acids in honey by capillary zone electrophoresis with direct ultraviolet detection. J Agric Food Chem 54(5):1541–1550
25. Karabagias IK, Badeka A, Kontakos S, Karabournioti S, Kontominas MG (2014) Characterisation and classification of Greek pine honeys according to their geographical origin based on volatiles, physicochemical parameters and chemometrics. Food Chem 146:548–557
26. Won S-R, Li C-Y, Kim J-W, Rhee H-I (2009) Immunological characterization of honey major protein and its application. Food Chem 113(4):1334–1338
27. Di Girolamo F, D'Amato A, Righetti PG (2012) Assessment of the floral origin of honey via proteomic tools. J Proteome 75(12):3688–3693
28. Manzanares AB, García ZH, Galdón BR, Rodríguez ER, Romero CD (2014) Physicochemical characteristics of minor monofloral honeys from Tenerife, Spain. LWT Food Sci Technol 55(2):572–578
29. Alqarni AS, Owayss AA, Mahmoud AA, Hannan MA (2014) Mineral content and physical properties of local and imported honeys in Saudi Arabia. J Saudi Chem Soc 18(5):618–625
30. Pontis JA, Costa LAMA, Silva SJR, Flach A (2014) Color, phenolic and flavonoid content, and antioxidant activity of honey from Roraima, Brazil. Food Sci Technol (Campinas) 34(1):69–73
31. Olaitan PB, Adeleke OE, Iyabo O (2007) Honey: a reservoir for microorganisms and an inhibitory agent for microbes. Afr Health Sci 7(3)
32. Escuredo O, Míguez M, Fernández-González M, Seijo MC (2013) Nutritional value and antioxidant activity of honeys produced in a European Atlantic area. Food Chem 138(2):851–856
33. Aznan MI, Khan OH, Unar AO, Sharif SET, Khan AH, Aziz SHSA, Zakaria AD (2016) Effect of Tualang honey on the anastomotic wound healing in large bowel anastomosis in rats-A randomized controlled trial. BMC Complement Altern Med 16(1):28
34. Mukai K, Komatsu E, Yamanishi M, Hutakuchi M, Kanzaka K, Uno Y, Yamazaki S, Kato S, Yamamoto T, Hattori M (2016) Effectiveness of changing the application of Japanese honey to a hydrocolloid dressing in between the inflammatory and proliferative phases on cutaneous wound healing in male mice. Wounds 29(1):1–9
35. Khoo YT, Halim AS, Singh KK, Mohamad NA (2010) Wound contraction effects and antibacterial properties of Tualang honey on full-thickness burn wounds in rats in comparison to hydrofibre. BMC Complement Altern Med 10(1):48
36. Zohdi R, Mukhtar S, Said S, Azmi N, Ali A (2014) A comparative study of the wound healing properties of Gelam honey and silver sulfadiazine in diabetic rats. In: Biomedical Engineering and Sciences (IECBES), 2014 IEEE Conference on IEEE. IEEE, Kuala Lumpur, Malaysia, pp 247–250
37. Molan PC (2001) Potential of honey in the treatment of wounds and burns. Am J Clin Dermatol 2(1):13–19
38. Oryan A, Alemzadeh E, Moshiri A (2016) Biological properties and therapeutic activities of honey in wound healing: a narrative review and meta-analysis. J Tissue Viabil 25(2):98–118
39. Raynaud A, Ghezali L, Gloaguen V, Liagre B, Quero F, Petit J-M (2013) Honey-induced macrophage stimulation: AP-1 and NF-κB activation and cytokine production are unrelated to LPS content of honey. Int Immunopharmacol 17(3):874–879
40. Hussein SZ, Mohd Yusoff K, Makpol S, Mohd Yusof YA (2012) Gelam honey inhibits the production of proinflammatory, mediators NO, PGE2, TNF-α,

and IL-6 in carrageenan-induced acute paw edema in rats. Evid Based Complement Alternat Med 2012:109636
41. Rossiter K, Cooper A, Voegeli D, Lwaleed B (2010) Honey promotes angiogenic activity in the rat aortic ring assay. J Wound Care 19(10):440–446
42. Nakajima Y, Nakano Y, Fuwano S, Hayashi N, Hiratoko Y, Kinoshita A, Miyahara M, Mochizuki T, Nishino K, Tsuruhara Y (2013) Effects of three types of Japanese honey on full-thickness wound in mice. Evid Based Complement Alternat Med 2013:504537
43. Molan PC (2002) Re-introducing honey in the management of wounds and ulcers-theory and practice. Ostomy Wound Manage 48(11):28–40
44. Boekema B, Pool L, Ulrich M (2013) The effect of a honey based gel and silver sulphadiazine on bacterial infections of in vitro burn wounds. Burns 39(4):754–759
45. Al-Jadi A-M, Enchang FK, Yusoff KM (2014) The effect of Malaysian honey and its major components on the proliferation of cultured fibroblasts. Turkish J Med Sci 44(5):733–740
46. Subrahmanyam M, Sahapure A, Nagane N, Bhagwat V, Ganu J (2001) Effects of topical application of honey on burn wound healing. Ann Burns Fire Disasters 14(3):143–145
47. Church D, Elsayed S, Reid O, Winston B, Lindsay R (2006) Burn wound infections. Clin Microbiol Rev 19(2):403–434
48. Atiyeh BS, Costagliola M, Hayek SN, Dibo SA (2007) Effect of silver on burn wound infection control and healing: review of the literature. Burns 33(2):139–148
49. Poon VK, Burd A (2004) In vitro cytotoxicity of silver: implication for clinical wound care. Burns 30(2):140–147
50. Pećanac M, Janjić Z, Komarčević A, Pajić M, Dobanovački D, Skeledžija-Mišković S (2013) Burns treatment in ancient times. Med Pregl 66(5–6):263–267
51. Choudhary K, Mohanty SK, Soni P (2016) A prospective randomized trial to compare the effectiveness of honey vs. silver sulfadiazine dressing in burn wound management. Int J Med Res Rev 4(1):67–74
52. Pannerselvam B, Jothinathan MKD, Rajenderan M, Perumal P, Thangavelu KP, Kim HJ, Singh V, Rangarajulu SK (2017) An in vitro study on the burn wound healing activity of cotton fabrics incorporated with phytosynthesized silver nanoparticles in male Wistar albino rats. Eur J Pharm Sci 100:187–196
53. Aziz Z, Hassan BAR (2017) The effects of honey compared to silver sulfadiazine for the treatment of burns: a systematic review of randomized controlled trials. Burns 43(1):50–57
54. Jull A, Walker N, Parag V, Molan P, Rodgers A (2008) Randomized clinical trial of honey-impregnated dressings for venous leg ulcers. Br J Surg 95(2):175–182
55. Kahle B, Hermanns H-J, Gallenkemper G (2011) Evidence-based treatment of chronic leg ulcers. Dtsch Arztebl Int 108(14):231–237
56. Gethin G, Cowman S (2008) Bacteriological changes in sloughy venous leg ulcers treated with manuka honey or hydrogel: an RCT. J Wound Care 17(6):241–244
57. Oluwatosin O, Olabanji J, Oluwatosin O, Tijani L, Onyechi H (2000) A comparison of topical honey and phenytoin in the treatment of chronic leg ulcers. Afr J Med Med Sci 29(1):31–34
58. Mohamed H, Salma M, Al Lenjawi B, Abdi S, Gouda Z, Barakat N, Elmahdi H, Abraham S, Hamza AH, Al Khozaei D (2015) The efficacy and safety of natural honey on the healing of foot ulcers: a case series. Wounds 27(4):103–114
59. Reiber G, Lipsky B, Gibbons G (1998) The burden of diabetic foot ulcers. Am J Surg 176(2):5S–10S
60. Kamaratos AV, Tzirogiannis KN, Iraklianou SA, Panoutsopoulos GI, Kanellos IE, Melidonis AI (2014) Manuka honey-impregnated dressings in the treatment of neuropathic diabetic foot ulcers. Int Wound J 11(3):259–263
61. Moghazy A, Shams M, Adly O, Abbas A, El-Badawy M, Elsakka D, Hassan S, Abdelmohsen W, Ali O, Mohamed B (2010) The clinical and cost effectiveness of bee honey dressing in the treatment of diabetic foot ulcers. Diabetes Res Clin Pract 89(3):276–281
62. Delshad E, Tavakkoli-Kakhki M, Motavasselian M (2016) Successful repair of diabetic foot ulcer with honey-based treatment: a case report. Iranian Red Crescent Med J (3):21–24
63. Insani IB, Widayanti N, Rifki A (2017) Honey as a treatment for diabetic foot ulcer: a systematic review. J Plast Rekonstr 3(2):45–51
64. Hillitt K, Jenkins R, Spiller OB, Beeton M (2016) Antimicrobial activity of Manuka honey against antibiotic resistant strains of the cell wall free bacteria Ureaplasma parvum and Ureaplasma urealyticum. Lett Appl Microbiol 64(3):198–202
65. Sherlock O, Dolan A, Athman R, Power A, Gethin G, Cowman S, Humphreys H (2010) Comparison of the antimicrobial activity of Ulmo honey from Chile and Manuka honey against methicillin-resistant Staphylococcus aureus, Escherichia coli and Pseudomonas aeruginosa. BMC Complement Altern Med 10(1):47
66. Halstead F, Webber M, Rauf M, Burt R, Dryden M, Oppenheim B (2016) In vitro activity of an engineered honey, medical-grade honeys, and antimicrobial wound dressings against biofilm-producing clinical bacterial isolates. J Wound Care 25(2):93–102
67. Brudzynski K, Abubaker K, Wang T (2012) Powerful bacterial killing by buckwheat honeys is concentration-dependent, involves complete DNA degradation and requires hydrogen peroxide. Front Microbiol 3:242

68. Kwakman PH, Te Velde AA, De Boer L, Vandenbroucke-Grauls CM, Zaat SA (2011) Two major medicinal honeys have different mechanisms of bactericidal activity. PLoS One 6(3):e17709
69. Mandal MD, Mandal S (2011) Honey: its medicinal property and antibacterial activity. Asian Pac J Trop Biomed 1(2):154–160
70. Oryan A, Alemzadeh E, Moshiri A (2017) Burn wound healing: present concepts, treatment strategies and future directions. J Wound Care 26(1):5–19
71. Emineke S, Cooper AJ, Fouch S, Birch BR, Lwaleed BA (2017) Diluted honey inhibits biofilm formation: potential application in urinary catheter management? J Clin Pathol 70(2):140–144
72. Sojka M, Valachova I, Bucekova M, Majtan J (2016) Antibiofilm efficacy of honey and bee-derived defensin-1 on multispecies wound biofilm. J Med Microbiol 65(4):337–344
73. Al-Waili NS, Salom K, Butler G, Al Ghamdi AA (2011) Honey and microbial infections: a review supporting the use of honey for microbial control. J Med Food 14(10):1079–1096
74. Brudzynski K (2006) Effect of hydrogen peroxide on antibacterial activities of Canadian honeys. Can J Microbiol 52(12):1228–1237
75. Loo AEK, Wong YT, Ho R, Wasser M, Du T, Ng WT, Halliwell B (2012) Effects of hydrogen peroxide on wound healing in mice in relation to oxidative damage. PLoS One 7(11):e49215
76. Dart A, Bischofberger A, Dart C, Jeffcott L (2015) A review of research into second intention equine wound healing using Manuka honey: current recommendations and future applications. Equine Veterinary Edu 27(12):658–664
77. Grainger MN, Manley-Harris M, Lane JR, Field RJ (2016) Kinetics of conversion of dihydroxyacetone to methylglyoxal in New Zealand mānuka honey: Part I–Honey systems. Food Chem 202:484–491
78. Majtan J (2011) Methylglyoxal—a potential risk factor of manuka honey in healing of diabetic ulcers. Evid Based Complement Altern Med 2011:295494
79. Majtan J, Bohova J, Prochazka E, Klaudiny J (2014) Methylglyoxal may affect hydrogen peroxide accumulation in manuka honey through the inhibition of glucose oxidase. J Med Food 17(2):290–293
80. Rabie E, Serem JC, Oberholzer HM, Gaspar ARM, Bester MJ (2016) How methylglyoxal kills bacteria: an ultrastructural study. Ultrastruct Pathol 40(2):107–111
81. Ilyasov R, Gaifullina L, Saltykova E, Poskryakov A, Nikolaenko A (2013) Defensins in the honeybee antiinfectious protection. J Evolutionary Biochem Physiol 49(1):1–9
82. Stewart JA, McGrane OL, Wedmore IS (2014) Wound care in the wilderness: is there evidence for honey? Wilderness Environ Med 25(1):103–110
83. Yaghoobi R, Kazerouni A (2013) Evidence for clinical use of honey in wound healing as an anti-bacterial, anti-inflammatory anti-oxidant and anti-viral agent: a review. Jundishapur J Natural Pharmaceut Prod 8(3):100–104
84. Bittmann S, Luchter E, Thiel M, Kameda G, Hanano R, Längler A (2010) Does honey have a role in paediatric wound management? Br J Nurs 19(15):19
85. Molan P (2001) Why honey is effective as a medicine: 2. The scientific explanation of its effects. Bee World 82(1):22–40
86. Malik KI, Malik M, Aslam A (2010) Honey compared with silver sulphadiazine in the treatment of superficial partial-thickness burns. Int Wound J 7(5):413–417
87. Alzahrani HA, Boukraâ L, Yuva Bellik FA, Bakhotmah BA, Kolayli S, Sahin H (2012) Evaluation of the antioxidant activity of three varieties of honey from different botanical and geographical origins. Glob J Health Sci 4(6):191
88. Kishore RK, Halim AS, Syazana MN, Sirajudeen K (2011) Tualang honey has higher phenolic content and greater radical scavenging activity compared with other honey sources. Nutr Res 31(4):322–325
89. Chung T-W, Moon S-K, Chang Y-C, Ko J-H, Lee Y-C, Cho G, Kim S-H, Kim J-G, Kim C-H (2004) Novel and therapeutic effect of caffeic acid and caffeic acid phenyl ester on hepatocarcinoma cells: complete regression of hepatoma growth and metastasis by dual mechanism. The FASEB J 18(14):1670–1681
90. Hämäläinen M, Nieminen R, Vuorela P, Heinonen M, Moilanen E (2007) Anti-inflammatory effects of flavonoids: genistein, kaempferol, quercetin, and daidzein inhibit STAT-1 and NF-κB activations, whereas flavone, isorhamnetin, naringenin, and pelargonidin inhibit only NF-κB activation along with their inhibitory effect on iNOS expression and NO production in activated macrophages. Mediat Inflamm 2007:45673
91. Majtan J (2014) Honey: an immunomodulator in wound healing. Wound Repair Regen 22(2):187–192
92. Kassim M, Achoui M, Mansor M, Yusoff KM (2010) The inhibitory effects of Gelam honey and its extracts on nitric oxide and prostaglandin E 2 in inflammatory tissues. Fitoterapia 81(8):1196–1201
93. Nagai T, Sakai M, Inoue R, Inoue H, Suzuki N (2001) Antioxidative activities of some commercially honeys, royal jelly, and propolis. Food Chem 75(2):237–240
94. Nayik GA, Nanda V (2016) Effect of thermal treatment and pH on antioxidant activity of saffron honey using response surface methodology. J Food Measure Characterization 10(1):64–70
95. Beretta G, Granata P, Ferrero M, Orioli M, Facino RM (2005) Standardization of antioxidant properties of honey by a combination of spectrophotometric/fluorimetric assays and chemometrics. Analytica Chim Acta 533(2):185–191
96. Habtemariam S (1997) Flavonoids as inhibitors or enhancers of the cytotoxicity of tumor necrosis factor-α in L-929 tumor cells. J Nat Prod 60(8):775–778

97. Kassim M, Achoui M, Mustafa MR, Mohd MA, Yusoff KM (2010) Ellagic acid, phenolic acids, and flavonoids in Malaysian honey extracts demonstrate in vitro anti-inflammatory activity. Nutr Res 30(9):650–659
98. Afroz R, Tanvir E, Paul S, Bhoumik NC, Gan SH, Khalil M (2016) DNA damage inhibition properties of Sundarban honey and its phenolic composition. J Food Biochem 40(4):436
99. Downe A (2014) How wound cleansing and debriding aids management and healing. J Comm Nurs 28(4):25–29
100. Shukla VK (2015) Honey debridement. Skin Necrosis Springer, Wien, pp 273–275
101. Molan PC (2011) The evidence and the rationale for the use of honey as wound dressing. Wound Pract Res 19(4):204–220
102. Gannabathula S, Krissansen GW, Bisson-Rowe L, Skinner M, Steinhorn G, Schlothauer R (2017) Correlation of the immunostimulatory activities of honeys with their contents of identified bioactives. Food Chem 221:39–46
103. Al-Waili N, Salom K, Al-Ghamdi AA (2011) Honey for wound healing, ulcers, and burns; data supporting its use in clinical practice. Sci World J 11:766–787
104. Gannabathula S, Krissansen GW, Skinner M, Steinhorn G, Schlothauer R (2015) Honeybee apisimin and plant arabinogalactans in honey costimulate monocytes. Food Chem 168:34–40
105. Chepulis LM (2007) The effects of honey compared with sucrose and a sugar-free diet on neutrophil phagocytosis and lymphocyte numbers after long-term feeding in rats. JCIM 4(1):1–7
106. Martinotti S, Ranzato E (2015) Propolis: a new frontier for wound healing? Burns Trauma 3(1):9
107. Wagh VD (2013) Propolis: a wonder bees product and its pharmacological potentials. Adv Pharmacol Sci 2013:308249
108. Ramos A, Miranda JL (2007) Propolis: a review of its anti-inflammatory and healing actions. J Venom Anim Toxins Trop Dis 13(4):697–710
109. De Castro S (2001) Propolis: biological and pharmacological activities. Therapeutic uses of this bee-product. Ann Rev Biomed Sci 3:49–83
110. Barroso PR, Lopes-Rocha R, Pereira EMF, Marinho SA, de Miranda JL, Lima NL, Verli FD (2012) Effect of propolis on mast cells in wound healing. Inflammopharmacol 20(5):289–294
111. Hozzein WN, Badr G, Al Ghamdi AA, Sayed A, Al-Waili NS, Garraud O (2015) Topical application of propolis enhances cutaneous wound healing by promoting TGF-beta/Smad-mediated collagen production in a streptozotocin-induced type I diabetic mouse model. Cell Physiol Biochem 37(3):940–954
112. de Almeida EB, Cordeiro Cardoso J, de Lima AK, de Oliveira NL, de Pontes-Filho NT, Oliveira Lima S, Souza IC, de Albuquerque-Júnior RL (2013) The incorporation of Brazilian propolis into collagen-based dressing films improves dermal burn healing. J Ethnopharmacol 147(2):419–425
113. Jacob A, Parolia A, Pau A, Amalraj FD (2015) The effects of Malaysian propolis and Brazilian red propolis on connective tissue fibroblasts in the wound healing process. BMC Complement Altern Med 15(1):294
114. Abreu AM, Oliveira DWD, Marinho SA, Lima NL, de Miranda JL, Verli FD (2012) Effect of topical application of different substances on fibroplasia in cutaneous surgical wounds. ISRN Dermatol 2012:282973
115. Abu-Seida AM (2015) Effect of propolis on experimental cutaneous wound healing in dogs. Vet Med Int 2015:672643
116. Jastrzębska-Stojko Ż, Stojko R, Rzepecka-Stojko A, Kabała-Dzik A, Stojko J (2013) Biological activity of propolis-honey balm in the treatment of experimentally-evoked burn wounds. Molecules 18(11):14397–14413
117. Takzaree N, Hadjiakhondi A, Hassanzadeh G, Rouini MR, Manayi A (2016) Synergistic effect of honey and propolis on cutaneous wound healing in rats. Acta Med Iranica 54(4):233–239
118. Henshaw FR, Bolton T, Nube V, Hood A, Veldhoen D, Pfrunder L, McKew GL, Macleod C, McLennan SV, Twigg SM (2014) Topical application of the bee hive protectant propolis is well tolerated and improves human diabetic foot ulcer healing in a prospective feasibility study. J Diabetes Complicat 28(6):850–857
119. Caparica-Santos C, Marcucci MC (2007) Quantitative determination of trans-10-Hydroxy-2-Decenoic Acid (10-HDA) in Brazilian royal jelly and commercial products containing royal jelly. J Apicultural Res 46(3):149–153
120. Nagai T, Inoue R (2004) Preparation and the functional properties of water extract and alkaline extract of royal jelly. Food Chem 84(2):181–186
121. Fujiwara S, Imai J, Fujiwara M, Yaeshima T, Kawashima T, Kobayashi K (1990) A potent antibacterial protein in royal jelly. Purification and determination of the primary structure of royalisin. J Biol Chem 265(19):11333–11337
122. Kerem Z, Chetrit D, Shoseyov O, Regev-Shoshani G (2006) Protection of lipids from oxidation by epicatechin, trans-resveratrol, and gallic and caffeic acids in intestinal model systems. J Agr Food Chem 54(26):10288–10293
123. Kramer KJ, Tager HS, Childs CN, Speirs RD (1977) Insulin-like hypoglycemic and immunological activities in honeybee royal jelly. J Insect Physiol 23(2):293–295
124. Kohno K, Okamoto I, Norie A, Iwaki K, Ikeda M, Kurimoto M (2004) Royal jelly inhibits the production of proinflammatory cytokines by activated macrophages. Biosci Biotech Biochem 68(1):138–145
125. Kim J, Kim Y, Yun H, Park H, Kim SY, Lee K-G, Han S-M, Cho Y (2010) Royal jelly enhances

migration of human dermal fibroblasts and alters the levels of cholesterol and sphinganine in an in vitro wound healing model. Nutr Res Pract 4(5):362–368
126. Gunaldi O, Daglioglu YK, Tugcu B, Kizilyildirim S, Postalci L, Ofluoglu E, Koksal F (2014) Antibacterial effect of royal jelly for preservation of implant-related spinal infection in rat. Turk Neurosurg 24(2):249–252
127. Romanelli A, Moggio L, Montella RC, Campiglia P, Iannaccone M, Capuano F, Pedone C, Capparelli R (2011) Peptides from Royal Jelly: studies on the antimicrobial activity of jelleins, jelleins analogs and synergy with temporins. J Peptide Sci 17(5):348–352
128. Shirzad M, Yousofi M, Zamanzad B, Sedaghat A, Hosseini M, Shahinfard N, Shirzad H (2014) Effects of royal jelly on sterile skin cut repair. J Herb Med Pharmacol 3(2):97–100
129. Fujii A, Kobayashi S, Kuboyama N, Furukawa Y, Kaneko Y, Ishihama S, Yamamoto H, Tamura T (1990) Augmentation of wound healing by royal jelly (RJ) in streptozotocin-diabetic rats. Jap J Pharmacol 53(3):331–337
130. Abdelatif M, Yakoot M, Etmaan M (2008) Safety and efficacy of a new honey ointment on diabetic foot ulcers: a prospective pilot study. J Wound Care 17(3):108–110
131. Khan S, Lari QH, Khan MA (2016) Therapeutic uses of Mom Zard (beeswax) in Unani system of medicine-a review. Int J Pharm Bio-Sci 1(1):1–4
132. Mendoza S, Noa M, Valle M, Mendoza N, Mas R (2013) Ameliorating effects of D-002, a mixture of beeswax alcohols, on monosodium iodoacetate-induced osteoarthritis in rats. Int J Pharm Sci Rev Res 19(1):10–15
133. Mendoza S, Noa M, Valle M, Mendoza N, Mas R (2013) Effects of D-002 on formaldehyde-induced osteoarthritis in rats. IOSR J Pharm 3:9–12
134. Moustafa A, Atiba A (2015) The effectiveness of a mixture of honey, beeswax and olive oil in treatment of canine deep second-degree burn. Glob Veterinaria 14:244–250
135. Fu H, Wang X-J, Lu H-F, Xu Q-W (2007) Experimental study on beeswax ointment in diabetic rabbit's model of wound healing. J Dalian Med Univ 4:003
136. Kroyer G, Hegedus N (2001) Evaluation of bioactive properties of pollen extracts as functional dietary food supplement. Innov Food Sci Emerging Technol 2(3):171–174
137. Almaraz-Abarca N (2004) Variability of antioxidant activity among honeybee-collected pollen of different botanical origin. Interciencia 29(10):574–578
138. Campos MG, Bogdanov S, de Almeida-Muradian LB, Szczesna T, Mancebo Y, Frigerio C, Ferreira F (2008) Pollen composition and standardisation of analytical methods. J Apicultural Res 47(2):154–161
139. Campos M, Frigerio C, Lopes J, Bogdanov S (2010) What is the future of Bee-Pollen. J ApiProd ApiMed Sci 2(4):131–144
140. Choi EM (2007) Antinociceptive and antiinflammatory activities of pine (Pinus densiflora) pollen extract. Phytother Res 21(5):471–475
141. Baltrušaitytė V, Venskutonis PR, Čeksterytė V (2007) Antibacterial activity of honey and beebread of different origin against S. aureus and S. epidermidis. Food Technol Biotechnol 45(2):201–208
142. Erkmen O, Özcan MM (2008) Antimicrobial effects of Turkish propolis, pollen, and laurel on spoilage and pathogenic food-related microorganisms. J Med Food 11(3):587–592
143. Pascoal A, Rodrigues S, Teixeira A, Feás X, Estevinho LM (2014) Biological activities of commercial bee pollens: antimicrobial, antimutagenic, antioxidant and anti-inflammatory. Food Chem Toxicol 63:233–239
144. Bogdanov S (2014) Pollen: production, nutrition and health: a review. Bee Product Science
145. Kanashiro A, Souza JG, Kabeya LM, Azzolini C, Elisa A, Lucisano-Valim YM (2007) Elastase release by stimulated neutrophils inhibited by flavonoids: importance of the catechol group. Zeit Naturforsch 62(5–6):357–361
146. Komosinska-Vassev K, Olczyk P, Kaźmierczak J, Mencner L, Olczyk K (2015) Bee pollen: chemical composition and therapeutic application. Evid Based Complement Alternat Med 2015:297425
147. Olczyk P, Koprowski R, Kaźmierczak J, Mencner L, Wojtyczka R, Stojko J, Olczyk K, Komosinska-Vassev K (2016) Bee pollen as a promising agent in the burn wounds treatment. Evid Based Complement Alternat Med 2016:8473937
148. Han SM, Lee KG, Park KK, Pak SC (2013) Skin sensitization study of bee venom (Apis mellifera L.) in guinea pigs and rats. Cutan Ocul Toxicol 32(1):27–30
149. Vasileiadou K, Pantazidis G, Papadopoulou K, Ligoudistianou C, Kourelis A, Petrakis S, Masmanidou E, Testa T, Kourounakis A, Hadjipetrou L (2010) α1-Acid glycoprotein production in rat dorsal air pouch in response to inflammatory stimuli, dexamethasone and honey bee venom. Exp Mol Pathol 89(1):63–71
150. Han SM, Park KK, Nicholls YM, Macfarlane N, Duncan G (2013) Effects of honeybee (Apis mellifera) venom on keratinocyte migration in vitro. Pharmacogy Mag 9(35):220–226
151. Amin MA, Abdel-Raheem IT (2014) Accelerated wound healing and anti-inflammatory effects of physically cross linked polyvinyl alcohol–chitosan hydrogel containing honey bee venom in diabetic rats. Arch Pharm Res 37(8):1016–1031
152. Han SM, Kim JM, Hong IP, Woo SO, Kim SG, Jang HR, Pak SC (2016) Antibacterial activity and antibiotic-enhancing effects of honeybee venom against methicillin-resistant staphylococcus aureus. Molecules 21(1):79
153. Kocyigit A, Guler EM, Kaleli S (2016) Anti-inflammatory, antioxidant and anti-genotoxic effects

of different doses of bee venom on adjuvant induce arthritis in rats. J Int Soc Antioxidants Nutr Health 3(1)
154. Gajski G, Čimbora-Zovko T, Rak S, Rožman M, Osmak M, Garaj-Vrhovac V (2014) Combined antitumor effects of bee venom and cisplatin on human cervical and laryngeal carcinoma cells and their drug resistant sublines. J Appl Toxicol 34(12):1332–1341
155. Badr G, Hozzein WN, Badr BM, Al Ghamdi A, Saad Eldien HM, Garraud O (2016) Bee venom accelerates wound healing in diabetic mice by suppressing activating transcription factor-3 (ATF-3) and inducible nitric oxide synthase (iNOS)-mediated oxidative stress and recruiting bone marrow-derived endothelial progenitor cells. J Cell Physiol 231(10):2159–2171

Reactive Oxygen Species Treatment in the Management of Wounds

Matthew S. Dryden

1 Introduction

Bacterial and fungal biofilms are a significant problem in many clinical settings particularly wounds and soft tissue lesions by virtue of their increased tolerance towards conventionally prescribed antimicrobials [1–3]. Antibiotic use in such conditions (chronic wounds, burns, chronic respiratory conditions and cystic fibrosis, recurrent cystitis) leads to intense selective pressure often resulting in further antibacterial resistance. Alternative therapeutic strategies that can improve antimicrobial efficacy towards biofilms, thereby limiting antibiotic use and reducing the development of further resistance would be of considerable benefit [4]. One such development may be the use of topical therapy with reactive oxygen species (ROS) in critically colonised lesions. Therapies involving ROS as a mechanism of action are already available in clinical use for wounds and are being developed for clinical use in other settings [5].

There is a global antibiotic resistance crisis which may limit therapeutic choices in the future [6, 7]. Governments and professional groups are developing (AMR) strategies that include programmes of antimicrobial stewardship [8, 9]. Such a programme has recently been published specifically for wound care [10]. The more widespread use of ROS in wounds to reduce bacterial bioburden may prevent extension of critical colonisation to deeper infection and reduce the requirements for systemic antimicrobials. The first entirely novel antimicrobial agent to reach early clinical use is one employing reactive oxygen species (ROS) as its mechanism of action, and this is specifically for wound treatment [11]. Current wound ROS therapy is in the form of a honey delivery mechanism—SurgihoneyRO (SHRO)—not to be confused with other pharmaceutical grade honeys. SHRO is engineered honey which delivers therapeutic levels of ROS at constant, steady concentrations over a prolonged period.

2 The Problem of Treating Infection in Wounds

The disease burden of skin and soft tissue care is huge throughout the world. In the UK alone, more than 100,000 new patients per year are estimated to develop leg ulcers at a cost to the UK health service in 2005/2006 of up to £198 million. Pressure ulcers were estimated to cost up to £2.64 billion at 2006 prices [12] and diabetic foot ulcers and amputations up to £662 million in 2010/2011 [13].

M.S. Dryden, M.D.
Hampshire Hospitals Foundation NHS Trust, Winchester, UK

University of Southampton Faculty of Medicine, Southampton, UK
e-mail: matthew.dryden@hhft.nhs.uk

Recent Clinical Techniques, Results, and Research in Wounds (2017)
DOI 10.1007/15695_2017_39, © Springer International Publishing AG
Published Online: 24 October 2017

Although skin and soft tissue infections are among the most common for which antibiotics are prescribed, there is little published guidance for prudent antimicrobial therapy practice for these patients. A recent position statement has reviewed the issues around antibiotic prescribing in this area [10]. The main problem is the diagnosis of infection, particularly in chronic wounds. All breaks in the skin get colonised with bacteria. It is not possible to rely on the results of microbiology swabs to determine infection. The difficulty is in knowing when there is a pathogenic combination of bacterial invasion and inflammation requiring antimicrobial treatment. Clinical evidence of inflammation surrounding a skin lesion is taken to mean invasive infection requiring systemic antibiotics. Colonised wounds and infected chronic wounds are frequently polymicrobial, and most wounds take many weeks (or even months) to heal. Some clinicians think that they should continue broad-spectrum antibiotic therapy until healing occurs, but no evidence supports this belief [14]. Furthermore, because wounds are frequently recurrently infected, these patients are often exposed to repeated courses of therapy. Additionally, while some wounds that show evidence of inflammation may not be infected, there is currently no universally accepted criterion standard for diagnosing infection. These factors frequently lead to antibiotic misuse among patients with both infected and uninfected wounds, ultimately leading to antibiotic-resistant infections [15].

A study in Sweden, where the consensus is to restrict antibiotic therapy of wounds, found that 27% of patients being treated via hospital care were receiving systemic antibiotic therapy, a rate of antibiotic therapy over ten times higher than that for the whole population of the study region [16]. Another report from Sweden, where a mandatory national registry of ulcer treatment was subsequently established [17], documented widespread unnecessary use of systemic antibiotics in the management of chronic wounds. Introduction of the registry led to a dramatic 40% reduction in patients receiving antibiotic [17].

3 The Use of Topical Antimicrobials in Wounds

The use of topical antimicrobials in wounds is controversial. While systemic antibiotic therapy is appropriate for most clinically infected acute wounds, topical antimicrobial (antibiotic and nonantibiotic) agents may have several potential benefits for superficial, mild infections [18]. A small amount of topical agent can achieve high levels directly at the site of infection; it avoids systemic adverse effects and allows the use of agents that cannot be administered systemically. There is much regional and geographical variation in the use of topical antibiotics and in resistance rates of pathogens to these agents. There is limited evidence of the effectiveness of topical antibiotics, and they often select for resistant colonising bacteria. Furthermore, topical treatment may cause periwound skin irritation, rash, eczema or impairment of wound healing [19]. Concerns also remain about possible cytotoxic effect of topical antimicrobials on the wound bed, especially with long-term treatment [20, 21]. A few topical antibiotics, e.g. fusidic acid, mupirocin and neomycin, may be appropriate to treat localised acute superficial skin infections, such as impetigo and folliculitis, but almost all other clinically infected wounds require systemic antibiotic therapy [20, 21]. Topical metronidazole may be beneficial in reducing wound odour, but the evidence is weak [22]. Generally, topical antibiotic use should be discouraged.

Nonantibiotic antimicrobials are widely used in wound care, notwithstanding the limited data supporting their usefulness. These include antiseptics (e.g. chlorhexidine, povidone or iodine), heavy metals (e.g. silver, mercury [mercurochrome]) and natural products (e.g. honey, charcoal). Topical antimicrobials may be helpful where there is limited localised infection of chronic wounds [19], although some antiseptics may delay healing [18, 20]. For wounds with secondary clinical signs of localised infection [23, 24], applying topical nonantibiotic agents after adequate debridement may be useful, perhaps by

Table 1 Potential benefits and limitations of topical agents and dressings in wounds

	Topical antibiotics	Hydrocolloid alginate	Silver agents/ dressings	Antiseptics (iodine, chlorhexidine)	Reactive oxygen agents
Reduction in bacterial load	+	−	+	+	+
Reduces/prevents biofilm	−	−	−	−	+
Avoids selection of antibiotic resistance	−	+	+	+	+
Nontoxic	−	+	−	−	+
Promotes wound healing at cellular level	−	−	−	−	+
Wound barrier	−	+	+	−	+
Wound nutrition	−	−	−	−	+
Odour control	+	−	−	+	+
Pain suppression	−	+	−	−	+

suppressing biofilm formation [23]. ROS could deliver all these functions and replace all topical antibiotics and antiseptics (Table 1).

4 What Is ROS?

The term 'ROS' applies to reactive oxygen radicals including superoxide anionO_2^-, peroxideO_2^{-2}, hydrogen peroxide H_2O_2, hydroxyl radicals OH and hydroxyl OH− ions [5]. ROS are directly antimicrobial. H_2O_2 appears to elicit its antimicrobial action by a reaction with thiol groups in enzymes and proteins, DNA and bacterial cell membranes. It possesses concentration-dependent activity and toxicity. H_2O_2 is unstable, rapidly breaking down to H_2O and O^-. While H_2O_2 can be used as a cleansing, antiseptic agent, the duration of its activity is too short to be of use as a therapeutic agent. However ROS gels have been manufactured to slowly release ROS over a prolonged period of time, allowing sustained continuous release of ROS to a target site [25]. ROS could be employed as a topical therapeutic antimicrobial agent not only on soft tissue lesions but also in cavities, prosthetic devices and by alternative delivery mechanisms to respiratory tract and uroepithelium.

In addition to their antimicrobial activity, ROS are pivotal in the normal wound-healing response. They act as secondary messengers to many immunocytes and non-lymphoid cells, regulation of angiogenesis and perfusion into the wound area [5]. ROS act in early host defence against infection through phagocytes and ROS burst. These immunomodulating roles could be exploited in clinical practice in addition to the direct antimicrobial activity to treat wounds and other sites of chronic inflammation, particularly when there is stalled healing, e.g. in chronic leg ulcers, pressure injury and infected/dehisced surgical wounds and burns and deeper structures of the respiratory tract, uroepithelium, peritoneum and prosthetic devices. Emerging concepts associated with ROS modulation and delivery mechanisms have the potential for novel strategies in clinical practice [5].

ROS has potent antimicrobial activity against bacteria, fungi and viruses. ROS is rapidly active in vitro against all Gram-positive and Gram-negative bacteria tested including multidrug-resistant (MDR) strains which are causing such infection control and therapeutic concern [26]. Even against those organisms that produce catalase such as *Staphylococcus aureus*, ROS is very effective presumably because the persistent production of ROS overwhelms the catalase [5]. MICs and MBCs are very consistent among isolates of the same bacterial species whether the isolates were MDR or highly sensitive. MICs and MBCs are well below concentrations that can be achieved with topical delivery. Cidal activity is very swift with threefold log reduction in colony-forming units in 30 min of exposure and complete eradication in 2 h when the lowest potency of ROS gel was used against *Staphylococcus aureus*.

The first ROS therapeutic agent was in the form of a pharmaceutical honey wound gel, SurgihoneyRO (SHRO). SHRO is a modified honey that has been engineered to provide a constant level of ROS over a prolonged period of time when applied to a wound [27]. The availability of ROS from SHRO, or indeed an alternative synthetic delivery system, can be enhanced and is scalable depending on the level of the engineered process [28]. Other ROS antibiotic agents and delivery systems, such as gels, sprays, nebulizers and infusions, employing this mechanism are being developed and may be particularly useful for delivery of ROS to other clinical sites.

5 ROS Activity In Vitro and in Clinical Practice

As well as being antimicrobial, ROS agents are effective at preventing the formation of and disrupting existing biofilm. SHRO and ROS prototypes of increased antimicrobial activity were compared to pharmaceutical grade honeys' five antimicrobial dressings (AMDs) in their ability to prevent biofilm formation in vitro by 16 bacterial isolates [28]. In serial dilution SHRO and ROS prototypes were most effective in disrupting established biofilm and in preventing the development of biofilm.

Antibiotics have greatest efficacy in acute infections. Acute infections are caused by planktonic bacteria invading blood or tissues which react with an innate inflammatory response characterised by polymorphonucleocytes. Antibiotics are usually effective in resolving such acute infections quickly and efficiently. In contrast biofilm infections do not respond well to antibiotics, although antibiotics in high dose and for prolonged periods are often used in an attempt to treat these conditions. This therapeutic approach is not very successful, and patients with biofilm infections tend to become progressively colonised with increasingly resistant bacteria.

Wounds, breaches in the normal skin epithelium, become contaminated with bacteria which are present as colonisers but which may become invasive causing infection. Infection occurs when bacterial growth and spread overwhelms local defences. There may be a state of critical colonisation where heavy bacterial bioburden and biofilm hinder normal healing [29, 30]. Other biofilm-related infections probably develop in a similar way to soft tissue biofilm pathology. These begin with colonisation, bacterial multiplication and biofilm formation with persistent low-grade inflammation. Antibiotics are poor at controlling this process, and low concentrations of antibiotic in biofilm help select progressively resistant bacteria. This is seen in chronic ulcers, burns and other biofilm pathologies such as chronic rhinosinusitis and otitis, chronic bronchitis, cystic fibrosis, bronchiectasis and chronic recurrent cystitis.

RO technologies may be the ideal agents to control and treat biofilm infections. ROS can be delivered topically to the site of biofilms via delivery mechanisms such as SHRO or RO gels for wounds, ears, operative sites, catheters and shunts and to many prosthetic devices. ROS agents can be added to douches and wash outs for rhinosinusitis or infiltrated in liquid form to catheters, shunts and bladders. It may be possible to develop ROS particles for inhalation to coat the respiratory tract in patients with chronic respiratory conditions or in ventilated patients. Slow continuous ROS production through such delivery mechanisms can control the bacterial load and break down the biofilm, probably reducing the need for systemic antibiotics and reducing the selection pressure which so often results in such patients acquiring MDR bacteria.

6 ROS in Skin and Soft Tissue

The disease burden of chronic soft tissue lesions is huge. Superficial wounds and skin ulcers are becoming increasingly common with the rising age of the population in many countries and the global epidemic of obesity and type 2 diabetes [31]. In the UK, community nurses spend as much as half their time dressing leg ulcers, and supervision by leg ulcer nurses is essential if standards are to be maintained in community leg ulcer services [32]. Most chronic breaks in the skin become colonised with bacteria [33–35]. It is difficult to know when and if these are pathogenic, but it is likely that even if overt infection is not present, bacterial colonisation plays a role in slowing tissue healing, establishing biofilm and resulting in wound slough and an offensive odour [36, 37].

The in vitro studies on the effects of SHRO and ROS prototypes on bioburden and biofilm [28] explain why SHRO and ROS gels may be so useful in these situations where antibiotics generally perform poorly. Early use of ROS in such lesions can control bioburden and biofilm, thus sparing conventional antibiotic use and supporting infection control [28, 38–40]. In addition, SHRO has all the properties of natural honey, providing healing properties (moist barrier, local nutrition, slough control, and possibly angio- and neurodegenerative properties) [41, 42].

In clinical studies ROS therapy through SHRO has demonstrated satisfactory safety and tolerance and clinical and cost-effectiveness in practice [26, 38–40], but most strikingly it has demonstrated dramatic clearance of bacterial bioburden and biofilm in chronic wounds best illustrated by its effect on the multidrug-resistant bacteria (*Pseudomonas aeruginosa*, methicillin-resistant *S. aureus* and vancomycin-resistant enterococci) present in an ischemic ulcer.

SHRO is the first ROS product available for topical use delivering sustained release of ROS as an entirely novel solution to controlling and eradicating bacteria [26]. It has perhaps not received as much clinical attention as it deserves as it is confused with other medical honeys which have a more limited effect in vitro. While there is good evidence that medical honey is effective in wound healing and burns [41, 42], medical honeys are very variable in potency, and being entirely natural products, their constituents are not standardised. This is not the case with ROS from SHRO which has a standard concentration of the enzyme glucose oxidase and can therefore deliver a precise concentration of ROS [25].

SHRO has been evaluated in a variety of chronic wounds in an open-label multicentre study and shown, through its ROS activity to reduce bacterial bioburden and biofilm and to support healing [11]. This study had a wide range of different chronic wounds and underlying pathologies and co-morbidities and was limited by the fact that it was an open-label study. However the study demonstrated the safety of the treatment and reduction in bacterial bioburden and chronic inflammatory material (Fig. 1). This should pave the way for

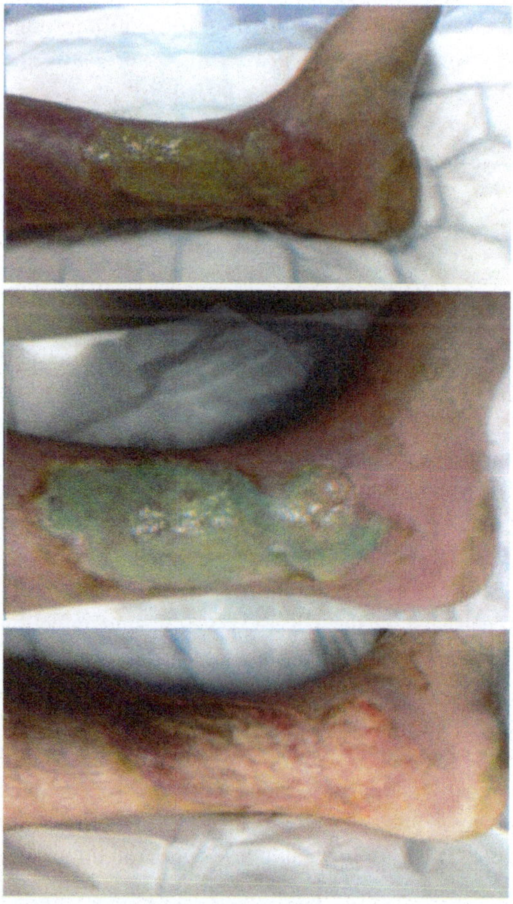

Fig. 1 Ischemic leg ulcer colonised with *Pseudomonas aeruginosa*, MRSA, mixed coliforms treated with topical SHRO. Days 1 (Top), 4 (Middle) and 10 (Bottom)

randomised controlled studies to look at the efficacy of SHRO or ROS gels in specific types of chronic wounds, particularly burns and diabetic ulcers. Key outcome criteria are healing time and prevention of deeper infection with important secondary outcome measures such as antibiotic use and colonisation with multidrug-resistant (MDR) bacteria. It has great potential to reduce inappropriate antibiotic use, support antimicrobial stewardship and reduce antimicrobial resistance in wound care [27]. It is simple to administer and can be applied to any healthcare system anywhere in the world. If SHRO can do this for wounds, then ROS by other delivery mechanisms could also do this for other mucosal biofilm and internal infections. The findings of all these clinical studies strongly support a role for SHRO in wound management, infection control, antimicrobial stewardship and preventing surgical site infections.

7 ROS and Soft Tissue Surgical Procedures

Antibiotic prophylaxis in surgery is well established, and in recent years there has been a tendency to reduce the duration of prophylaxis to single dosing where practical. Nevertheless some surgical procedures still have high rates of post-operative surgical site infection. For example, there has been a national increase in caesarean section (CS) wound infection (8–24.6%) [43, 44] and a wide variation across NHS hospitals (13.6–31.9%) associated with the 147,726 cases of CS each year in the UK [45]. CS wound infection results in prolonged hospital stay, resource consumption, as well as other morbidities and mortality [45]. Recovery from CS is more difficult for women who develop postoperative wound infection, and the burden on healthcare resources is huge [46]. A study to investigate the potential of SHRO to prevent CS wound infection was designed as a temporal study comparing surgical site infection (SSI) rates in CS wounds before and after an intervention with a single application of SHRO at wound closure [39].

This open-labelled service evaluation compared SSI rates for 3 months before the intervention, a single application of SHRO to the CS wound at closure, and for the 3 months of using the intervention [39]. There was a striking reduction in CS wound infection rates, from 5% prior to the intervention to 2% using SHRO. While this study has significant limitations, it nevertheless paves the way for future randomised controlled trials of ROS in surgical prophylaxis. Considering the fact that SSIs are a leading cause of healthcare-associated infection leading to increased mortality, prolonged duration of hospital stay and increased use of resources, further SSI preventative measures are required [47, 48]. SHRO application to all soft tissue surgery could reduce infection rates and the use of antibiotics and possibly even improve healing times, particularly when extensive soft tissue debridement or manipulation has occurred in plastic or breast procedures.

SHRO or ROS infiltration may also benefit deeper surgical procedures such as abscess drainage or intra-abdominal surgery where there has been peritoneal contamination. SHRO has been used in a small number of complex revisions of prosthetic joints [49]. Topical application of SHRO directly onto the prosthetic joint has been shown to be safe and to suppress infection for up to a year and possibly eradicate biofilm-associated infection. If such a simple and cheap intervention can reduce SSI to such a degree, its potential for more widespread surgical use needs urgent investigation.

8 ROS to Support Infection Prevention and Antimicrobial Stewardship

ROS has been successfully used in infection prevention [38]. This report highlighted the efficacy of SHRO in clearing methicillin-resistant *S. aureus* from wounds and carbapenemase-producing bacteria from a colonised line site and intravascular line care [40]. In vitro work has additionally demonstrated greater anti-MRSA biofilm efficacy for ROS than mupirocin, suggesting a possible role for topical clearance of MRSA-colonised patients [4].

Antimicrobial stewardship as a solution for the global antibiotic resistance crisis requires a reduction or indeed even an eradication of inappropriate antibiotic use. Antibiotics are frequently used in biofilm-based infections in wounds, burns and chronic respiratory conditions with generally poor efficacy, and it is notable that the organisms found in these chronic inflammatory conditions are frequently multiresistant, selected by antibiotic pressure. ROS has great potential for the control of bioburden and biofilm at many sites, thus providing an alternative to systemic antibiotics on epithelial/mucosal surfaces.

9 Other Therapeutic Possibilities for ROS

ROS antimicrobial activity is activated by contact with water [9], so if ROS can be delivered directly or in a protected format to the site of bacterial load in respiratory or uroepithelium or deep surgical sites, then there is potential for antimicrobial control. Novel delivery mechanisms such as nanoparticles, emulsions and nebulised aspirate may help with delivery. It may therefore be possible to use ROS in chronic respiratory, urinary and surgical sepsis (Table 2).

Table 2 ROS technology—clinical uses and therapeutic potential

Clinical applications of ROS	Therapeutic benefits	Evidence
Wounds, skin and soft tissue	Reduction in bacterial load and biofilm. Healing promotion	Large observational study [11]. In vitro studies [4, 5, 26–28]
Surgical prophylaxis	Reduction in rates of surgical site infection	Temporal observation study [39]. RCTs required
Infection prevention	Eradication of multiresistant and pathogenic organisms	Observational reports describing effective eradication and control [38, 40]
Antimicrobial stewardship	Great potential for antibiotic sparing around the world, particularly early use in soft tissue lesions May have potential in respiratory and urinary mucosa to prevent colonisation with MDR bacteria and requirement for last resort antibiotics	Large observational study [11]. Further studies required
Prosthetic joint infection	Use as topical suppression therapy on joint	Small series of case reports demonstrate efficacy and safety. Further studies required [49]
Infected surgical cavities	Potential use in infected cavities—peritoneum, thorax, deep wounds, abscesses	No studies as yet
Upper respiratory tract	Reduction in bacterial load and biofilm. Healing promotion in sinusitis	In vitro and clinical studies in progress [4]
Chronic lower respiratory tract conditions	Potential to reduce bacterial load and biofilm and prevent exacerbations in chronic obstructive airway disease, bronchiectasis, cystic fibrosis, ventilator-associated infection	Limited in vitro data and anecdotal clinical cases [4] Further studies required
Recurrent urinary tract infection	Potential for ROS use via urinary/nephrostomy catheters to reduce bacterial load and biofilm and eradicate MDR organisms	No studies as yet. In vitro efficacy of ROS against MDR pathogens [26, 28]

Conclusions

With a pressing need for solutions to the crisis of global antibiotic resistance, ROS has emerged as the only antibiotic alternative to date to reach clinical use in skin and soft tissue infection and with a large range of potential clinical therapeutic uses at other sites in early development. Early clinical data supports ROS treatment in skin and soft tissue lesions to reduce bacterial bioburden and biofilm in critical colonisation and in preventing surgical site infection. This review has demonstrated the mechanism, the efficacy and the wide range of existing and potential clinical applications for ROS technology. The applications of ROS technology for global health could be immense, as the agents are relatively simple to produce, safe to use, economical, simple to transport, store and administer to colonised, infected and biofilm-affected structures. As such this technology could be applicable to all health economies, developed and developing. New mechanisms of delivery should allow ROS to be applied to sites other than topical wounds, such as deep surgical cavities, and the respiratory tract and uroepithelium where multiresistant organisms may cause chronic inflammation. ROS therapy may reduce the requirement for systemic antibiotics and thus reduce the selection pressure on microbes from antibiotics. ROS may suppress MDR organisms and thereby reduce transmission of these strains. ROS technology requires much further research but has the potential to deliver exciting novel therapeutic options.

Acknowledgements The author wishes to thank the following colleagues for their contributions to work on ROS presented at a symposium on ROS at the University of Birmingham, 2016 [4].

Hampshire Hospitals Foundation NHS Trust: Kordo Saeed, Amy Dickson, Gemma Lockyer

Southampton University: Rami Salib, Sylvia Pender, Ray Allan, Ali Salamat, Timothy Biggs

Birmingham University: Fenella Halstead, Beryl Oppenheim. Manchester University: Jonathan Cooke, Malcolm Richardson. Cardiff University and Swansea University: Rodri Williams, Rhidian Morgan-Jones

References

1. Davis S, Martinez L, Kirsner R (2006) The diabetic foot: the importance of biofilms and wound bed preparation. Curr Diab Rep 6:439–434
2. Mertz PM (2003) Cutaneous biofilms: friend or foe? Wounds 15:129–132
3. Percival SL, Bowler PG (2004) Biofilms and. their potential role in wound healing. Wounds 16:234–240
4. ROS Symposium link (2016) http://www.reactiveoxygen.co.uk/videos_archive.asp. Accessed 27 July 2016
5. Dunnill C, Patton T, Brennan J, Barrett J, Dryden M, Cooke J, Leaper D, Georgopoulos NT (2017) Reactive oxygen species (ROS) and wound healing: the functional role of ROS and emerging ROS-modulating technologies for augmentation of the healing process. Int Wound J 14(1):89–96
6. WHO (2014) Antimicrobial resistance: global report on surveillance. http://www.who.int/drugresistance/documents/surveillancereport/en/. Accessed 30 Dec 2016
7. Davies S (2016) Annual Report of the Chief Medical Officer. Volume Two. Infections and the Rise of Antimicrobial Resistance. http://www.dh.gov.uk/health/2013/03/cmo-vol2/. Accessed 30 Dec 2016
8. O'Neil J (2016) Tackling drug-resistant infections globally. http://amr-review.org/sites/default/files/160525_Final%20paper_with%20cover.pdf. Accessed 30 Dec 2016
9. Department of Health and Department for Environment, Food and Rural Affairs (2016) UK Five Year Antimicrobial Resistance Strategy 2013 to 2018. https://www.gov.uk/government/uploads/system/uploads/attachment_data/file/244058/20130902_UK_5_year_AMR_strategy.pdf. Accessed 30 Dec 2016
10. Lipsky BA, Dryden M, Gottrup F, Nathwani D, Seaton RA, Stryja J (2016) Antimicrobial stewardship in wound care: a Position Paper from the British Society for Antimicrobial Chemotherapy and European Wound Management Association. J Antimicrob Chemother 71(11):3026–3035
11. Dryden M, Dickinson A, Brooks J, Hudgell L, Saeed K, Cutting K (2016) A multi-centre clinical evaluation of reactive oxygen topical wound gel in 114 wounds. J Wound Care 25:140–146
12. Posnett J, Franks PJ (2008) The burden of chronic wounds in the UK. Nurs Times 104(3):44–45
13. NHS Diabetes Factsheet No 37 (2012) Foot care for people with diabetes in the NHS in England: The economic case for change
14. Abbas M, Uckay I, Lipsky BA (2015) In diabetic foot infections antibiotics are to treat infection, not to heal wounds. Expert Opin Pharmacother 16(6):821–832
15. Howell-Jones RS, Price PE, Howard AJ, Thomas DW (2006) Antibiotic prescribing for chronic skin wounds in primary care. Wound Repair Regen 14(4):387–393

16. Tammelin A, Lindholm C, Hambraeus A (1998) Chronic ulcers and antibiotic treatment. J Wound Care 7(9):435–437
17. Oien RF, Forssell HW (2013) Ulcer healing time and antibiotic treatment before and after the introduction of the Registry of Ulcer Treatment: an improvement project in a national quality registry in Sweden. BMJ Open 3(8):e003091
18. Lipsky BA, Hoey C (2009) Topical antimicrobial therapy for treating chronic wounds. Clin Infect Dis 49(10):1541–1549
19. Gottrup F, Apelqvist J, Bjarnsholt T, Cooper R, Moore Z, Peters EJ et al (2013) EWMA document: antimicrobials and non-healing wounds – evidence, controversies and suggestions. J Wound Care 22(5 Suppl):S1–92
20. Holder IA, Boyce ST (1999) Assessment of the potential for microbial resistance to topical use of multiple antimicrobial agents. Wound Repair Regen 7(4):238–243
21. Wilkinson JD (1998) Fusidic acid in dermatology. Br J Dermatol 139(Suppl 53):37–40
22. Castro DL, Santos VL (2015) Controlling wound odor with metronidazole: a systematic review. Rev Esc Enferm USP 49(5):858–863
23. Leaper D, Assadian O, Edmiston CE (2015) Approach to chronic wound infections. Br J Dermatol 173(2):351–358
24. Cutting KF, White RJ, Mahoney P, Harding KG (2005) Clinical identification of wound infection: a Delphi approach. Identifying criteria for wound Infection. In: European Wound Management Association (EWMA). Position document: identifying criteria for wound infection. MEP Ltd, London
25. Cooke J, Dryden M, Patton T, Brennan J, Barrett J (2015) The antimicrobial activity of prototype modified honeys that generate reactive oxygen species (ROS) hydrogen peroxide. BMC Res Notes 8:20
26. Dryden M, Lockyer G, Saeed K, Cooke J (2014) Engineered honey: in vitro antimicrobial activity of a novel topical wound care treatment. J Glob Antimicrob Resist 2(3):168–172
27. Cooke J (2014) When antibiotics can be avoided in skin inflammation and bacterial colonization: a review of topical treatments. Curr Opin Infect Dis 27:125–129
28. Halstead FD, Webber MA, Rauf M, Burt R, Dryden M, Oppenheim BA (2016) In vitro activity of an engineered honey, medical-grade honeys, and antimicrobial wound dressings against biofilm-producing clinical bacterial isolates. J Wound Care 25:93–102
29. Woo KY, Alam T, Marin J (2014) Topical antimicrobial toolkit for wound infection. Surg Technol Int 25:45–52
30. Abbass M, Uçkay I, Lipsky BA (2015) Diabetic foot infection, antibiotics are to cure infection, not to heal wounds. Expert Opin Clinical Pharmacother 16:821–828
31. Diabetic foot problems: inpatient management of diabetic foot problems (2011) NICE Clinical Guidelines, No. 119. Centre for Clinical Practice at NICE (UK)
32. Simon DA, Dix FP, McCollum CN (2004) Management of venous leg ulcers. BMJ 328(7452):1358–1362
33. Gjødsbøl K, Christensen JJ, Karlsmark T, Jørgensen B, Klein BM, Krogfelt KA (2006) Multiple bacterial species reside in chronic wounds: a longitudinal study. Int Wound J 3(3):225–231
34. Renner R, Sticherling M, Rüger R, Simon J (2012) Persistence of bacteria like Pseudomonas aeruginosa in non-healing venous ulcers. Eur J Dermatol 22(6):751–757
35. Leaper DJ, Schultz G, Carville K, Fletcher J, Swanson T, Drake R (2012) Extending the TIME concept: what have we learned in the past 10 years? Int Wound J 9:1–19
36. Scali C, Kunimoto B (2013) An update on chronic wounds and the role of biofilms. J Cutan Med Surg 17(6):371–376
37. Percival SL, Hill KE, Williams DW, Hooper SJ, Thomas DW, Costerton JW (2012) A review of the scientific evidence for biofilms in wounds. Wound Repair Regen 20(5):647–657
38. Dryden M, Milward G, Saeed K (2014) Infection prevention in wounds with Surgihoney. J Hosp Infect 88(2):121–122
39. Dryden M, Goddard C, Madadi A, Heard M, Saeed K, Cooke J (2014) Bioengineered Surgihoney as an antimicrobial wound dressing to prevent Caesarean wound infection: a clinical and cost-effectiveness study. Br J Midwifery 22:23–27
40. Dryden M, Tawse C, Adams J, Saeed K, Cooke J (2014) The use of Surgihoney to prevent or eradicate bacterial colonisation in dressing oncology long vascular lines. J Wound Care 23:338–341
41. Al-Waili N, Salom K, Al-Ghamdi AA (2011) Honey for wound healing, ulcers, and burns; data supporting its use in clinical practice. ScientificWorldJournal 11:766–787
42. Cooper R, Jenkins R (2012) Are there feasible prospects for manuka honey as an alternative to conventional antimicrobials? Expert Rev Anti-Infect Ther 10(6):623–625
43. National Collaborating Centre for Women's and Children's Health (UK) (2008) Surgical site infection prevention and treatment of surgical site infection. In: National Institute for Health and Clinical Excellence: Guidance. RCOG Press, London
44. Paranjothy S, Frost C, Thomas J (2005) How much variation in CS rates can be explained by case mix differences? BJOG 112:658–666
45. Bragg F, Cromwell DA, Edozien LC, Gurol-Urganci I, Mahmood TA, Templeton A, Van der Meulen JH (2010) Variation in rates of caesarean section among English NHS trusts after accounting for maternal and clinical risk: cross sectional study. BMJ 341:c5065
46. Wloch C, Wilson J, Lamagni T, Harrington P, Charlett A, Sheridan E (2012) Risk factors for surgical site infection following caesarean section in England: results from a multicentre cohort study. BJOG 119:1324–1333

47. Wloch C, Lamagni T, Conneely J, Harrington P, Elgohari S, Jan Van Hoek A, Wilson J, Sheridan E (2012) Estimating the healthcare costs of post-surgical infection in patients undergoing caesarean section in England. Health Protection Agency, London
48. Abbas M, Pittet D (2016) Surgical site infection prevention: a global priority. J Hosp Infect 93:319–322
49. Khan W, Williams R, Metah A, Morgan-Jones R (2015) Surgihoney as a novel antimicrobial coating in salvage revision total knee arthroplasty. Orthop Proc 97-B:66

The manufacturer's authorised representative in the EU is Springer Nature Customer Service Centre GmbH, Europaplatz 3, 69115 Heidelberg, Germany. If you have any concerns regarding our products, please contact ProductSafety@springernature.com

Printed and bound by CPI Group (UK) Ltd, Croydon, CR0 4YY
22/09/2026
02221056-0008